In describing and explaining the sexes, medicine and science participated in the delineation of what was "feminine" and what was "masculine" in the Middle Ages. Hildegard of Bingen and Albertus Magnus, among others, writing about gynecology, the human constitution, fetal development, or the naturalistic dimensions of divine Creation, became increasingly interested in issues surrounding reproduction and sexuality. Did women as well as men produce procreative seed? How did the physiology of the sexes influence their healthy states and their susceptibility to disease? Who derived more pleasure from sexual intercourse, men or women?

The answers to such questions created a network of flexible concepts which did not endorse a single model of male–female relations but did affect views of the health consequences of sexual abstinence for women and men and the allocation of responsibility for infertility – problems with much social and religious significance in the Middle Ages. Sometimes at odds with and sometimes in accord with other forces in medieval society, medicine and natural philosophy helped to construct a set of notions which divided significant portions of the world – from the behavior of animals to the operations of astrological signs – into "masculine" and "feminine." Even cases which seemed to exist outside the definitions of this duality, such as hermaphrodite features or homosexual behavior, were brought under control by the application of gendered labels, such as "masculine women."

Meanings of sex difference in the Middle Ages

Cambridge History of Medicine

Edited by

CHARLES WEBSTER, Reader in the History of Medicine, University of Oxford, and Fellow of All Souls College

CHARLES ROSENBERG, Professor of History and Sociology of Science, University of Pennsylvania

For a list of titles in the series, see end of book.

Meanings of sex difference in the Middle Ages

Medicine, science, and culture

JOAN CADDEN
Kenyon College

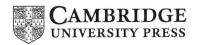

CAMBRIDGE
UNIVERSITY PRESS

Published by the Press Syndicate of the University of Cambridge
The Pitt Building, Trumpington Street, Cambridge CB2 1RP
40 West 20th Street, New York, NY 10011-4211, USA
10 Stamford Road, Oakleigh, Melbourne 3166, Australia

© Cambridge University Press 1993

First published 1993
First paperback edition 1995

Printed in the United States of America

Library of Congress Cataloging-in-Publication Data is available.

A catalogue record for this book is available from the British Library.

ISBN 0-521-34363-1 hardback
ISBN 0-521-48378-6 paperback

To
Vivian Liebman Cadden
Mater and *Alma Mater*

CONTENTS

ILLUSTRATIONS

ACKNOWLEDGMENTS

For medieval Aristotelians, the most basic functions of living creatures are nutrition, growth, and reproduction. Because I had already worked on medieval theories of nutrition and growth, I might well have found my way to a book on medieval theories of reproduction without the help of Will Scott and Clark Dougan, colleagues in the history department at Kenyon College – but it would not have been this book. At a department meeting in 1979, they took the position that our curriculum ought to include something about the history of women. Predictably, all eyes turned to the only woman in the department. The initial result was a fairly unsatisfactory course called History of Biological Ideas of Female and Male; the long-term result was a reorientation of my research, in both subject and approach (as well as a reorientation of our history curriculum). The evolution of the project has depended at every stage upon the advice and support of others, who have patiently and generously helped me with paleography, feminist theory, English prose, and innumerable other elements of the work.

For years I inhabited (or haunted) manuscript, rare book, and microfilm collections, and I am thus immeasurably indebted to those libraries' staff members, only some of whom I know by name. I am grateful to those who facilitated my use of the Latin manuscript collections at the Bibliothèque Nationale, the British Library, and Trinity College, Cambridge, and I wish to credit in particular Godfrey Waller at Cambridge University Library, Timothy Hobbes at Gonville and Caius, Albinia de la Mare and C. Starks at the Bodleian Library, and Frau Renner at the Bayerische Staatsbibliothek. For their helpfulness and expertise with early printed books, I owe thanks to Salli Morgenstern of the Rare Book Room at the New York Academy of Medicine, Glen Jenkins of the Rare Book Room at the Allen Medical Library in Cleveland, and Richard Eimas of the Martin Room at the University of Iowa Medical School. At the Vatican Film Library of Saint Louis University, Charles Ermatinger kindly made arrangements for me to use films; at the Hill Monastic Manuscript Library at Saint John's University, Wilfred Theisen was my guide; and Jack Noordhoorn at Columbia University Library located some uncatalogued films made by Lynn Thorndike. Closer to home, the staffs of the Ohio State University Library and the Kenyon College Library kept me well supplied with the bread of scholarship. At Kenyon, Nadine George, Jami Peelle, Allen Bosch, and the interlibrary loan department – Carol Marshall, Deborah McCann, Joan Pomajevich, and Sandra Wallace – have been resourceful and indefatigable.

In dealing with the manuscripts I received special assistance from three scholars whose generosity is matched only by their learning. Marie Thérèse d'Alverny cheerfully deciphered the apparently indecipherable in several manuscripts at the Bibliothèque Nationale and introduced me into hidden reaches of the library, where endless *fichiers* yielded valuable codicological data. Also at the BN, Danielle Jacquart unreservedly made available to me her notes on Latin medical manuscripts in the collection, the product of years of careful and expert labor. In Munich, Eleanor Roach collected and forwarded to me from the Bayerische Staatsbibliothek information about a large number of manuscripts in which I was interested.

All along the way, many people – many of whom saw or heard parts of this work as it was taking shape – made suggestions, contributed bibliographical references, offered conceptual approaches, advised about organization, and generally enriched the experience of researching and writing the book. Among these I wish especially to thank Mary Martin McLaughlin, Monica Green, Ellen Furlough, Rita Kipp, Caroline Bynum, Wendy Cadden, Michael McVaugh, Katharine Park, Linda Voigts, and Mary Wack. Several colleagues have been kind enough to permit me to see and benefit from the unpublished results of their research: Helen Lemay, Joyce Salisbury, James Brundage, Margaret Schleissner, and Monica Green, who, from the very beginning, has been tireless in her willingness to consider and criticize my work in an informed, frank, and constructive manner. In posing serious challenges on matters of method and conceptualization, Bert Hansen has earned my collegial gratitude. I am especially indebted to Nancy Siraisi and Joyce Salisbury for their careful and learned readings of the manuscript. Pamela Bruton made many helpful suggestions and spotted errors in half a dozen languages; Mary Hopper's keen editorial eye, her computer expertise, and her day-to-day support were invaluable. Margaret Zimansky devoted more time to this book than anyone but myself.

Anyone familiar with the work of these individuals will find the conventional disclaimer amusingly superfluous: not only the errors but any weakness, mediocrity, obscurity, or omissions are, of course, my own. All translations are my own unless otherwise noted.

Moral as well as material support came from the institutions which saw fit to fund various aspects of this project. It is a pleasure to acknowledge the generosity of the National Science Foundation, the George A. and Eliza Gardner Howard Foundation, the American Philosophical Society, and Kenyon College.

INTRODUCTION

When we pronounce the phrase "the facts of life," we are aware of being rhetorically coy, of using a euphemism to avoid even such Latinate and therefore cool locutions as "sexual intercourse," not to speak of blunter terms. Yet there is another, less visible but no less significant rhetorical strategy contained in the naive expression: the aura of neutrality and objectivity that glows around the word "facts" obscures at least part of the agenda. When parents begin an earnest talk with their child, "When a man and a woman love each other very much . . ." the prescriptive messages they are conveying about heterosexuality and monogamy are not far beneath the surface. Woody Allen dressed up as "Sperm No. 2" in *Everything You Always Wanted to Know about Sex* reminds us of the courage, fortitude, and adventurousness our culture expects of male gametes.[1] Nor is it only our colloquial accounts which offer glimpses of the society behind the science: even fairly specialized and technical treatments convey cultural assumptions.[2] A 1961 endocrinological text, for example, reports a hypothesis about the relationship of a specific hormone to libido, based on the "fact" that although males without testes exhibit decreased libido, females without ovaries do not. The author acknowledges that "definitive reports on eroticism in treated hypogonadal females are lacking in the literature." Furthermore, we learn that in one relevant study libido has been measured by "end organ sensitivity."[3] The studies and therefore the proposed explanations have focused on male sexual response and have been extended to females by

---

1 Woody Allen (director), *Everything You Always Wanted to Know about Sex, but Were Afraid to Ask* (United Artists, 1972).
2 For a wealth of examples, see Laurel Richardson Walum, *The Dynamics of Sex and Gender: A Sociological Perspective* (Chicago: Rand McNally College Publishing, 1977), pp. 70–87; and Winifred W. Doane and Barbara K. Abbott, *Pocketbook Profiles: (Sexism Satirized:) Quotes from the Biological Literature* (n.p.: Society for Developmental Biology, 1976).
3 John W. Money, "Sex Hormones and Other Variables in Human Eroticism," in William C. Young, ed., *Sex and Internal Secretions*, 3d ed. (Baltimore: Williams and Wilkins, 1961), vol. 2, pp. 1390–1.

extrapolation or analogy. This practice and the anatomical isolation of eroticism suggest something about our culture's conceptualization of sexuality and its models of male and female.

If modern science, with its ideals of objectivity and value neutrality and with its linguistic and professional isolation from other kinds of knowledge, bears the stamp of its times, can medieval science fail to do so? This study explores medieval answers to just such questions as "Where do babies come from?" and "Are men's and women's sexual pleasure similar?" and gleans from them insights into medieval gender constructs – into what were understood to be the distinguishing characteristics of women and men, femininity and masculinity. Although there were clear distinctions in the Middle Ages between natural philosophy and moral philosophy, between the study of health and the study of salvation, these were not domains of incommensurable discourse, and they often shared both methods and meanings. The very term "natural philosophy," as distinguished from the modern term "science," suggests that the investigation of natural phenomena was part of a network of systematic knowledge, not an isolated endeavor. The theoretical dimensions of medieval medicine also had a place in that network, and the more practical dimensions were shaped as well by the interests and expectations of patients. Thus when medieval authors explained sterility or explicated the ancient tenet that males are warmer than females, they left clues from which we may extract some insight into the social and cultural meanings of "female" and "male." The assumption on which this book is founded is that medieval natural philosophical theories and medical notions about reproduction and about sexual impulses, actions, and experiences will intersect at many points with ideas about such matters as the social roles of women and men, the purpose of marriage, and the road to salvation – in short, that scientific ideas about sex differences in the later Middle Ages participated in the broader culture's assumptions about gender.

Both the content and the dynamics of this participation were multivalent, thus revealing the extent to which medical and scientific learning operated within the medieval power structures and, at the same time, the variety and intricacy of the interactions. Medieval society in western Europe was not homogeneous: it was peasant and noble; north and south; rural and urban; Christian, heretic, and Jew. Furthermore, in the period from the late eleventh through the fourteenth century, with which this study is concerned, it underwent enormous economic, social, and cultural changes. There is no coherent set of concepts that can be said to constitute the medieval gender framework. Similarly, the vast and evolving body of knowledge which constituted medieval medicine and natural philosophy – the repository of much of what we would call "science" – did not offer a single model of the sexes, much less one which could be said to shape or to be derived from a clear system of gender roles. Not only did medicine and natural philosophy draw ideas from a variety of differing sources, but medical authors and natural philosophers applied their ideas in a wide range of contexts, not all of which could be encompassed under a single theory. The research presented here shows that just as we would be betraying the evidence if we took Eve to be the paradigm of women in the Middle Ages, so we would be unjustified in representing the Aristotelian opposition between male and female natures as the scientific model of sex difference. Indeed, we would be doing only a little better if we asserted that medieval concepts of women were contained within the conflict between the idea of Eve and the idea of the Virgin Mary or that concepts of sex were contained within the conflict between Aristotelian duality and a Galenic system of sex parallels. This analysis differs from that of Thomas Laqueur, whose recent work argues that before the eighteenth century male and female were in various ways regarded as manifestations of a unified substratum. Though there is much evidence in the present study that fits his "one sex" model, medieval views on the status of the uterus and the opinions of medieval physiognomers about male and female traits suggest evidence of other models not reducible to Laqueur's.[4]

The interactions of concepts in medicine or natural philosophy with other facets of medieval society and culture are likewise not reducible to a formula, whether of impact or complicity or conflict. On many points and in many contexts the relationship has elements of both congruence and tension. Christian doctrine and medical opinion might agree, for example, that sexual intercourse was a good thing for married couples, but that very real agreement cannot mask their disagreement about why it was or their consequent disagreement about satisfying the sexual appetites of unmarried persons. Nor did medicine and natural philosophy always agree with each other, especially in cases in which practical remedies were called for, as in the treatment of sterility. Although it is tempting to ask whether the role of medicine and natural philosophy in medieval gender constructs was good or bad for women, the question, if answerable at all, cannot be answered by the evidence assembled here. Ways of looking at reproduction that assigned women a certain level of responsibility at once accorded them the dignity of activity in a positive outcome and the burden of blame in a negative one. In a more subtle sense, the participation of medical and natural philosophical opinion about sex differences in the culture of the later Middle Ages reflects on the character of medieval society. On the one hand, the recovery of ancient wisdom, the resurgence of medical learning, the elaboration of scholarly methods, as well as such specific developments as a heightened interest in the subject of sexual pleasure and the personal tone of some discussions of sterility, all suggest why the centuries with which this book is concerned are

4 Thomas Laqueur, *Making Sex: Body and Gender from the Greeks to Freud* (Cambridge: Harvard University Press, 1990).

traditionally crowned in textbooks with such labels as "renaissance," "spring," and "summer." On the other hand, the period from the twelfth through the fourteenth century (which I shall be referring to as the "later Middle Ages," since the term "late Middle Ages" usually excludes the twelfth century) has been suspect too. According to some recent scholarship, European culture and society became increasingly inflexible, intolerant, and closed, due in part to some of the very developments previously celebrated – reason, reform, institutionalization. The Crusades, the codification of laws, the rise of the universities, the suppression of heresies, the increased persecution of Jews, and the end of the reclamation of new lands have all been cited as manifestations of the new dogmatic, authoritarian, intolerant spirit.[5] Attitudes toward women and sexuality were not exempt from the trend: ecclesiastical policy on contraception and abortion formed and hardened; and homosexual inclinations and acts came under fire.[6] The persistence with which medical writers and natural philosophers applied the terminology of sex difference, particularly in situations or cases, such as sodomy, which did not fit the binary structure of sex distinctions, suggests that knowledge about nature was one element in the enforcement of narrower norms. The diversity of medical and natural philosophical opinion can weigh in favor of both perspectives on the period: neither dogma nor dogmatism is visible in discussions relating to sex difference, yet the very variety of concepts gave medicine and philosophy a flexible and consequently powerful set of tools with which to approach any project.

This book is, among other things, about diversity, eclecticism, and alternatives, and its approach mirrors the habits of medieval natural philosophers and medical writers in gleaning questions, information, and methods from many kinds of sources. Some of the authors cited were prominent and influential, like the natural philosopher and theologian Albertus Magnus and the medical professor Bernard of Gordon, whose prominent careers as teachers and scholars are attested in their writings (many of which have been edited and printed) and in the modern scholarly attention they have commanded. Others are anonymous or forgotten, unprinted and unstudied. Some of the works on which this study is based are comprehensive; some

---

5 Friedrich Heer, *The Medieval World: Europe, 1100–1350*, trans. Janet Sondheimer (Cleveland: World, 1962); R. I. Moore, *The Formation of a Persecuting Society: Power and Deviance in Western Europe, 950–1250* (Oxford: Basil Blackwell, 1987); Jeremy Cohen, "Scholarship and Intolerance in the Medieval Academy: The Study and Evaluation of Judaism in European Christendom," *American Historical Review* 91 (1986): 592–613; and idem, *The Friars and the Jews: The Evolution of Medieval Anti-Judaism* (Ithaca: Cornell University Press, 1982).

6 John T. Noonan, Jr., *Contraception: A History of Its Treatment by the Catholic Theologians and Canonists* (Cambridge: Belnap Press, Harvard University Press, 1965); John Boswell, *Christianity, Social Tolerance, and Homosexuality: Gay People in Western Europe from the Beginning of the Christian Era to the Fourteenth Century* (Chicago: University of Chicago Press, 1980), esp. pt. IV.

are original; many are fragmentary and derivative. These less impressive, less well documented, and less examined sources are harder to place in precise contexts and harder to interpret, but they make up a significant proportion of the works on natural philosophy and medicine that have come down to us from the Middle Ages.

Most of the sources examined are in Latin and were thus the products of a small learned elite largely dominated by men. They are not masquerading here as evidence of popular medicine. Yet the Latin traditions were not as closed and narrow as their origins and status might seem to imply. Many of the Latin texts themselves were neither sophisticated nor elaborate. They often contained bits of medical lore gleaned from a variety of sources and assembled in a form – for example, a small format – that suggests they were carried around and used by practitioners, who need have had no contact with university medical faculties. Such a text could therefore be translated into concrete acts by the practitioner, who performed an examination or pre-scribed a diet according to its precepts, and who was at the same time familiar with the expectations and practices of the patient's family. In addition, learned male authors sometimes mentioned women as their informants. They re-ported variously what midwives, Frenchwomen, Saracen women, and prosti-tutes said or did. Not all of these references are reliable – some may be made up to achieve one effect or another – but they suggest the likelihood that the ideas and practices of the individuals and groups outside a small elite could have made their way into the writings of the educated. Finally, the many layers and varieties of health care practice were not without opportunities for mutual contact. The country woman who practiced herbal healing in addi-tion to her agricultural and household duties was not likely to meet up with a professor of medicine from an urban university. Nevertheless, the herbalist might supply an apothecary in a nearby town who worked with practitioners who, though they might not themselves know Latin, were anxious to acquire knowledge and prestige by attending a physician called in from the city to treat or advise a member of the local elite.[7] Not all those who rose in the educational system were of exalted birth, not all readers and writers of Latin had institutional ties with the Church, and not all experts were men. Both Latin and vernacular texts refer to the apparently renowned medical practitio-ners known as "the women of Salerno" and to a celebrated expert called

7 Ernest Wickersheimer, *Dictionaire biographique des médecins en France au Moyen Age*, 2 vols. (Paris: Droz, 1936); and Danielle Jacquart, *Le milieu médical en France du XIIᵉ au XVᵉ siècle: En annexe 2ᵉ supplément au* Dictionaire d'Ernest Wickersheimer, Centre de recherches d'histoire et de philologie de la IVᵉ section de l'Ecole practique des hautes études V, Hautes études médiévales et modernes 46 (Geneva: Droz, 1981). Wickersheimer illustrates and Jacquart analyzes the diversity of types of health care practice. Jacquart examines practitioners' educa-tion and their contacts with humble patients. She also demonstrates that a decreasing propor-tion of practitioners were attached to great patrons during this period, leaving more to seek a broader clientele.

"Trotula."[8] Hildegard of Bingen, whose anthropological, physiological, and medical ideas figure significantly in this study, was by no means typical, but neither was she entirely alone. Scholars are just beginning to evaluate the character and extent of women's learning and practice in these areas.[9] Thus, though largely limited by the Latin language and by the urban environment, ideas contained in works of medicine and even of natural philosophy were not entirely inaccessible or impermeable, and were by no means monolithic.

The diversity of sources makes the project of investigating the meanings of sex difference more complicated but also more significant. The concepts "female" and "male" come into play at a variety of levels in a variety of contexts. "What are the male and female roles in reproduction?" "Which sex enjoys intercourse more?" "How can you distinguish a male embryo from a female?" "How can you have a son?" "What features distinguish the female body from the male?" "What dispositions and behaviors distinguish a male from a female?" Although medieval authors did not investigate the general subject of sex difference directly, they did pose questions such as these and, in the course of answering them, generated fields of understanding. Not only were they interested in addressing topics that reflected on the distinction between female and male, but they also abstracted and extended those distinctions in their applications of the terms "masculine" and "feminine" to many parts of nature: leopards are feminine, lions are masculine; the planet Mars is masculine, the planet Saturn is feminine; the mandrake plant comes in feminine and masculine forms. Indeed, this way of dividing the world sometimes entailed the designation of "masculine woman" or "feminine man." These extensions, along with the conviction that disposition and mores are based in female and male nature in the same way as beards and wombs, are part of the process by which, from a modern point of view, the medieval world – physical, social, spiritual – becomes gendered. From the medieval point of view, however, it would make no sense to draw a line between the application of sex-distinguishing terms to sexually reproducing animals and their application to the trait of generosity or the job of spinning wool.

In whatever contexts they appear, ideas of this sort are always, at some important level, about women and men, and thus this book belongs to the tradition of feminist scholarship, which began with literary historians' studies of the depiction of medieval women and evolved under the influence of social and cultural history to incorporate consideration of ways in which images, language, and doctrine inhered in and represented women's experiences and perceptions. The history of medicine is an especially promising

---

8 John Benton, "Trotula, Women's Problems, and the Professionalization of Medicine in the Middle Ages," *Bulletin of the History of Medicine* 59 (1985): 30–53, illustrates some of the processes and problems involved in the transmission of knowledge.

9 See Monica H. Green, "Women's Medical Practice and Health Care in Medieval Europe," *Signs* 14 (1989): 434–73.

lode for such work, since it encompasses a body of articulated knowledge and a well identified (if not always easily accessible) domain of practice with women as both subjects and objects. Monica Green's work, including her study of the transmission of gynecological ideas, is a paradigm of the way in which traditional methods of intellectual history and philological analysis can be reoriented by a feminist approach, yielding, for example, such previously unattended subjects as the conceptual relationship between women's health and their reproductive function.[10] The present study is not about women, but it does point up the numerous contexts in which medieval authors made a special issue of women or of femininity, as in their discussions of menstruation or sexual appetite or the Creation.

In order to explain and to establish the significance of the sense of the feminine and the masculine conveyed by medical and scientific sources, the book suggests specific relationships and interactions among medicine, natural philosophy, Christian theology and doctrine, secular social concerns, and other dimensions of the medieval world. It therefore draws upon a wide range of recent scholarship on women, sexuality, gender, and family[11] to remedy the narrowness of more traditional works on the history of embryology and gynecology.[12] The goals of this study differ considerably from works on related subjects, such as the history of sexuality. Michel Foucault, for example, a pioneer in the field, is not interested in sex differences; indeed, his *History of Sexuality* is almost entirely a history of male sexuality. His work is significant for its formulation of sexuality as an object of historical investigation. The history of sexuality has influenced the present work, which includes extensive consideration of medieval texts on the subject of sexual pleasure. However, like the words "science" and "gender," the word "sexuality" (and also the words "homosexuality" and even "orgasm") occurs infrequently here, in order to avoid any implication that those concepts were or correspond to medieval intellectual categories. Medieval authors spoke frequently about such subjects as sexual contact between members of the same sex (which they sometimes named or included under the heading of "sodomy"), nocturnal emissions by men and women, and whether prostitutes experienced pleasure in intercourse. They even talked about libido and "the flesh." We can learn something about the complexity, fragmentation, and difference of what we call "sexuality" in the Middle Ages when we

10 Monica H. Green, "The Transmission of Ancient Theories of Female Physiology and Disease through the Early Middle Ages" (Ph.D. diss., Princeton University, 1985).
11 E.g., Caroline W. Bynum, *Holy Feast and Holy Fast: The Religious Significance of Food to Medieval Women* (Berkeley and Los Angeles: University of California Press, 1987); and James A. Brundage, *Law, Sex, and Christian Society in Medieval Europe* (Chicago: University of Chicago Press, 1987).
12 E.g., Joseph Needham, *A History of Embryology*, 2d ed., rev. with Arthur Hughes; History, Philosophy and Sociology of Science (Cambridge: Cambridge University Press, 1959; reprint, New York: Arno, 1975); Paul Diepgen, *Frau und Frauheilkunde in der Kultur des Mittelalters* (Stuttgart: Georg Thieme, 1963).

refrain from lending coherence to this multiplicity by our use of unifying terminology. From the late eleventh century on, medieval Latin writers employed the terms "masculinity" and "femininity," indicating the properties of being male or female, and it is concepts such as these and their relation to one another, referred to as "sex difference," that this book sets out to identify and interpret.[13]

Foucault used the Middle Ages mainly as a foil, highlighting his characterization of Greek attitudes toward pleasure by contrasting them with later Christian attitudes, which he saw as legalistic, negative, and narrowly tied to procreation.[14] This view contains no acknowledgment of the medieval medical opinion that intercourse could promote health or of scholastic interest in nonreproductive sexual behavior.[15] Danielle Jacquart and Claude Thomasset's *Sexuality and Medicine in the Middle Ages* is far more sensitive to the variety of forces at work and to the ambivalence and tensions which infused medieval attitudes and opinions. For example, it lays out some of the interplay between the impulse to regulate and the desire to explain. Besides containing an excellent summary of medieval medical ideas about the anatomy and physiology of human sexuality, about sexual hygiene and the erotic, about varieties of sexual expression, and about disorders associated with sexual activities, this work, which is based on some of the same sources as the present study, explores the relationship of medical views to other aspects of the culture, such as the influence of Arabic traditions and the formulation of ideas of courtly love. Because the authors' goals lie elsewhere, they do not systematically apply their materials to the question of differences between males and females, nor do they address the topics of reproduction or sex determination, except as related to the central subject of sexuality. Taking medicine as their protagonist, Jacquart and Thomasset tend to see medical and philosophical ideas as more distinct than the present study does and to picture medicine as a liberating force, in contrast to natural philosophy and theology.[16] Their work, which, like this one, concentrates on the period from the late eleventh through the fourteenth century, and Monica Green's, which deals with the transmission of ancient gynecological ideas to the Latin West in the earlier Middle Ages,[17] convey the continuity and malleability of medieval medical learning.

---

13 Constantinus Africanus, *Liber de coitu: El tratado de andrología de Constantino el Africano*, ed. and trans. Enrique Montero Cartelle, Monografias de la Universidad de Santiago de Compostela 77 (Santiago de Compostela: Universidad de Santiago, 1983), ch. 7, p. 106.

14 Michel Foucault, *The Use of Pleasure*, trans. Robert Hurley, vol. 2 of *The History of Sexuality* (New York: Random House, 1985), e.g., pp. 138–9.

15 Monica Green reviews the literature concerned with medieval women in "Female Sexuality in the Medieval West," *Trends in History* 4 (1990): 127–58.

16 Danielle Jacquart and Claude Thomasset, *Sexuality and Medicine in the Middle Ages*, trans. Matthew Adamson (Princeton: Princeton University Press, 1988). The translation contains material and an index not included in the 1985 French edition.

17 Green, "Transmission."

The goals of this book are both vertical and horizontal. On the one hand, it aims at understanding the origins and evolution of medieval notions about sex differences over a period of several centuries during which changes occurred both in the ideas themselves and in the ways they were learned, organized, and used. This goal is addressed by a chronological approach in the first part of the book. On the other hand, it aims at integrating scientific and medical notions with each other and with elements of the larger context, such as secular ideas about marriage and religious ideas about the flesh. This goal is addressed by a thematic approach in the second part of the book.

Part I deals with the evolution of medieval medical and natural philosophical ideas about sex difference, starting with the ancient sources which influenced the Middle Ages at various stages and culminating with university discussions of the thirteenth and fourteenth centuries. It focuses closely on the contents of concepts about sex difference, taking into account only the immediate environment – the genres of writing and the settings in which they were expressed. This development itself is not simple or linear. First of all, the questions and emphases shift: at first, characterizations of female and male were elaborated in the context of their roles in reproduction; later that context was joined (not replaced) by a set of questions about their experience of sexual pleasure and its function. Second, the ways in which scholars accommodated differences of opinion and new authoritative sources changed, though in general the effect was an accumulation rather than a succession of ideas and methods. Finally, although medicine and natural philosophy shared many principles and practices, they did not always deal with issues in the same way or agree substantively.

Part II scrutinizes the learned ideas which had evolved and accumulated, in order to bring together those elements of the discussions about reproduction, about the formation of female and male children, and about the natures and functions of sexual pleasures which suggest what was womanly and what was manly, what pertained to the feminine and what pertained to the masculine. It does this, first, by looking directly at the way in which texts characterize the male and the female – both what the two sexes are and how they got to be that way – and, second, by seeing how men and women figure in discussions of two concrete and practical problems – how to overcome infertility and how to handle situations in which sexual abstinence is expected. In these chapters the varieties and ambiguities within medicine and natural philosophy interact with other aspects of medieval society, such as ecclesiastical interest in regulating sexual behavior and the preference of the laity for sons over daughters. What emerges is not a grand synthetic scheme that captures the medieval concept of gender but rather a cluster of gender-related notions, sometimes competing, sometimes mutually reinforcing; sometimes permissive, sometimes constraining; sometimes consistent, sometimes ad hoc. The plot of this account, therefore, does not consist in the discovery of the essence of medieval views on sex difference and the logic of their relation to a gender system; instead it consists in the unfolding of relations among various distinct but overlapping sets of theories, values, and interests. Thus, if it is, in one sense, a contribution to our understanding of medieval perspectives on the meanings of femaleness and maleness, it is, in another sense, a case study of the ways in which scientific and medical ideas developed in specifically medieval settings (in monasteries and medical faculties, in compilations and commentaries) and also of the ways in which those ideas, institutions, and genres of writing made up a part of a larger culture.

PART I

Seeds and pleasures: The evolution of learned opinions

INTRODUCTION: THE CHARACTER AND EXTENT OF
MEDIEVAL DEPENDENCY

The medieval intellectual landscape was dominated by towering formations of the past. Scripture and Patristic writings were the rocks upon which Christian thought was founded, but in other areas as well – from rhetoric to geography – a person of even modest education could name the one or two giants of antiquity in whom authority resided. Indeed, important aspects of the history of medieval thought can be traced by the succession of ancient figures who held sway: that the title of "The Philosopher" passed from Plato to Aristotle in the thirteenth century tells us both about the shift in philosophical orientation and about the stability of medieval reverence for ancient authority. The discovery, transmission, and assimilation of ancient texts in the later Middle Ages are thus crucial to the development of medieval science and medicine in general and to notions of sex difference and reproduction in particular. Yet to portray medieval thought simply as derivative – as passively dependent on a set or even a succession of ancient ideas – is to misrepresent the dynamism and creativity of the period. Nor was respect for the ancients in constant conflict with flexibility and resourcefulness. Rather, though reverence for authority may sometimes have constrained the medieval imagination, it also fueled it.

The recourse to authority was real, but it was anything but static. For example, medieval authors used the word "seed" (*semen*) so flexibly that it is not always easy to place them squarely in the camp of Aristotle, who taught that reproduction involved one seed, or in the camp of Galen and others, who taught that reproduction involved two seeds. If Virgil was held in the highest regard by the literate public in the later Middle Ages, he was also remolded to function within medieval culture. Indeed, he took two new forms: that of the proto-Christian, the pagan equivalent of the Hebrew Patriarchs; and that of the magus, the repository of secret and powerful wisdom. When Dante honored him in the *Divine Comedy*, he did so within limits defined by the medieval Christian hierarchy of salvation. And if Chaucer borrowed from the late Roman authority Macrobius not only his cosmological picture but also his literary device for revealing it, he nevertheless subverted and parodied it when he placed his persona soaring to great heights in the claws of an eagle pontificating on scholastic physics.[1] The power exerted by ancient authors upon medieval views of sex difference and reproduction was by no means trivial, but it was far from absolute.

1 Geoffrey Chaucer, "House of Fame," in *The Complete Works*, ed. Walter W. Skeat (Oxford: Clarendon Press, 1894), vol. 3, pp. 1–64. For the scholastic eagle, see bk. II, ll. 729–863, pp. 22–6.

1

Prelude to medieval theories and debates: Greek authorities and their Latin transformations

THE ORIGINS OF MEDIEVAL ALTERNATIVES: ANCIENT
GREEK AUTHORITIES

The authorities of antiquity appear in this chapter as they did to medieval thinkers, as inhabitants of an abstract past without full context, relationships, or connections; as texts surrounded with an aura of dignity and authority. They do, of course, have a history of their own: they belonged to different worlds, were subject to various influences, represented and reacted to crosscurrents of contemporary thought. But here their own histories are set aside, and they make their appearance only as sources of late medieval beliefs about sex difference and reproduction. Indeed this account even distorts the shape of their ideas, to the extent that the emphasis is upon those elements of ancient thought that were available and influential later. The most important of these sources are a number of gynecological and general medical works from the Hippocratic corpus; Aristotle's work on animal reproduction and, to a lesser extent, his other works on animals; and Galen's general works on the body and on medicine. The work of Soranus, of less importance to later medieval thinkers, has a place here because his views on gynecology were widely disseminated in the Latin West before the full introduction of Galenic and Aristotelian ideas.

Medieval authors had direct or indirect access to far more Greek and Roman sources than are mentioned here. Like Scripture and the writings of the Church Fathers, many influential classical works that addressed other subjects – metaphysical, ethical, political, etc. – contained material about procreation or sex differences or sexual desire. Thus, for example, scholastic natural philosophers will quote Ovid as well as Aristotle on the subect of sexual pleasure. But medieval authors do not always cite (or indeed always know) the sources of their opinions, and the precise influence of such works is difficult to gauge not only because their influence is diffuse but also because they themselves are often borrowing and echoing both learned and popular tenets.

The views of Plato are a case in point. His philosophy marginalized medicine and natural science, so he was less interested in reproduction as a physical than as a spiritual process.[1] Furthermore, the only passage in which he seriously discussed reproduction as a phenomenon in nature was not translated into Latin during the Middle Ages.[2] Plato's account of reproduction occurs at the end of the *Timaeus*, as part of an extended creation myth. He begins by saying that those men who failed to attain the higher life – the cowardly and those who lived badly – returned to the world as women in their second life. Once there were women, the gods created a new animal, sexual desire, of which there are two kinds. The desire for sexual intercourse in men is aroused when a special type of marrow, the sperm, descends from the brain through passages opened for it by the gods, through the neck and down the spine, joining the vessel through which liquids are expelled. This sperm, which has a vital soul, desires release, which in turn produces the reproductive *eros*. Hence the male's penis is willful and uncontrollable, a living creature which rebels against reason. The female equivalent is the uterus, which is also like an animate being, possessed of the second, female desire: to produce children. Like that of the male seed, the uterus's desire is forceful and petulant. If not satisfied by pregnancy and childbirth, the uterus will roam about the abdominal cavity and cause all kinds of trouble, especially by obstructing airways, making breathing difficult. The problems are resolved when the man's erotic impulse and the woman's desire unite to conceive offspring.[3]

A number of the ideas expressed by Plato occur in other ancient and medieval contexts. There is the notion that males are superior to females, that in some sense females are fallen or failed males.[4] Although this specific version of the origins of inequality was not widely accepted, the value hierarchy in general played an important role in ancient and medieval discus-

---

1 Plato, *Le banquet* [*Symposium*], ed. and trans. Léon Robin, vol. 4, pt. 2 of *Oeuvres complètes*, Collections des Universités de France, Association Guillaume Budé (Paris: Société d'Edition "Les Belles Lettres," 1962), 206B–207A, pp. 60–2. In the *Timaeus* he appends his discussion of reproduction to an exposition of the highest form of *eros* of which humans are capable. See Francis MacDonald Cornford, trans. and comm., *Plato's Cosmology: The* Timaeus *of Plato* (London: Routledge and Kegan Paul, 1937), pp. 291–3.
2 Plato's succinct account is at *Timaeus*, 90E–91D: Albert Rivaud, ed. and trans., *Timée, Critias*, vol. 10 of *Oeuvres complètes*, Collections des Universités de France, Association Guillaume Budé (Paris: Société d'Edition "Les Belles Lettres," 1963), pp. 226–7. The *Timaeus* was in fact the most influential Platonic work of the Middle Ages and the only one available before the twelfth century, but the Latin version (which was accompanied by the commentary of Chalcidius) omitted the whole last part of the dialogue, in which the passage in question occurs.
3 Cornford (*Plato's Cosmology*, p. 357, n. 2) emphasizes Plato's distinction between male and female passion by attributing *eros* to the male and *epithumia* to the female. Rivaud (*Timée*, p. 226) sees love and lust as applying equally to both sexes at this point (91D).
4 Plato presents an alternative myth of the history of the sexes and sexuality in *Symposium*, 189D–193C.

sions of male and female. On a more concrete level, Plato's account of the male and female generative parts contained elements which related to contemporary medical thought and which persisted in later writings. The notions that the semen originates from the head and is related to the matter of which the brain and nerves are made, that near the kidneys it joins up with vessels leading to the penis, and that it has some sort of spirit which impels it, all are pieces of a picture frequently alluded to by other authors. The attribution of soul and will to the seed or penis and to the uterus has a more problematic relationship to common traditions. The representation of the uterus as having a desire to produce children and a tendency to make trouble if unsatisfied is more often repeated or alluded to than is the personification of the penis. On the other hand, the attribution of some sort of spirit or soul to the semen is a common way of explaining its apparent mobility and of expressing its perceived ability to communicate life to offspring. And even though many later authors reject the notion of a moving womb, the idea that it is subject to particular pathological conditions was widespread: the uterus could create pressures which in turn gave rise to serious illness, including what is called "uterine suffocation" or (from *hystera*, "the womb") "hysterical suffocation." The idea that emptiness caused these disorders and that intercourse leading to pregnancy is the solution shared some currency with the description of uterine suffocation and served as the most striking evidence both that women had a set of illnesses all their own and that women's health was dependent upon the reproductive functions.

Plato's specific ideas on these subjects were not universally shared. Galen denied that the womb wandered, and Soranus saw no such radical separation between male and female health. But the case of Plato underscores the extent to which the issues that Hippocrates, Aristotle, Soranus, and Galen took up were framed in terms with which the educated elite of the ancient world was broadly familiar. His incorporation of this material and the extent to which it is linked to the discourse of philosophers and medical writers concerned with reproductive theory, gynecology, and related subjects suggests a resonance between specialized and more widely held views. Such resonance will again be apparent in the later Middle Ages and will help explain some of the conjunctions and tensions between ideas and their social context in that period.

Hippocratic balance

The Hippocratic corpus – the vast collection of fifth- and fourth-century Greek medical texts, of which few if any were written by the renowned physician Hippocrates of Cos – contains a number of works on gynecology, obstetrics, and embryology that made their way into the medical literature of the Middle Ages.[5] The work known as the *Aphorisms*, a loosely organized set of dicta on a much wider range of medical subjects, also exerted considerable influence, especially because it was transmitted to western Europe adorned with a commentary by Galen.[6] In contrast to many of Aristotle's works, which take the form of arguments and center on the development of a theoretical framework, these gynecological and obstetrical works are of a more practical nature and contain information and instructions directly related to diagnosis, prognosis, and treatment. The material lends itself to selective borrowing and rearrangement and often does not appear to take an explicit stance on theoretical issues. Thus the Hippocratic writings on subjects related to sex differences and reproduction represented a rich mine of knowledge that could be exploited by itself or in conjunction with material from other sources. For example, medieval medical writers frequently repeated the assertion that because semen passes down from the brain through veins behind the ears, cutting those veins renders a man sterile.[7]

The texts that touch on sex difference and reproduction are not, in fact, free from theoretical substance. Like many other tracts in the Hippocratic corpus, they are based on a general understanding of the body and its functions, of health and disease, that is, on the idea of balance. The recognition of imbalance and the maintenance and restoration of balance were among the most important tasks of the physician, who worked in conjunction with the natural processes that promoted temperateness, especially the mild cooking and blending in which the body engaged. The notion of balance was a relative one: men and women had different appropriate equilibria, as did the young

5 This group of works, though by several authors, belongs to the Cnidian school and has a common vocabulary and set of assumptions about medicine, in general, and about gynecology, obstetrics, reproduction, and embryology, in particular. The standard edition of the Hippocratic corpus is Emile Littré, ed., *Les oeuvres complètes d'Hippocrate*, 10 vols. (Paris: J. B. Baillière, 1839–61), and includes the relevant works *On the Nature of Woman, On the Seven-Month Fetus, On the Eight-Month Fetus, On Generation,* and *On the Nature of the Child,* all in vol. 7 (1851), pp. 310–543; *Diseases of Women* I and II, *On Sterile Women, On the Diseases of Young Women, On Superfetation,* and *On Embryotomy,* vol. 8 (1853). Some of these are available in more recent versions: *De la génération, De la nature de l'enfant, Des maladies IV, Du foetus de huit mois,* ed. and trans. Robert Joly, vol. 11 of *Oeuvres,* Collection des Universités de France (Paris: Société d'Edition "Les Belles Lettres," 1970); Iain M. Lonie, *The Hippocratic Treatises* On Generation, On the Nature of the Child, Diseases IV: *A Commentary,* Ars medica: Texte und Untersuchungen zur Quellenkunde der alten Medizin 2. Abteilung, Griechisch-lateinische Medizin 7 (Berlin: Walter de Gruyter, 1981) (with translations); Tage U. H. Ellinger, trans., *Hippocrates on Intercourse and Pregnancy: An English Translation of* On Semen *and* On the Development of the Child (New York: Henry Schuman, 1952); Ann E. Hanson, trans., "Hippocrates: *Diseases of Women,* I," *Signs* 1 (1975): 567–84.

6 This work, from the school of Cos, is not closely related to the gynecological texts but does not differ from them radically on the points discussed here. See *Aphorisms,* esp. bk. V, 28–63 (Littré, vol. 4 [1844; repr. 1962], pp. 458–609; Hippocrates, *Works,* ed. and trans. W. H. S. Jones, E. T. Witherington, and Paul Potter, 6 vols., Loeb Classical Library [Cambridge: Harvard University Press; London: William Heinemann, 1923–88], vol. 4 [1931], pp. 97–221).

7 Hippocrates, *Airs, Waters, Places* (*Works,* ed. Jones, ch. xxii, pp. 126–8).

and the old; different geographical places and different times of the year affected the balance of the individual and might require an adjustment in what constituted health. This balance was a version of the Greek notion of moderation and incorporated concerns about behavior and patterns of living into medicine: one should work to achieve moderate sexual activity, moderate diet, and moderate exercise, just as one should be moderate in one's ethical and political life.[8] The medical concept of balance, like the general notion of moderation, presupposed the existence of polarities and sets of extremes between which a mean must be sought. Some of these were very specific, such as too little or too much menstrual flow; some were more general and were often the cause of the more specific: hot and cold, moist and dry, were the critical polar principles in almost every aspect of what we would call physiology. Hippocratic works sometimes represented these principles in the more concrete terms of the four humors – cholera (mostly hot), phlegm (mostly cold), black bile (mostly dry), and blood (mostly moist) – but in the language of the gynecological, obstetrical, and embryological works, the more abstract qualities prevail.

The Hippocratic system of polarities, it should be noted, is not hierarchical. That is, it does not, like the polarities of the Pythagorean school, ascribe positive value to one pole and negative value to the other or, as Aristotle would later do, assign higher value to one and lower value to the other. Since the value of a particular quality, say heat, is contextual, depending on the individual, on the weather, and on innumerable other conditions, heat cannot regularly be valued more highly than cold. It is necessary as a principle of life; it is potentially fatal as a principle of fevers. Furthermore, heat is not invariably associated with the male in the Hippocratic writings. *Diseases of Women, I* represents women as hotter than men, because of the loose and porous quality of their flesh.[9] From the point of view of the history of ideas about sex difference, the nonhierarchical character of Hippocratic polarities is significant because it does not invite ranking the sexes on physiological grounds. True, these polarities were formulated in an ancient culture and transmitted to a medieval culture that were both familiar with the value associations making right better than left and warm better than cold, but the presentation of these categories in the Hippocratic writings on obstetrics and gynecology does not advance the devaluation of the female. The male fetus may tend to the right side of the womb, the female to the left, the typical male balance may rest at a drier point than the typical female balance, but those differences do not themselves imply the superiority of the male.[10]

Likewise, the theory of reproduction contained in these Hippocratic writ-

---

8 See Foucault, *Use of Pleasure*, pp. 99–108.
9 Hippocrates, *Diseases of Women*, I (Littré, vol. 8, pp. 12, 13).
10 Hippocrates, *Aphorisms*, V, 38 and 48 (Littré, vol. 4, pp. 544, 550; Jones, vol. 4, pp. 166, 170).

ings does not contain a value difference or even an important functional difference between the sexes in the conception of a child. The authors of the Hippocratic gynecological texts were not concerned with providing an explanation of the process of generation, so evidence of a theory is scattered and sometimes indirect. Still, a general picture emerges, which is confirmed by other works in the Hippocratic corpus and which was perceived by later readers.[11] Both parents contribute seed drawn from all parts of their bodies, a process known as "pangenesis"; family resemblance and sex difference are explained in terms of the generative contributions of both parents. (This version of reproduction has the advantage of providing a ready explanation for the resemblance of the offspring to both parents and their families, though, as Aristotle pointed out in his critique of pangenesis, it has a set of problems related to the sorting of characteristics.)[12] For any given feature, the seed may come more from the mother's side or the father's: with respect to that feature, the child will resemble the parent whose contribution is greatest. Each parent has both male and female emissions; thus both the mother and the father have the seed (*gone, sperma*) to produce male and female offspring. The child's sex is determined by the interactions of the parents' emissions. If they are not in agreement, one – not necessarily the son-producing seed or the father's seed – will prevail.[13]

Although many of the details of this presentation of the reproductive process were not directly accessible in the Middle Ages (*On the Seed* was apparently not translated into Latin), the association of Hippocrates with a two seed system was familiar. The treatise *On the Nature of the Child*, for example, which was translated in the thirteenth century, opens with the words, "If the sperm of both [parents] makes its way into the woman's womb. . . ."[14] What this Hippocratic account offered to future scholars and practitioners was a model of reproduction that minimized differences in the areas of conception and heredity. It suggested parallel functions of female and male and used the basic polarities of quality without denigrating the female partner. Yet the Hippocratic heritage was not without ambiguities. Not only because the corpus was composed by various authors at various times but also because of the secondary importance of systematic, theoreti-

11 Two articles on the ancient conversation about conception summarize the competing theories: Anthony Preus, "Galen's Criticism of Aristotle's Conception Theory," *Journal of the History of Biology* 10 (1977): 65–85; Michael Boylan, "Galenic and Hippocratic Challenges to Aristotle's Conception Theory," *Journal of the History of Biology* 17 (1984): 83–112.

12 Aristotle, *Generation of Animals*, ed. and trans. A. L. Peck, Loeb Classical Library (Cambridge: Harvard University Press; London: William Heinemann, 1953), I, xvii–xviii.

13 Hippocrates, *On Generation*, V-VII (Joly, pp. 48–50); and *On Regimen*, I, 7–21 (Robert Joly, ed. and trans., *Du régime*, vol. 6, pt. 2 of *Oeuvres*, Collection des Universités de France [Paris: Société d'Edition "Les Belles Lettres," 1972], pp. 21–5).

14 Pearl Kibre, *Hippocrates Latinus: Repertorium of Hippocratic Writings in the Latin Middle Ages*, rev. ed. (New York: Fordham University Press, 1985), XL, pp. 189–91: "Si sperma ab utrisque permansit in matrice mulieris. . . ." On the unity of this cluster of Hippocratic texts, see Lonie, *Hippocratic Treatises*, pp. 43–51.

cal analysis and, perhaps too, because of a real ambivalence on the subject of sex difference, the works also project views of female and male that do emphasize differences and imply the primacy and superiority of the male. With respect to the value placed on the male, the fact that son-producing seed is sometimes characterized as stronger (even though it does not necessarily prevail) and the daughter-producing seed is called weaker is sufficient sign that these works are by no means egalitarian. The exposition of differences is both implicit and explicit. The word "seed" is by far more frequently associated with the male than with the female, and the production of seed does not play a significant role in the many Hippocratic discussions of female reproductive disorders, where the emphasis is upon the uterus and menstruation.[15] Indeed the functional equivalence of male and female contributions is much less prominent in the Hippocratic writings than is the homology between male semen and female menstrual flow. Thus, for example, sexual maturity is associated with the opening up of the passageways for semen in the male and for menstrual flow in the female.[16] This parallel between the sexes is far more frequently alluded to in the Hippocratic writings than the functional parallel represented by the two-seed theory of reproduction, but both came to be associated with the Hippocratic tradition in later eras.

The identification of female physiology with menstruation is linked to the Hippocratic interest in the womb, both as an important element in the health and sickness of women and as an instrument of generation. Many of the conditions discussed and many of the treatments suggested in the Hippocratic treatises on the diseases of women are associated with the regularity or irregularity of menstruation or with the positions or motions of the uterus. Women's general health, as well as their reproductive health, depended on regular and moderate menstruation (a purgation necessary to avoid the accumulation and putrefaction of superfluous fluids) and on the proper placement and complexion of the uterus (which might shift about or dry out, causing trouble). Therapies were thus often aimed at the regulation of menstruation or the realignment of a uterus which had dangerously risen, causing suffocation, or fallen, causing urinary obstruction, called "strangury,"[17] and they might even involve a prescription of intercourse or pregnancy. According to the treatise *On Generation*, for example, "if [women] have intercourse with men their health is better than if they do not. . . . Intercourse by heating the blood and rendering it more fluid gives an easier passage to the menses; whereas if the menses do not flow, women's bodies become prone to sickness."[18] (See Figure 1.)

15 E.g., *Diseases of Women*, I and II (Littré, vol. 8, pp. 10–407), and *On Sterile Women* (ibid., pp. 408–63).
16 Hippocrates, *On Generation*, II (Joly, p. 46).
17 See especially *Diseases of Women*, I, 7 (Littré, vol. 8, pp. 32–5).
18 Hippocrates, *On Generation* (Lonie, *Hippocratic Treatises*, p. 4). See also *On Virgins* (Littré, vol. 8, pp. 466–71). The translation given here is Lonie's.

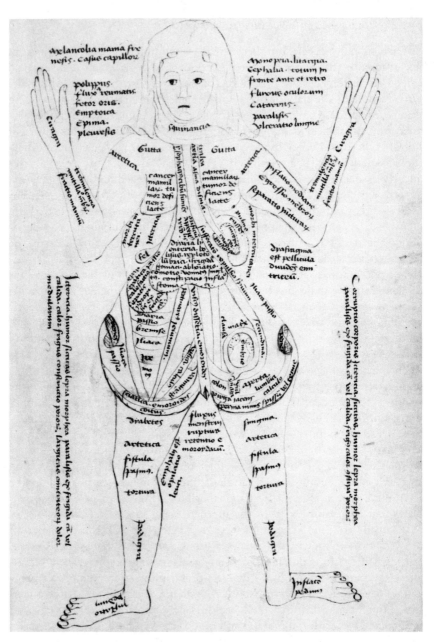

Figure 1. Disease woman, a relatively uncommon variation on male figures labeled with diseases specific to particular parts of the body and for the most part common to the two sexes. This female figure emphasizes conditions, from breast tumors to swollen feet, which were often discussed in treatises on the diseases of women. In this fourteenth-century example, the woman is pregnant with twins. (Paris, Bibliothèque Nationale, MS lat. 11229, fol. 31r. Phot. Bibl. Nat. Paris. Reproduced by permission of the Bibliothèque Nationale.)

The contribution of Hippocratic medicine to later discourse on the subjects of sex difference, sexuality, and reproduction is thus a composite one. It involves an abstract theory of balance and a set of concrete instructions, many but not all of which are clearly related to the notion of balance. It offers both a view of conception in which the sexes are on a par with each other and a massive amount of material based on the premise that female health is bound up with organs and functions that have no significant counterpart in the male. For if there are functional parallels between the female and the male in the process of conception, there are differences between the sexes which are crucial to the medical intentions of the Hippocratic treatises on gynecology and obstetrics. Later authors drew on many aspects of this contribution, fascinated, for example, by the challenge of a two-seed reproductive theory and grateful for the wealth of detail about menstrual and uterine disorders. Some of the ideas and information contained in the Hippocratic treatises came to the Latin West directly, some indirectly, some early, some late. The *Aphorisms*, for example, was available in Latin as early as the sixth century; obstetrical and gynecological fragments are found in manuscripts from the eighth and ninth centuries, but the works from which they were excerpted were not retranslated until the sixteenth century; and the treatise *On the Nature of the Embryo*, also available in Latin in the early Middle Ages, was translated again in the thirteenth century.[19] The broad dissemination and influence of Hippocratic ideas in antiquity ensured that much of the Greek and, later, Arabic heritage from which the Latin West drew was infused with Hippocratic assumptions and material.

Aristotelian oppositions

In his work *Generation of Animals*, Aristotle agreed with and may have been indebted to certain principles found in Hippocratic works. He endorsed the notions of balance and moderation, for example, not just as general cultural axioms but as specific rules for the functioning of living creatures. Like many of the Hippocratic treatises, his works invoke pairs of opposing qualities, especially hot and cold, moist and dry, though he connected them with the four elements more than with the four humors. And like the Hippocratic authors he attributed roles both to seed and to environmental conditions in his discussions of reproduction. But Aristotle differed from them both in his goals and in his specific convictions. For Aristotle was writing as a natural philosopher, not as a physician, and his goal was to provide a

---

19 Kibre, *Hippocrates Latinus*, III, pp. 29–33; XXXIX, p. 188; and XL, pp. 189–91; and Pearl Kibre, "Hippocratic Writings in the Middle Ages," *Bulletin of the History of Medicine* 18 (1945): 371–412.

systematic explanation of the natural phenomena connected with reproduction that was consistent with his broader philosophy. He did not, like the medical writers, limit himself to *human* reproduction, nor was he much concerned with the pathological or the therapeutic aspects of his subject, except insofar as they provided evidence and examples of his points. Furthermore, the substance of Aristotle's view of reproduction differed from the views reflected in the Hippocratic treatises about, among other things, the reproductive roles of female and male.

Like the medical opinions of the Hippocratic works, Aristotle's theory of generation fits into a larger framework of understanding. Specifically, his ideas about form and matter and his concept of causation underlie his representation of sex difference and reproduction. All natural objects, according to Aristotle, are defined and shaped by their *form*, which is an essence and a principle of actualization: it makes a thing what it is. But form cannot exist alone in nature. It must always inhere in some *matter*, indeed in some particular matter appropriate to the character of the form – you cannot make a bed out of bananas. Any proper account of natural objects or processes must focus on the forms; any complete account will also consider the matter. In reproduction, the communication of the form (by the male) is central, but the provision of appropriate (and therefore not entirely formless) material by the female is nonetheless necessary. Form and matter are among the *causes* of things and events. To these Aristotle adds efficient and final causes, to complete the set of analytical categories of natural explanation. In the production of semen, for example, Aristotle saw the heat of the father's heart as the efficient cause, the moving force of reproduction. It was the heart that converted digested food into useful blood, and the male heart that effected the refinement of a portion of useful blood into a white, spiritous substance subsequently stored in the testicles. Efficient causes are thus often the present and visible (or palpable) causes with which modern science is concerned. Final causes, like forms (or formal causes), to which they are closely related, are more important to Aristotle, since they embody the purpose, the direction, the goal of an object or process – and its place in the fabric of nature. A final cause of reproduction, for example, is the accomplishment of eternal existence for the kind or species – a goal unattainable for the individual.[20] Medieval authors applied these ideas of causation as they explored, for example, the mechanisms responsible for sexual pleasure (i.e., its efficient causes) and the purposes for which sexual pleasure existed in nature (i.e., its final causes).

Aristotle's treatment of sex difference and reproduction is infused with such teleological considerations. Small details of a particular animal's structure, as well as prominent features of the natural world – like the existence

---

20 Aristotle, *Generation of Animals*, II, i, 731b31–732a1.

of sexual specialization – serve nature's purpose. And they do so through the mediation of efficient causes. Heat, for example, effects such processes as digestion and the refinement of semen.

Through his insistence on a high standard of thoroughness and consistency, Aristotle's works on living things set a strong and influential example for the rational analysis of nature; through his omnivorous incorporation of empirical information gleaned from observation, the work of earlier writers, and common lore, he provided a store of specific knowledge which could be (and was) separated from its theoretical context by later readers. Thus, like the Hippocratic corpus, the works of Aristotle provided more than one model and more than one set of opportunities for posterity. His complex and synthetic method could be borrowed whole, or it could be dismantled and used in parts – the rationalism appealing to some, the body of empirical information to others. And his notions of form and matter and of cause, which he himself applied flexibly, invited application in new ways and to new subjects.

The dynamics of reproduction start, for Aristotle, with the four qualities, especially hot and cold. As in the Hippocratic writings, the balance between opposites is a crucial feature of Aristotle's view of living bodies. Hot organs, like the heart, and cold organs, like the brain, counterbalance one another, preventing excess. But Aristotle, more than the authors of the Hippocratic texts, tended consistently to read values in the poles: warm is better than cool, even though it is possible to be too warm; the heart is superior to the brain, even though the brain is necessary. Thus when he applied the polarities to sex differences, they served to indicate the superiority of the male over the female. Not only is the female cooler than the male – a fact which in itself would earn her a lower place in the natural order of things – but the inadequacy of her warmth is the cause of the difference between her reproductive role and that of the male. Males, by their heat, are able to refine surplus nutriment not merely to the stage at which it becomes blood (which is what happens to most useful nutriment) but beyond that to the point where it becomes semen – pure, white, and spiritous. Females, however, lacking sufficient heat, are unable to make semen and produce instead just more blood – menstrual blood – with the proper characteristics to become a fetus. The difference in degree of heat produces a qualitative difference between the two fluids: the semen is able to shape and communicate the male parent's form to the blood contributed by the female; and that blood can, in turn, receive form and nourish the fetus, which the male principle has defined.[21] Thus, in Aristotle's system, warm and cold translate into superiority and inferiority, ability and inability, activity and passivity.

Modern scholars have noted Aristotle's comment in this connection that

---

21 Ibid., I, 2 and 17–23; II, 1–3.

females are in a sense monstrosities, deformed males.[22] He does indeed suggest that female offspring represent a failure in the reproductive process: either the weakness of the father's seed or the intractability of the mother's material or some external condition has, by default, produced a daughter – a naturalistic version of Plato's moral fall.[23] Physiologically she will lack sufficient heat to produce seed, and anatomically (also for lack of heat) her reproductive organs will be internal rather than external. But neither Aristotle's teleological concept of nature nor his information about the specific facts of reproduction permitted him to stop at that, to dismiss the female as a useless by-product of male self-replication. Nature does nothing in vain, and females do, after all, bear young. In analyzing any situation, Aristotle distinguished that which is "for the better" from that which is merely "necessary." The production of a male child is for the better, in the sense that it represents the fullest and most successful actualization of the reproductive process; the production of a female child was a result of necessity, that is, of a natural process constrained by conditions. Furthermore, even the matter contributed by the mother is not completely devoid of form. Indeed it must be (and by the female's modicum of heat is prepared to be) appropriate for the formation of a human being similar to the mother. This form and this potential, though not definitive, can nevertheless be influential. Daughters are thus disappointing but not unnatural. Although each individual female is an imperfection, the existence of two sexes, and thus the segregation of the formal and material principles of generation, are for the better. From the point of view of parenthood, fathers' contributions are superior, for it is their seed which provides the defining essence, the actualizing form for the offspring, whereas mothers' contributions are inferior, for the incompletely processed surplus nutriment which they produce is the more passive matter out of which the more active, form-bearing seed shapes the offspring. And though it is not true that females *have* no souls, they cannot *effect* them.[24]

The polarization of female and male is much more pronounced in the Aristotelian representation than in the Hippocratic. Hot and cold, perfect and imperfect, ability to produce semen and inability to do so, contributor of form and contributor of matter, active and passive: in spite of the fact that Aristotle understood these pairs in relative terms, they create a radical contrast between the sexes. The contrast contains unambiguous value implications, since in Aristotle's system active is clearly better than passive, form

---

22 Ibid., IV, vi, 775a15–16; see also II, iii, 737a25–30. Maryanne Cline Horowitz, "Aristotle and Women," *Journal of the History of Biology* 9 (1976): 183–213, for example.

23 Aristotle, *Generation of Animals*, IV, ii, 367a23–35.

24 Ibid., I, i; II, i–iii. See David M. Balme, trans. and comm., *Aristotle's De partibus animalium I and De generatione animalium I with Passages from II.1–3*, Clarendon Aristotle Series (Oxford: Clarendon Press, 1972), notes, pp. 127–9 and 155–65; and idem, "Ανθρωπος ἄνθρωπον γεννᾷ: Human Is Generated by Human," in G. R. Dunstan, ed., *The Human Embryo: Aristotle and the Arabic and European Traditions* (Exeter: Exeter University Press, 1990), pp. 20–31.

better than matter. Furthermore, except for hot and cold, the extremes cannot meaningfully be mediated, so neither the Hippocratic principle of balance, to which Aristotle in general subscribed, nor the Hippocratic notion of parallelism between the sexes, which Aristotle rejected, mitigated the value-laden opposition between female and male.[25]

Aristotle offered the heirs of antiquity alternatives to Hippocratic views not only in regard to specific theories of reproduction (one seed versus two seeds) and in conceptualization (value-laden polarities versus limited analogies) but also in regard to the domains emphasized and deemphasized. Aristotle went much farther in integrating his account of generation into a systematic natural philosophy based on a clearly articulated metaphysical foundation, but he left unaddressed many questions about sexual and reproductive function and dysfunction that were of crucial interest to medical writers. Thus what might be called Aristotle's "gynecology" is scant, his "obstetrics" scantier. Menstrual blood is an essential element in Aristotle's form–matter view of reproduction, and like the Hippocratic authors, he treated menstruation as the emission of superfluous matter and associated menarche with sexual maturity. During pregnancy this superfluity constitutes the material upon which the form (provided through the seed of the father) operates. But in most of his discussions of generation Aristotle did not concern himself with the relationship between menstruation and female health or with the existence of – much less the causes and cures for – menstrual retention or excessive menstrual flow. Nor did he give much attention to the uterus, although he identified it as the female reproductive organ. How much is there to say about this simple receptacle? Since it is passive, it would not make much sense to think of it as influential, much less as a semiautonomous quasi-animate entity. This is not to say that Aristotle denied the existence of the malady known as suffocation of the womb, or hysteria; it was a widely accepted diagnosis which he had no reason to question.[26] But his concept of the womb combined with his focus on natural philosophy rather than medicine led him to neglect the uterine and menstrual subjects that were at the center of so much ancient gynecology and obstetrics. The one significant exception to this lack of interest is in the tenth and last book of the *History of Animals*, where several chapters are devoted to the causes and diagnosis of sterility, in the course of which uterine and menstrual disorders are mentioned. Aristotle's authorship of this section is not certain, but it was taken as genuine in the Middle Ages.[27]

---

25 On balance, see, e.g., Aristotle, *Generation of Animals*, IV, ii, 767a14–35. Aristotle's rejection of the idea that both female and male produce seed is embedded in his argument against pangenesis (ibid., I, xvii–xviii).

26 Ibid., I, xi, 719a18–21.

27 Aristotle, *History of Animals*, bk. X (trans. Jonathan Barnes, in Jonathan Barnes, ed., *The Complete Works of Aristotle,* 2 vols., rev. Oxford translation, Bollingen Series 71/2 [Princeton: Princeton University Press, 1984], vol. 1, pp. 984–93). See Balme, "Human Is Generated by Human," p. 21.

The difference in emphases meant, among other things, that the Aristotelian and Hippocratic traditions opened up very different paths for the expression of later misogyny. From Aristotle came the hierarchical formulation which represented females as consistently inferior and specifically cool, weak, and passive. From the Hippocratic writers – and no doubt the popular conceptions represented by Plato – came the womb-centered version, according to which females (still likely to be cool and weak) were subject to the erratic influence of a powerful and active organ that affected health and disposition and was the repository of a formidable sexual appetite.

Soranus and the reduction of difference

Medical writers of later antiquity shared with the Hippocratic writers an interest in gynecology and obstetrics not central to the concerns of natural philosophers like Aristotle, but they did not always agree with the substance of Hippocratic opinion. Soranus of Ephesus, a successful Greek physician in second-century Rome, wrote on a range of medical subjects, including medical biography and etymology, as well as on acute and chronic diseases, surgery, and medicines. His main surviving work is his *Gynecology*, which treats many of the same topics as the Hippocratic works but which differs from them in nature and in content.[28] Soranus, like Galen slightly later, profited from the rich contributions of Alexandria, which was a center of medical research and teaching from the fourth century B.C.E. to his own time. And Soranus, like Galen, reflected critically upon the history of medicine and upon the various medical sects, with their different assumptions and methods in medical theory and practice.

The Methodist school, with which Soranus was associated by training and general approach, offered a model of health and disease that served especially well those areas of gynecology and obstetrics concerned with the womb. The Methodist notion that tension and laxity were the keys to understanding the state of the body and its parts applied easily and productively to that organ whose muscularity and elasticity are among its most remarkable properties. Soranus also expressed other aspects of sexuality and reproduction in terms of looseness and constriction. He identified a disorder in both women and men to which he applied the generic term "gonorrhea" – the frequent emission of semen without sexual arousal. It results in pallor and weakness of the body as a whole, and is a clear example of the ill effects of too much laxity or insuffi-

---

28 Soranus, *Gynaeciorum libri iv, De signis fracturarum, De fasciis, Vita Hippocratis secundum Soranum*, ed. Johannes Ilberg, Corpus medicorum Graecorum 4 (Leipzig and Berlin: B. G. Teubner, 1927), pp. 3–152; *Soranus'* Gynecology, trans. Owsei Temkin with Nicholson J. Eastman, Ludwig Edelstein, and Alan F. Guttmacher, Publications of the Institute of the History of Medicine, Johns Hopkins University, 2d ser., Texts and Documents 3 (Baltimore: Johns Hopkins University Press, 1956). The latter contains a general introduction to Soranus, his *Gynecology*, and its fate (pp. xxiii–xlix). See Green, "Transmission," pp. 23–36.

cient tension. Soranus therefore prescribed constrictives to remedy the condition, including placing a thin sheet of lead under the hips overnight and local applications to strengthen the relevant bodily parts. (The patient – female in this work – should also be shielded from the causes of sexual excitement, such as pictures of good-looking men and stories about sexual intercourse.)[29]

This example illustrates several aspects of Soranus's outlook. First, like the Hippocratic writers, he viewed health and disease in terms of general notions of balance and imbalance. Unlike them, however, and unlike Aristotle, he represented the body's temperament not in terms of qualities or humors but rather in terms of physical states related to the constriction and relaxation of tiny pores. Second, and consequently, his remedies, whether for gastrointestinal, respiratory, or sexual disorders, sought to restore the proper balance of tension and laxity. Third, with some exceptions, Soranus tended to treat male and female as essentially and structurally similar – in this case both subject to a disorder of the same sort as "pollutions" (nocturnal emissions), which, like "gonorrhoea" (involuntary emissions), had sometimes been associated only with men.[30]

The male–female parallel reflects Soranus's implicit agreement with the Hippocratic model of reproduction, according to which both parents contribute active seed to the formation of offspring. He did not, however, lay out a theory which would provide a fully developed alternative to Aristotle's position that only the male provides seed with formative power. Rather, as in the case of gonorrhea, Soranus alluded to the similarities of the sexes in the course of discussing more specific concerns. He mentioned female testes (the Greek medical term for what we call "ovaries"), seminal ducts, and seed, for example.[31] But neither medieval nor modern students of Soranus have been able to say with certainty how he understood the role of the female semen, since his treatise *On the Seed*, which no doubt contained the answer, is lost. When he traced the anatomy of the semen's pathway from the female testes, he commented that the semen's position outside the uterus makes it seem as though the female semen is useless in the creation of young.[32] Soranus did sometimes speak as though it was the

---

29 Soranus, *Gynaecia*, III, xii, 45–6 (Ilberg, pp. 124–5; Temkin, pp. 168–70). See also satyriasis in men and women: III, iii, 25 (Ilberg, p. 109; Temkin, p. 148).

30 E.g., Celsus, *De medicina*, ed. and trans. W. G. Spencer, 3 vols., Loeb Classical Library (Cambridge: Harvard University Press; London: William Heinemann, 1935), bk. IV, ch. 28 (vol. I, pp. 450, 452).

31 Soranus, *Gynaecia*, I, iii, 12 (Ilberg, p. 9; Temkin, pp. 11–12). The Greek is *didymoi*, which the Latin versions render as *testiculi mulierum* (women's testicles). Caelius Aurelianus, *Gynaecia: Fragments of a Latin Version of Soranus' Gynaecia from a Thirteenth-Century Manuscript*, trans. Miriam F. Drabkin and Israel E. Drabkin, Supplements to the Bulletin of the History of Medicine 13 (Baltimore: Johns Hopkins University Press, 1951), I, 15–16, p. 5; Muscio, *Sorani Gynaeciorum vetus translatio Latina*, ed. Valentine Rose (Leipzig: B. G. Teubner, 1882), I, 16–17, p. 10.

32 Soranus, *Gynaecia*, I, iii, 12 (Ilberg, p. 9; Temkin, p. 12).

menstrual blood, not the female semen, that was the female analogue of the male semen, but his general view of menstruation plays down its reproductive role.[33] Although Soranus identified menstruation as the natural flow of superfluous blood or fluid by which the body is purged, he did not attribute to it the essential role in female health upon which some Hippocratic writings insisted.[34] In fact, he argued explicitly against those who held such a view. If nature had any purpose in creating menstruation, it was for reproduction, not health – witness the fact that women too young or too old to conceive do not menstruate and can nevertheless be perfectly healthy.[35] Unlike the Hippocratic writings, which treat amenorrhea per se as a pathological condition, Soranus remarked that women who engage in moderate exercise, such as singing or walking around, sometimes do not menstruate and that the superfluity may be consumed in several ways consonant with health: not only by exercise but also by a young girl's growth or by the nutritional needs of the healthy uterus.[36] Although he did believe that the failure to menstruate was sometimes the result of disease (of the uterus or of another part of the body), it was not a disease in itself. He therefore introduced his discussion of pathological amenorrhea with a reminder that the same symptom can result from perfectly healthy conditions, which should be ruled out before addressing the absence of menstruation as a disorder.[37] Menstrual blood is thus not so much a purgation of harmful superfluities as it is one of several means by which the body manages an excess of healthy blood. Indeed, menstruation is positively harmful, though its ill effects are readily visible only in weaker women.[38]

One effect of Soranus's attitude toward menstruation was to displace it from the central position it holds in Hippocratic diagnosis and therapy. A second effect was to downplay the uniqueness of female function in favor of a stronger analogy between the sexes. This analogy is sustained in Soranus's discussion of the uterus, virginity, and the effects of childbirth. Because he was writing a treatise on gynecology, Soranus had to take the uterus more seriously than Aristotle did. At the opening of the work he described its position and anatomy in some detail, and he introduced the subjects that follow – menstruation, conception, pregnancy, and childbirth – as functions of the uterus.[39] Later in the work, he addressed a wide range of medical problems related to the condition and position of the uterus and prescribed

33 See Wolfgang Gerlach, "Das Problem des 'Weiblichen Samens' in der antiken und mittelalterlichen Medizin," *Sudhoffs Archiv für Geschichte der Medizin und Naturwissenschaften* 30
   (1938): 186.
34 Soranus, *Gynaecia*, I, iv, 19 (Ilberg, p. 13; Temkin, pp. 16–17). See Green, "Transmission,"
   pp. 23–36.
35 Soranus, *Gynaecia*, I, vi, 28 (Ilberg, pp. 18–19; Temkin, p. 24–5).
36 Ibid., iv, 22–3 (Ilberg, p. 15; Temkin, pp. 18–20).
37 Ibid., III, i, 6–9 (Ilberg, pp. 97–9; Temkin, pp. 132–5).
38 Ibid., I, vi, 29 (Ilberg, p. 19; Temkin, pp. 25–7).
39 Ibid., iii, 6–15 (Ilberg, pp. 6–10; Temkin, pp. 8–14).

treatments, some of which were mechanical manipulations and many of which were designed to promote greater laxity or constriction, depending upon the character of the disorder.[40] In other words, he applied the general principles of Methodist medicine, and he did not appeal to special physiological characteristics of the female body either to explain or to resolve gynecological and obstetrical problems. Although he did discuss diseases of the womb such as suffocation (hysteria), understood to have an impact on the whole body and even on the mind, Soranus showed no inclination to make the uterus the center of female health and disease.[41] On this score he was more restrained than some of the authors of the Hippocratic writings, and he directly attacked those who regarded the uterus as an animal.[42] (Soranus's tone suggests that this belief, expressed by Plato, was widely held.) He thus retained his tendency to minimize differences between the sexes.

Soranus's positions on menstruation and the uterus are linked in turn to his view of intercourse, both in the maintenance of a parallel between female and male and in the deemphasis of the purgative nature of the emission of sexual or reproductive fluids. Intercourse is necessary for reproduction, and reproduction is necessary for the perpetuation of the species, but from the point of view of the individual – female or male – virginity is a healthy state.[43] The emission of seed, like the emission of menstrual blood, does not play an essential role in the maintenance of health. Indeed, intercourse is essentially unhealthy in both women and men. Nor do women need to produce children to achieve individual equilibrium. On the contrary, pregnancy and childbirth strain and endanger. There are specific reasons why certain women are at risk,[44] but even mature, healthy women are subject to a number of woes. They suffer from the general heaviness of pregnancy and from *kissa*, a disorder encompassing nausea, cravings for strange foods, and other symptoms of early pregnancy.[45] And since the food sufficient for one is now partly siphoned off by the uterus to provide not just for the fetus's nourishment but for its growth, the woman herself is deprived – hardly a healthy situation. For this reason, pregnancies, although certainly not in themselves pathological, cause wasting of the body, weakness, and the onset of old age.[46] Soranus was consciously opposing himself to those (including, presumably, the Hippocratics) who held that childbearing was healthy and even curative. The theory underlying Soranus's reservations about men-

---

40 Ibid., III and IV, xv.
41 On suffocation see ibid., III, iv (Ilberg, pp. 109–13; Temkin, pp. 149–54).
42 Ibid., I, iii, 8 (Ilberg, p. 7; Temkin, p. 9).
43 Ibid., vii (Ilberg, pp. 20–2; Temkin, pp. 27–30).
44 Ibid., viii (Ilberg, pp. 22–3; Temkin, pp. 30–2).
45 Ibid., xv (Ilberg, pp. 35–9; Temkin, pp. 49–54).
46 Ibid., xi (Ilberg, pp. 29–30; Temkin, pp. 40–2); Caelius Aurelianus, *Gynaecia*, I, 52, pp. 16–17.

struation and pregnancy seems to have been that they both represent states of disequilibrium; they promote health only if they act as correctives for a previously existing imbalance or malady, but they have adverse effects upon women whose bodies are well tuned to begin with. He compared them with phlebotomy (bleeding): just because it can help remedy certain diseases does not make it healthy in and of itself.[47] In addition, he often observed that pregnancy, miscarriage, and abortion are the causes of uterine disorders. For Soranus a woman's health, like a man's, was defined and experienced independently of reproductive function.

Of the ancient authors considered here, Soranus's influence upon the thought of the later Middle Ages was the most fragmentary and indirect.[48] Yet Soranus's outlook traveled along with his specific descriptions and prescriptions into the medical literature of the later Middle Ages. Gynecological therapies deriving from the principles of constriction and laxity or reflecting Soranus's perspective on the uterus, menstruation, and childbearing continued to be collected and disseminated, spreading – if only indirectly – his dissenting views on these subjects. Although his long argument on the question of whether women have their own special diseases[49] was not rendered into Latin by his translators, who apparently saw their job as getting down to the brass tacks of anatomy, diagnosis, and treatment, the sorts of specific positions cited here on the uterus, menstruation, and intercourse perpetuated the message that Soranus had laid out systematically in the Greek text: women and men are essentially the same with respect to health and disease.

Galen's critical eclecticism

Like Soranus, Galen was a Greek physician from Asia Minor who was trained at several medical centers in the eastern Mediterranean and whose successful career took him to Rome, heart of the empire. He was born in about 130 C.E., around the time of Soranus's death, and lived till the end of the century. Like Soranus, he was versed in the medical advances of the Alexandrian school and conscious of the intricate doctrinal differences among the competing medical sects of his day. More than Soranus, he entered into the debates about goals and methods, employing at times a fierce polemical tone that suggests inflexibility and dogmatism. In fact, although Galen dismissed the beliefs of many of his predecessors and contemporaries, he borrowed selectively even from those whose general positions he rejected. Thus he served his medieval successors both as an example

47 Soranus, *Gynaecia*, I, xi (Ilberg, pp. 29–30; Temkin, pp. 40–2).
48 On the transmission of ancient gynecological thought to the Latin West and through the early Middle Ages, see Green's "Transmission."
49 Soranus, *Gynaecia*, III, [Prologue], 1–5 (Ilberg, pp. 94–7; Temkin, pp. 128–32).

of creative eclecticism and as a repository of information and ideas from a variety of sources. Not only did he draw together specific insights from his predecessors' work, he also synthesized the styles and methods of the authors upon whom he drew, creating a systematic, theoretical, and philosophical medicine. In his work *On Seed* for example, he often alluded to the importance of dissections for medical demonstrations, and his work *On the Use of Parts* is devoted to the praise of nature's art and economy. Galen was not the only medical writer of antiquity to consider the epistemological foundations of his art or to discuss the metaphysical implications of the relationship between physiology and anatomy, but he was the most influential in his own time and in the later Middle Ages.

Galen shared with Aristotle, then, a desire to place biological knowledge on a firm philosophical foundation and to present that knowledge systematically within a rational framework. He held that the best physician is also a philosopher, wrote works which he intended as contributions to both medicine and natural philosophy, and declared his intellectual heroes to be Hippocrates and Plato.[50] Works ascribed to Hippocrates in Galen's time were revered both by Empiricists (members of a medical sect that shunned theoretical and speculative medicine and emphasized the observational and even experimental basis of true medical knowledge) and by Dogmatists (members of a medical sect that insisted upon the importance of systematic theoretical reasoning as the basis of medical knowledge). Galen saw and subscribed to both views in the Hippocratic writings and thus took a position closely related to Aristotle's on the proper investigation of nature: his work is rich in observation, both general and clinical, and it is often structured by analytical categories and deductive logic. In *On Seed*, for example, he employed what he ostentatiously labeled Aristotelian syllogism on his way to the non-Aristotelian conclusion that females have active seed.[51] Although interested in matter and in efficient causes, Galen shared with Plato a strict opposition to the emphasis of ancient atomists and others upon matter as the essence of nature and upon chance as its source of order. He was thus adamantly opposed to Methodism, the tradition in which Soranus was trained, because he saw its assumptions as mechanistic and materialistic. (He did not, however, call Soranus's authority into question and cited him on pharmacological points.)[52] Following Aristotle's formulation, he held that the examination of form is crucial to scientific analysis and that nature does

---

50 On Galen's general medical theory and on his status as a medical philosopher, see Owsei Temkin, *Galenism: Rise and Decline of a Medical Philosophy*, Cornell Publications in the History of Medicine (Ithaca: Cornell University Press, 1973), pp. 10–50; Glen W. Bowersock, *The Greek Sophists in the Roman Empire* (Oxford: Oxford University Press, 1969), pp. 59–75.

51 Galen, *On Seed*, in *Opera omnia*, ed. Carl Gottlob Kühn, 20 vols. in 22 (Leipzig: C. Cnobloch, 1821–33; repr., Hildesheim: Georg Olms, 1964–5), vol. 4 (1922), II, ii, pp. 607–8.

52 Temkin, Introduction, in *Soranus' Gynecology*, p. xxxvi.

everything for a purpose, and he was indebted to other philosophical schools, including the Sophists, for other aspects of his method.[53]

Unlike the Hippocratic writers and Soranus, Galen did not devote works to gynecology or obstetrics, with the exception of an early tract on the anatomy of the uterus; unlike Aristotle, he did not write a separate treatise on reproduction.[54] He expressed his views on these subjects in a number of works – for the most part without reference to clinical concerns.[55] Sometimes, especially in his works *On the Use of Parts* and *On the Natural Faculties*, his opinions are at least as much a reflection of his general outlook on medicine as they are an independently developed representation of sex difference, sexual function, and reproduction. In this respect, he differs from the Hippocratics and Soranus, who devoted extended attention specifically to women's health, and from Aristotle, for whom the case of generation was a matter of direct concern, as well as a central example of an argument for his broader natural philosophy.

Hippocrates, Aristotle, and indeed many other authors provided Galen with the principles of his physiological understanding. He embraced the notion of balance, and he collected and ordered the various formulations of the qualities and substances to be balanced. Aligning ideas of the humors, the elements, the qualities, and the temperaments, Galen wove schemata present in many earlier schools of natural philosophy and medicine into a larger system of health and disease.[56] He agreed with Aristotle in seeing semen as the product of successive refinements but rejected Aristotle's view of the heart as the seat of physiological activity and adopted instead a more decentralized view of sexual arousal and semen, according to which the liver and its powers are involved in the production of blood and appetite; the brain and its powers are involved in the production of spirit and sensitivity; and the testes and their vessels contribute to the final refinement of the seed. His system incorporated, among other things, the polarities employed by

53 Bowersock, *Greek Sophists*, pp. 68ff.
54 Galen, *On the Dissection of the Uterus* (Kühn, vol. 2, pp. 887–908); and Charles Mayo Goss, trans., "On the Anatomy of the Uterus," *Anatomical Record* 144 (1962): 77–83.
55 Galen, *On Seed* (Kühn, vol. 4, pp. 512–651); *On the Use of Parts* (Kühn, vol. 3); *On the Usefulness of the Parts of the Body: Peri chreias morion: De usu partium*, trans. Margaret Tallmadge May, 2 vols., Cornell Publications in the History of Science, (Ithaca: Cornell University Press, 1968); and, less informative, *On the Natural Faculties*, ed. and trans. Arthur John Brock, Loeb Classical Library (Cambridge: Harvard University Press; London: William Heinemann, 1916). For a survey of Galen's ideas on these subjects, see Johann Lachs, *Die Gynaekologie des Galen: Eine geschichtlich-gynaekologische Studie*, Abhandlungen zur Geschichte der Medicin 4 (Breslau: J. U. Kerns, 1903). On Galen's relation to his predecessors, see Preus, "Galen's Criticism," and Boylan, "Galenic and Hippocratic Challenges."
56 See, e.g., *The Art of Medicine* (Kühn, vol. 1, pp. 306–412, esp. ch. IV–XVIII); *On the Elements after Hippocrates* (Kühn, vol. 1, pp. 413–508); and *On the Temperaments*, (Kühn, vol. 1, pp. 509–694); all of which were translated into Latin during the Middle Ages.

his predecessors. He agreed with Hippocratic sources, for example, that women were moister and men drier, and with Aristotle that women were cooler and men warmer.[57] He also adopted and adapted the polarity of left and right found here and there in Hippocratic and Aristotelian works and employed the traditional association of right with male, left with female.[58] Most of the pairs of opposites with which Galen deals admit of mediation, and he frequently emphasizes the provident moderation of nature. Thus, the uterus is hard enough to provide proper space and protection for the seed, yet soft enough to be able to expand and contract appropriately.[59]

In contrast to Aristotle, Galen did not emphasize the differences between the sexes: his use of polarities does not suggest radical contrariety. But following Aristotle, though to a lesser extent, he used evaluative language in discussing sex difference. Females are less perfect than males, according to Galen, because they are less warm, and heat is a crucial factor in natural processes. He compared female reproductive organs, which are internal and therefore not quite perfected, to moles' eyes, for example.[60] Galen was more explicit than Aristotle, however, about the physiological benefits for the species which result from this individual imperfection. If the female were warmer, the excess nutriment in her body would be dispersed by the heat, and she would have no nutriment to provide for the growth of an embryo. Indeed, seen in the light of the reproductive process, the female enjoys a perfectly appropriate moderation: she is warm enough to concoct the extra nutriment necessary, but not so warm that it is rendered inaccessible to the fetus.[61] So in fact, Galen asserts, female genitals are better than moles' eyes, which do the creatures no good.

In defining the female temperament in terms of its reproductive function, Galen's view contrasts with Soranus's in two respects. First, he suggested that the healthy female state differs significantly from the healthy male state. Second, he centered his characterization of female physiology on her reproductive role. Yet whereas Aristotle used female lack of heat as an explanation for female inability to produce semen, thus reasserting the contrary natures of the sexes and underscoring the value hierarchy, Galen once again

---

57 For ancient opinions on the relative warmth of the sexes, see *On the Usefulness of the Parts of the Body*, trans. May, vol. 1, p. 382, n. 78.
58 E.g., Galen, *Use of Parts*, XIV, iv (Kühn, vol. 3, p. 154; May, vol. 2, p. 626); Hippocrates, *Aphorisms*, sec. V, 48 (Littré, vol. 4, pp. 550, 551); Aristotle, *Parts of Animals*, ed. and trans. A. L. Peck, Loeb Classical Library (Cambridge: Harvard University Press; London: William Heinemann, 1937), II, ii, 648a 11–13, pp. 120, 121.
59 Galen, *Use of Parts*, XIV, iii (Kühn, vol. 3, pp. 148–50; May, vol. 2, p. 624).
60 Ibid., vi (Kühn, vol. 3, pp. 159–60; May, vol. 2, pp. 629–30); *On Seed*, II, v (Kühn, vol. 4, p. 640).
61 Galen, *Use of Parts*, XIV, vi. Aristotle does, of course, see a purpose for sexual differentiation and therefore, by implication, for female imperfection (*Generation of Animals*, II, i, 731b18–732a12).

diminished the contrast, taking the Hippocratic position that females do produce semen, but that it is cooler, moister, and less plentiful than that of males, which is warmer, thicker (i.e., less watery), and more plentiful.[62]

For Galen, the physiological similarities and differences between the sexes were necessarily closely related to the anatomical similarities and differences, for the design and economy of nature ensure that structure and function are suited to each other. He took great pains to demonstrate that the reproductive parts of females and males were anatomically equivalent – with the small difference that the female organs are internal – and that the anatomical equivalence necessarily implied functional equivalence. On the basis of this argument and others, he insisted that females, like males, not only produced semen but produced semen capable of communicating motion to the fetus and influencing its character and appearance. Thus, although he acknowledged a limited role for the constituent material in shaping the child, he explicitly rejected the opinion that any resemblance a child bears to its mother is due merely to her having provided the matter from which the fetus was made.[63] In short, the two semens operate according to the same principles. However, the fact that the female's semen results from less heat (and therefore does not bear as great motive potential as the male's) makes the two seeds sufficiently different that a mixture is necessary for generation. Galen also noted that the path of the female semen from the female testes to the uterus differs from the path of the male semen. Because of the anatomical difference in the path and the physiological difference in degree of warmth, he assigned distinct roles to the female semen – it is perfected by the male semen; because of its close similarity to the male semen, it supplies it with excellent nutriment; it forms the allantoid membrane; and it "provides for" the male semen.[64] On this point as elsewhere, Galen struggled with two conflicting interpretations of sex difference and reproduction. On the one hand, he wished to follow Hippocrates, whose two-seed theory had led him to observe with admiration the homologies between female and male and to argue that these parallel structures were designed to accommodate parallel functions. On the other hand, he wished to honor Aristotle and perhaps to acknowledge the medical attention commanded by the uterus, and thus he drew attention to the differences and argued that nature, purposeful and economical, would not have created two sexes to accomplish only one function. This tension, born of Galen's eclecticism, was later to become an opportunity for debate and a locus of revision and choices.

Galen's tendency to collect explanations from disparate sources may have derived in part from a respect for ancient authorities, but it was probably also a result of his appreciation of the complexity of the issues with which he

62 Galen, *Use of Parts*, XIV, vi (Kühn, vol. 3, pp. 163–5; May, pp. 631–2). See also *On Seed*, II, i.
63 A good part of the treatise *On Seed* is devoted to these and related arguments.
64 *On Seed*, II, i (Kühn, vol. 4, p. 600): "*pareskevakenai*"; I, vii (Kühn, vol. 4, pp. 536–7).

was dealing and of the multiplicity of questions which needed to be answered. Thus, although the supposition that two active semens went into the creation of a fetus could account for the existence of parallel anatomical structures in males and females and could explain how a child might resemble either parent, it did not provide a satisfactory explanation of sex determination. For, as Galen observed, sons who resembled their mothers and daughters who resembled their fathers could not result simply from the dominance of one of the constituent semens. So he incorporated the Hippocratic notion that the fetal environment influences the development of the child. Enter, therefore, the uterus.

For Galen, the uterus, like the male and female semen, was an active participant in the process of generation. Drawing on the concern of medical writers for this organ (even though he had downplayed its uniqueness by pressing the parallels between male and female anatomy), he accorded it positive functions, including a role in sex determination. Citing Hippocrates, he associated the production of male offspring with the right side of the uterus (or, as he says, the right uterus, representing it as two separate compartments) and the production of female offspring with the left.[65] For anatomical reasons having to do with the putative origins of the blood vessels which feed them, the left uterus and the left male testis receive less purified blood and are therefore less warm than their counterparts on the right. If the semen from the male's left testis is stronger, it will contribute to the production of a female; if from the right, to the production of a male. But the uterine environment is critical, for it may either augment or override the influence of the father's semen. Hence a fetus which rests to the right will be influenced by greater heat in the course of its development: it will be more fully perfected; it will be a male.[66] Galen combined the two left–right pairs in an account of sex determination that left the calculus of influence unclear.

In shifting his attention to the uterus, Galen temporarily set aside the male testis/female testis parallel in favor of a male testis/uterus analogy. In doing so, he partially undermined his argument that male and female are essentially similar in structure and function, though he did not thereby adopt the Aristotelian opposition according to which the female principle is passive. Rather he reintroduced and tamed the earlier medical and philosophical views that represented the uterus as an erratic and potentially dangerous feature of the female body: he took it to be active but declined to give attention to the reproductive or systemic effects of uterine activity or dysfunction, and he brought its powers within a general scientific theory of bodily functions – the idea of the natural faculties.

The natural faculties are a critical dimension of Galen's physiology, for,

65 *Use of Parts*, XIV, iv (Kühn, vol. 3, pp. 153–4; May, vol. 2, p. 626).
66 Ibid., vi (Kühn, vol. 3, pp. 170–5; May, vol. 2, pp. 635–8).

along with heat, they represent the dynamic principle of his system and they link the physiological substances, whether seen in terms of elements and humors or in terms of the production of successive coctions, with the broader purposes of physiological function. They are the forces by which the parts of the body accomplish their teleological goals.[67] Some of these powers, such as the blood-making faculty, are specific to one part of the body; others are manifested in a number of parts. Prominent among the latter are the faculties of attraction, retention, and expulsion, all of which the uterus possesses. Like all parts of the body, the uterus has the power to attract blood for nourishment, to retain it while assimilating what is appropriate for its sustenance or growth, and to expel the waste and surplus. In addition these faculties carry out its specific reproductive functions. The uterus attracts both the male and the female semen and (nature ever artful) is specifically constructed to do so, the cervix providing the passageway for the male semen, and what we call the Fallopian tubes constituting the passageway for the female semen.[68] Galen used the uterus as his prime illustration of the retentive faculty, because it holds its contents (the embryo) for so long compared with the other organs that serve as vessels, especially the bladder and the stomach.[69] During gestation the tight closure of the cervix and the snugness with which the uterus surrounds the embryo are manifestations of its retentive power. Likewise, at birth the dilation of the cervix and the propulsive actions of the uterine muscles demonstrate its expulsive faculty, immoderate exercise of which can cause a prolapsed uterus.[70]

The uterus is thus one organ among many with the structures and powers necessary to accomplish its specific ends. The faculties it possesses are closely related to those of other parts of the body, and its motions are closely suited to its reproductive function. In short, Galen attributed to the uterus a role and a set of characteristics that gave it moderate significance in his decentralized system of anatomy and physiology, which featured the heart, the brain, and the liver, as well as the reproductive organs. Yet aspects of this picture allowed later interpreters of Galen to place his account in a different light. He seemed to be abandoning the male–female parallels upon which he had so vigorously insisted. Not only did he make no attempt to develop the structure and role of the scrotum, putative male analogue to the uterus, in ways that would preserve the appearance of equivalence, but he also spoke of menstrual blood as a surplus which, during gestation, the embryo attracts for its nourishment[71] and even sometimes spoke of the

---

67 Galen is aware that there is a problem of tautology in his postulating a faculty for each bodily activity and hastens to say that the concept stands in for the real cause when the real cause is unknown (*Natural Faculties*, I, iv).
68 Galen, *Use of Parts*, XIV, xi (Kühn, vol. 3, pp. 192–3; May, vol. 2, p. 646).
69 Galen, *Natural Faculties*, III, ii, pp. 226–9.
70 Ibid., iii, pp. 228–37.
71 E.g., Galen, *Use of Parts*, XIV, viii (Kühn, vol 3, pp. 177–8; May, vol. 2, pp. 638–9).

complementary roles of semen and menstruum, appearing to retreat from functional as well as structural parallels.[72] The shift does not necessarily reveal an inconsistency. (Galen may, for example, have been using the word "seed" [*sperma*] at one point for the separate seminal contributions of the male and female parents and at another point for the combined seeds of male and female after conception. In any case, the contexts of his remarks vary, and he was constrained by his interest in observation to account for the particular features of the uterus and menstruation.) It did, however, offer a measure of flexibility and choice to medieval authors attempting to reconstruct Galenic views on the question. In particular, ambiguities arising from the complexities of Galen's thought, the variety of perspectives he took on sex difference and reproduction, the tensions between theories and observations, and, perhaps too, the changes and inconsistencies in his ideas left room for later authors to assimilate Galen's views to those of other authorities. For example, the pairing of semen and menstruum – both blood products, one more fully processed than the other – suggests affinities with Aristotle's view (which Galen in fact opposes) that male semen and menstruum provided respectively the active and nutritive elements of reproduction. And the attribution of motions and an attractive faculty to the uterus suggests connections with Hippocratic notions of an active organ with an appetite and a significant role in reproduction.

Ancient issues and choices

The ancient precedents surveyed here, as well as many not mentioned, offered a range of options to later centuries. First, they illustrated the variety of purposes that investigation of sex difference and reproduction could serve: to understand the structure and dynamics of the natural world, to account scientifically for specific natural phenomena, to assist in the normal process of childbirth, or to treat diseases and dysfunctions related to sexuality, reproductive organs (especially the uterus), and female physiology. Second, they suggested many formats for the discussion of these subjects, from short specialized treatises to inclusion in more comprehensive works, from expositions structured as extended rational arguments to collections of information (diagnostic signs or therapies) conveniently subdivided for clinical use. And third, through disagreement or ambiguity, they left open certain substantive questions – invitations to debate, flexibility, or compromise in later eras.

The issues that engaged later medieval authors were often drawn from those left open by ancient authorities, but they were not always those with which ancient authors were most urgently concerned. Thus although the

---

72 E.g., *Natural Faculties*, II, iii, p. 134; *On Seed*, II, ii (Kühn, vol. 4, pp. 612–15).

substance of the arguments may at points be closely related to those earlier traditions, the proportions and emphases are often not. Aristotle and Galen, for example, went to great lengths to discredit the arguments of certain schools which proposed materialistic and mechanistic interpretations of living creatures. Large portions of Aristotle's *Generation of Animals* are devoted to refuting theories of reproduction that ignore form, soul, and final cause; likewise, Galen's *On Natural Faculties* is aimed at discrediting such notions as the one that vacuums, not vital attractions, draw fluids into the parts of the body which need them. By the beginning of the Middle Ages, materialism and mechanism, as manifested in such previously successful doctrines as atomism, had been largely defeated, and the rise of Christianity in the West reinforced the victory of those committed to form, soul, final cause, and the purposefulness of creation. Combating materialism had lost its urgency in the Middle Ages. Conversely, medieval intellectuals identified and developed problems which had not seriously concerned natural philosophers and medical writers in antiquity. Although Foucault makes medical notions about regimen one of the pillars of his analysis of "the use of pleasure" in antiquity, he acknowledges that medical writers gave sexual activities no special place in their work.[73] Sexual pleasure figures only occasionally in ancient medicine and natural philosophy.[74] A brief passage in the Hippocratic work *On Generation* provides the most extensive medical discussion of the subject, explaining that a woman's pleasure, incited by friction and heat, ends either when she experiences emission or when the man ejaculates (whichever occurs first) and that the man feels greater pleasure because his secretion is more sudden.[75] But from the twelfth century on, Latin scholars expounded at length on pleasure within their scientific debates about reproduction and within their medical reflections on sterility.

The unresolved issues of antiquity that medieval thinkers did find worthy of their urgent attention were of several kinds. Some had to do with specific elements of theories of reproduction. The existence of the female seed was one such problem: because it revealed a specific discrepancy between influential sources, it had broad implications for the way in which sex difference was conceptualized. Others had to do with emphasis and deemphasis, such as the implicit question of the significance to be placed upon the specifically female features of the uterus and menstruation. Still others concerned concepts of health and disease, such as the gap between the Hippocratics and Soranus on the natural state of the female body or on the roles of sexual

---

73 Foucault, *Use of Pleasure*, pp. 99–139, esp, pp. 109–14. In his treatment of dietetics Foucault therefore relies mostly upon authors from outside the sphere of natural science, such as Plato and Xenophon.

74 Foucault exaggerates the significance of pleasure per se by translating *aphrodisia* (which he has previously defined as "the acts, gestures, and contacts that produce a certain form of pleasure" [ibid., p. 40]) simply as "pleasure" (e.g., p. 119).

75 Hippocrates, *On Generation* (Lonie, *Hippocratic Treatises*, pp. 2–3).

activity and childbirth in the balance of health. By no means all of the richness of ancient opinion on these subjects was to reach the Middle Ages, but a sufficient array of disagreements, ambiguities, and alternative perspectives, of language, concepts, and implications, was accessible to preclude any serious suggestion that medieval thinkers were severely constrained in their own formulations of sex difference and reproduction. On the contrary, what they received from the antiquity which they revered was a wide range of choices in the substance, format, and uses of knowledge about females and males and their roles in the production of offspring. What the Middle Ages constructed was thus its own, in the same way that medieval architecture, though it borrowed motifs and even stone from ancient buildings, was far more than a mere extension of or variation on the Roman.

EARLY TRANSLATIONS, USES, AND FORMS:
THE TRANSMISSION OF ANCIENT IDEAS TO THE LATIN WEST

If nothing else, the means by which the works and views of antiquity reached the Latin West of the twelfth through the fourteenth century and the form in which they arrived there constitute sufficient assurance that medieval society did not simply reiterate opinions created centuries earlier in an entirely different context. At first only small portions of the ancient writings on generation and on gynecology, obstetrics, and embryology made their way into Latin; those that did were often excerpted and abbreviated; and even when a whole work was made available in Latin, the nature of the translation, the accompanying commentaries, its place in the constellation of knowledge, and the uses to which it was put gave it a specifically medieval character. The centuries-long process by which medieval Europe accumulated and assimilated these materials was guided sometimes by the choices of medieval authors, institutions, and patrons, sometimes by the circumstances of medieval geography, resources, and communications, so that by the later Middle Ages the corpus of ancient scientific and medical works and the heritage of ancient scientific and medical ideas had a structure, content, and cast characteristic of the Latin West. This is not to say that the translations were generally poor or that the interpretations were invariably ill founded; rather it is to suggest that the various choices, revisions, constructions, and applications added up to something unique to that period of history.

The story of the transmission of ancient Greek wisdom to the medieval West is embedded in a long and complicated process, within which the transmission of notions of sex difference and reproduction is a subplot.[76]

76 Marie-Thérèse d'Alverny, "Translations and Translators," in *Renaissance and Renewal in the Twelfth Century*, ed. Robert L. Benson and Giles Constable (Cambridge: Harvard University Press, 1982), pp. 421–62, with a bibliographical note encompassing more than the

Translation and assimilation took place in two broad phases: the first during the centuries that preceded and followed the disintegration of the Roman Empire – especially in the fourth through the sixth century; the second during the period of renewal from the late eleventh through the thirteenth century. During each, choices and reinterpretations, as well as contexts and accidents, reshaped the classical traditions in specific ways. In particular, the first period was characterized by a condensation of earlier learning and an emphasis on handy access and on practical or literary utility, and included material on obstetrics and gynecology; the later period, deeply colored by the influence of Arabic scholarship, was characterized by an impulse to extend and broaden knowledge and to reintegrate general principles, and included material on theoretical medicine and on the natural philosophy of sexuality and reproduction.[77]

Even before the migrations and invasions which accelerated the demise of the Roman Empire, the process of translating the fruits of classical learning from Greek into Latin was well under way. Galen and Soranus addressed their Roman audiences – from philosophers to midwives to patricians – in Greek in the second century C.E., but the trends toward Latin, practicality, and eclecticism that were to become dominant in the following centuries

twelfth century; idem, "Les traductions d'Avicenne (Moyen Age et Renaissance)," in *Avicenna nella storia della cultura medioevale: Relazioni e discussione (15 aprile 1955)*, Problemi attuali di scienza e di cultura 40 (Rome: Accademia Nazionale dei Lincei, 1957), pp. 71–87; Augusto Beccaria, "Sulle trace di un antico canone latino di Ippocrate e di Galeno, I," *Italia medioevale e umanistica* 2 (1959): 1–56; idem, "II. Gli *Aforismi* di Ippocrate nella versione e nei commenti del primo medioevo," ibid. 4 (1961): 1–75; idem, "III. Quattro opere di Galeno nei commenti della scuola di Ravenna all'inizio del medioevo," ibid. 14 (1971): 1–23; Hermann Diels, *Die Handschriften der antiker Arzte*, 2 pts., Philosophische und historische Abhandlungen (Berlin: Akademie der Wissenschaften, 1905–6); supplemented by Richard J. Durling, "Corrigenda and Addenda to Diels' Galenica, I: Codices Vaticani," *Traditio* 23 (1967): 463–76; Green, "Transmission"; Charles Homer Haskins, *Studies in the History of Mediaeval Science,* 2d ed. (Cambridge: Harvard University Press, 1927; repr. New York: Frederick Ungar, 1960); Pearl Kibre, *Hippocrates Latinus*; idem, "Hippocratic Writings"; Georges Lacombe, Aleksander Birkenmajer, and Lorenzo Minio-Paluello, *Aristoteles Latinus: Codices*, 3 vols.: vol. 1, rev. ed., Union académique internationale: Corpus philosophorum Medii Aevi (Bruges and Paris: Desclée de Brouwer, 1957); vol. 2 (Cambridge: Academia, 1955); [vol. 3], *Supplementa altera* (Bruges and Paris: Desclée de Brouwer, 1961); Temkin, *Galenism*, esp. ch. III; Moritz Steinschneider, *Die europäischen Uebersetzungen aus dem arabischen bis Mitte des 17. Jahrhunderts*, Sitzungsberichten der Kaiserlichen Akademie der Wissenschaften, philosophisch-historische Klasse 149 (1904) and 151 (1905) (Vienna: Kaiserlichen Akademie der Wissenschaften, 1905–6; repr., Graz: Academische Druck- und Verlagsanstalt, 1956); Heinrich Schipperges, *Die Assimilation der arabischen Medizin durch das lateinische Mittelalter*, Sudhoffs Archiv für Geschichte der Medizin und der Naturwissenschaften, 48, suppl. 3 (Weisbaden: F. Steiner, 1964); Lynn Thorndike, "Translations of Works of Galen from the Greek by Niccolô da Reggio (c. 1308–1345)," *Byzantina Metabyzantina* 1 (1946): 213–35.

77 On the general shift to a more theoretical outlook, see Paul Oskar Kristeller's classic, "The School of Salerno: Its Development and Its Contribution to the History of Learning," *Bulletin of the History of Medicine* 17 (1945): 138–94, reprinted in his *Studies in Renaissance Thought and Letters*, Storia e letteratura 54 (Rome: Edizioni de Storia e Letteratura, 1956), pp. 495–551.

had already begun a century earlier. In natural philosophy, Lucretius made a point of presenting an easy-to-swallow, popularized Latin version of the technical Greek philosophy of Epicurus (including a materialist account of sexual pleasure and reproduction). In medicine, Celsus (first century), probably not a physician himself, gathered from many Greek and Latin sources a diverse and useful body of knowledge, which he presented in a convenient encyclopedic format. This tendency to borrow, condense, and reorder is most fully illustrated by Pliny the Elder's *Natural History*, also from the first century. This mammoth work contains all the facts about the natural world the author deemed worthy of consideration. His indifference to theory and even consistency and his willingness to appropriate something of interest from any source serve as a paradigm of the process by which Roman scholars transformed and transferred the contributions of their predecessors.[78] Pliny's nephew reports that his uncle believed any book, no matter how bad, had something to offer him, and his research method apparently was to make extracts of everything he read (or had read to him).[79] The first book of the *Natural History*, an elaborate table of contents, announces the number of facts and observations to be found in each book and lists for each book the dozens of Greek and Roman authorities from whose works they have been drawn. Since he is not interested in theory, he does not address the principles of generation per se, but in the course of a brief discussion of menstruation, he does assert, following Aristotle, that menstrual blood is the matter from which generation occurs and that the male semen causes it to coagulate (as rennet produces cheese), animating it.[80] Yet when he is discussing the appearance and character of the offspring, he refers more to the influence of the mother than to that of the father. Among the bits of information he picks up and imparts are that the male fetus tends to rest in the right side of the uterus, the female in the left; that the male fetus starts to move after forty days, the female after ninety; that a female child is harder to carry and deliver than a male; and that men are fertile sometimes as late as their eighties, women into their forties or fifties.[81] He devotes considerable attention to the ill effects of menstruation – not upon the woman but upon the world – and is no doubt the source of many later misogynistic claims.

78 William Harris Stahl devotes a chapter to Pliny's theoretical science in which he catalogue's Pliny's theoretical assertions on a number of topics, but he argues in general that theory was Pliny's weakest area: *Roman Science: Origins, Development, and Influence to the Later Middle Ages* (Madison: University of Wisconsin Press, 1962), ch. 7.
79 C. Plinius Caecilius Secundus, *Epistolarum libri decem*, ed. R. A. B. Mynors, Scriptorum classicorum bibliotheca Oxoniensis (Oxford: Oxford University Press, 1963), III, v, 10–11; p. 73, ll. 18–22.
80 Pliny, *Natural History*, ed. and trans. H. Rackham, W. H. S. Jones, and D. E. Eicholz, 10 vols., Loeb Classical Library (Cambridge: Harvard University Press; London: William Heinemann, 1938–62), VII, xv, 66; vol. 2 (1942), pp. 548, 549. Aristotle had used the same simile (*Generation of Animals*, I, xx, 729a10–14; pp. 108, 109).
81 Pliny, *Natural History*, VII, vi–xiv.

Menstrual blood can, for example, cause wine to sour, mirrors to grow dull, metal to rust, and bees to die.[82] In keeping with the practical orientation of Roman science, much of Pliny's work is devoted to the medicinal uses of the various plants, animals, and minerals he describes. Remedies for sexual and reproductive disorders are scattered here and there among these. Violets, for example, can be used in a remedy for a prolapsed uterus and to promote menstruation or reduce menstrual flow (two apparently Hippocratic concerns), as well as to cure epilepsy in children and to counteract scorpion stings.[83]

The works of Pliny and Celsus illustrate the Roman inclination to extract and collect, to minimize theory (and even consistency) in favor of the practical uses of specific, sometimes incompatible, units of knowledge – an inclination, therefore, that predates the transition to medieval society and culture. This tendency coexisted in the Roman Empire with the Greek alternative: the theoretical, systematic, and even grandiose vision of medicine and natural philosophy, represented by Galen. The two strands of Roman science have in common an indebtedness to Greek culture and a marked eclecticism; however, they differ not only in language but also in the commitment of one to philosophical principles and the other to information. Therefore, they also differ in their organization, the one taking the form of discursive exposition, of logical and empirical demonstration, the other taking the form of classified lists of information and anecdotal, empirical cases.

Thus the medieval heirs of ancient knowledge about nature and medicine were faced, once again, not with a monolithic authority to follow but with a choice of sources and models. As the Roman Empire, still expanding geographically, began to decline in terms of the social, institutional, and economic base for the production of knowledge, the model provided by Pliny gained ascendancy over the model provided by Galen. And to the propensity for the Latin language, practicality, and eclecticism, the early Middle Ages added an inclination to brevity: even the encyclopedic example of Pliny – the most extensive single work on the natural world to come down to us from antiquity – was scaled down, so that later compendious works were far more selective and abbreviated.

The condensed encyclopedia was not the only genre consistent with the needs and preferences of the late Roman Empire and early Middle Ages. As the field of medicine illustrates, specialized works showed the same signs of disregard for extended reflection on theoretical foundations and the same signs of concern for practicality, convenience, brevity, and, to a certain extent, eclecticism. In fifth- and sixth-century North Africa and parts of Italy,

---

82 Ibid., xv. Aristotle mentioned the mirror-clouding gaze of a menstruating woman in *On Dreams* (*On the Soul, Parva naturalia, On Breath*, ed. and trans. W. S. Hett, rev. ed. [Cambridge: Harvard University Press; London: William Heinemann, 1957], II, 459b28–31).

83 Pliny, *Natural History*, XXI, lxxvi.

where the cultural and intellectual traditions of the East lasted longer than in most of western Europe, Latin versions of Greek medical works reflected choices of both substance and genre. In obstetrics and gynecology choices of both kinds were deliberate and reflected the climate of the period.[84]

First, in terms of substance, there was a persistent interest in making Soranus's gynecological work available to Latin readers. Two authors, Caelius Aurelianus and Muscio (or Mustio), produced Latin versions of the *Gynecology* in the fifth and sixth centuries, and a third, Theodorus Pricianus, incorporated significant portions into a larger work. This interest in Soranus reveals the period's decided preference for the mild and practical strain of Methodism, represented by Soranus, over the polemical and theoretical bent of Galen and over the other array of approaches still accessible to readers of Greek at that time.[85] There may also have been other reasons for this preference for Soranus, having to do with attitudes toward women and reproduction or with the organization of gynecological and obstetrical care in late antiquity, but such connections have not yet been investigated. Thus the Latin tradition of the early Middle Ages came to be influenced by Soranus's views of sexuality and reproduction, including the possibility that amenorrhea and virginity might be healthy, and coitus, pregnancy, and childbirth harmful. The dominance of Galenic medicine characteristic of the Arabic East and the later Latin Middle Ages was, in the case of early Latin views on gynecology and reproduction, largely absent. There was, however, no long-term and consistent adherence to Methodism as a system of medical knowledge highlighting constriction and laxity. Even in these early translations, the views of Soranus (not himself wedded to fixed principles) were sometimes displaced by others, such as the Hippocratic notion, which apparently enjoyed strong currency, that uterine suffocation was the result of a wandering womb.[86]

The second direction taken by the authors of these versions of Soranus's *Gynecology* – and the one that encouraged the later lack of fidelity to Soranus and Methodism – had to do with the form of these works. The material contained in them was selected, excerpted, and abbreviated from the Greek original. The authors' goal was to present gynecological knowledge in what they considered a practical form, meaning in this case a work that included material with direct applications and excluded most general matters and theoretical speculation. Furthermore, works of this kind were

---

84 Green, "Transmission," pp. 131–40.
85 Caelius Aurelianus, *Gynaecia*; Muscio, *Sorani Gynaeciorum vetus translatio*; Theodorus Priscianus, *Euporiston libri III cum Physicorum fragmento et additamentis pseudo-Theodoreis*, ed. Valentin Rose, Bibliotheca scriptorum Graecorum et Latinorum Teubneriana (Leipzig: B. G. Teubner, 1894), bk. III, "Gynaecia," pp. 224–48. See also Vindicianus Afrus (4th c.), *Gynaecia*, in ibid., pp. 428–62. A number of manuscripts of each survive, and Muscio is frequently referred to by later authors and compilers.
86 Green, "Transmission," p. 137.

one route through which the genre of the pedagogical dialogue was communicated to the medieval world: the *Gynecology* of Muscio was presented in a question-and-answer format, which not only illustrates the commitment to convenience, simplicity, and practicality but also suggests the role that such texts were to play in medical education. This genre of medieval medical text – sometimes a single question followed by its answer, sometimes a series of questions and answers, sometimes just a list of questions (the answers to which were presumably passed on orally) – came to be associated with the thriving medical community in Salerno.[87] The form of these works suggests a pattern of recitation – questions and answers memorized and rehearsed, probably by a group of students – for the purpose of mastering what were considered basic medical facts and principles. Perhaps such exercises formed part of the general learning of nonpractitioners; they were almost certainly used to supplement the training of young apprentices. The format suggests in turn both the value and the limits placed on book learning and theory in early medieval medicine. On the one hand, the existence and nature of such texts attest to the conviction of at least part of the learned and medical community that the wisdom of accumulated experience should be joined with at least something of the opinions of the authorities, including theories (explicit or implied) as well as practical information. On the other hand, the brevity of the responses ensured that the information communicated was cursory and that no theoretical principles were significantly developed or rationalized. And since the questions, although sometimes loosely grouped by subject, were essentially discrete and isolated from each other, they provided no occasion for recognizing and confronting theoretical problems or for constructing a coherent systematic foundation for medical and scientific understanding.

Thus the format of the Soranus translations in particular and of the question literature generally had an effect on the character of medical thought. Not only did those who transmitted ancient knowledge sometimes omit extended discussions of theoretical matters – such as Soranus's concern to establish that women suffered from the same kinds of disorders as men – but in making the material accessible and practical – as in the creation of simple medical catechisms – they also narrowed the opportunity for debate, speculation, and system building. The theories were there – the elements, the humors, and the principles of hot and cold in diagnosis and treatment – but their components were scattered, and their significance was not fully manifest.

At about the same time as Soranus's *Gynecology* was being translated, similar versions of Hippocratic and Galenic works were being prepared in Italy, probably at Ravenna, most significant among them the Hippocratic works on the diseases of women and the *Aphorisms*.[88] The presence of these works in the Latin West diluted somewhat the prominence of the Latin versions of Soranus. The eclecticism and disinclination to pursue theoretical systems, characteristic of the early Middle Ages, minimized implicit tensions, so that, in the words of Henry Sigerist, "in the field of gynecology, as in other fields, the dogmatic [Hippocratic–Galenic] and the methodic [Soranian] traditions went side by side, with the latter in the foreground."[89]

By the later Middle Ages, however, although the name of Soranus was still being invoked frequently in the medical literature, most of his works had been lost, and his influence is more difficult to discern. On the one hand, his gynecology was the only one of his treatises to survive more or less intact; on the other hand, its status as a source of systematic understanding was minimal. The waning of Soranus's prominence may be due in part to the circumstances of medical and educational institutions and the accidents of manuscript transmission. It is probably linked to the association of Methodist medicine with Epicurean materialist philosophy, which, in spite of the eclecticism and negligence of systematic philosophy discernible in the period's science and medicine, was generally suspect. The notions of tension and laxity seemed to constitute a distinctly mechanistic approach to human life, and the attribution of a significant role to minute pores and the particles that fill them smacked of atomistic materialism. Such views ebbed in relation to Hippocratic and Galenic influences[90] and in the face of the rising tides of Neoplatonism in late antiquity and of Christianity in the late Middle Ages, thus according an advantage to scientific and medical works which made a place for forms, faculties, souls, and vital forces. Soranus had made fun of the sort of teleological arguments at the heart of the dominant antimaterialist philosophy: if Providence could create menstruation to expel harmful excesses, why couldn't it just design a way to prevent the development of harmful excesses?[91] In some ways, Soranus's ideological disabilities are ironic, given some of the prominent concerns of the Christian Middle Ages. It was Soranus, for example, not Hippocrates or Galen, who was in a position to provide medical justification for virginity and sexual abstinence.

At the time of the early translations, however, Latin renderings of Hippo-

---

88 Beccaria, "Sulle trace," I, II and III; Kibre, *Hippocrates Latinus*, pp. 29–33, 187–8; Green, "Transmission," pp. 140–55.
89 Henry E. Sigerist, "Early Mediaeval Medical Texts in the Manuscripts of Vendôme," *Bulletin of the History of Medicine* 14 (1943): 108. See also Beccaria, "Sulle trace, I," pp. 42–3.
90 Green, "Transmission," esp. pp. 209–18, 252–5.
91 Soranus, *Gynaecia*, I, vi, 28 (Ilberg, p. 18; Temkin, p. 24). This passage is not rendered into Latin by either Muscio or Caelius Aurelianus, probably simply because it is part of a long academic argument of the sort they were wont to skip.

cratic works reinforced some of the characteristics, if not the philosophy, of the Soranus translations, for they too were compiled by shortening and excerpting. Thus, in addition to the pattern of encyclopedic compilation presented by Pliny in the area of natural history and natural philosophy, the early Middle Ages inherited two patterns set by specialized medical treatises. One was the medical handbook, which communicated only the gist of the practical suggestions contained in earlier, more expansive, and in some cases more systematically grounded works. The other pattern was the pedagogical dialogue, which communicated only the essentials surrounding discrete and particular medical circumstances. These literary genres had in common a respect for ancient wisdom and a distance from ancient philosophies or methods, an emphasis on the factual and the practical, and a lack of development of the theoretical. The shorter treatises, like the gynecological excerpts and to a greater extent the fragments found in several early manuscripts,[92] exemplify an impulse for brevity; the earlier, more comprehensive works, like those of Celsus and Pliny, illustrate a penchant for inclusiveness. Both of these tendencies appeared in later works, although for the most part, fragmentation outstripped accretion in the early Middle Ages.

The changes which accelerated the adoption and abbreviation of these genres – the encyclopedia, the handbook, the pedagogical dialogue – were many and complex. They involved demographic, social, economic, political, cultural, and religious transformations by which the Latin West of the Middle Ages came into being. Here we can merely note a few of them, which occurred in stages and over a period of centuries. Increasing isolation from centers of learning in the East left the Latin- and Germanic-speaking West reliant on what was translated and borrowed from Greek sources and on the Roman habits of compilation. Late exceptions to this rule illustrate its force. In the early sixth century, the Roman patrician Boethius announced his intention to translate as many works of Plato and Aristotle as he could, adding commentaries to show that they were in agreement. When he was executed for political reasons, he was in his forties and had accomplished only a small part of his program. (His translation of some of Aristotle's logical works made an important contribution to the intellectual life of subsequent centuries.) We might say that the failure of Aristotle's theories of reproduction to reach the Latin West in their full form – and thus the absence of an important model for scientific demonstration in the area of reproduction and sex difference – was the unhappy result of a political incident. But by the sixth century Boethius's plan was an anomaly. His project had no social foundation – no institution, no patron, no disciples. It was an

---

92 See, e.g., Ferdinand Paul Egert, *Gynäkologische Fragmente aus dem frühen Mittelalter nach einer Petersburger Handschrift aus dem VIII.–IX. Jahrhundert*, Abhandlungen zur Geschichte der Medizin und der Naturwissenschaften 11 (Berlin: Emil Ebering, 1936; repr. Nendeln, Liechtenstein: Kraus, 1977).

isolated individual effort, for which the skill, rationale, and appetite had all faded by Boethius's time. Boethius himself, with his intention to bring Aristotle and Plato together, hinted at the strong tendency among his contemporaries to minimize differences among authorities in favor of an agglomeration of various ancient opinions.

A process of demographic and administrative decentralization undermined what institutional and social support there had been for sustained philosophical and theoretical investigation, or even for the active study and preservation of the considerable body of knowledge transmitted by such authors as Lucretius and Cicero. Later, when monastic communities emerged as the repositories of classical learning, the trend in science and medicine away from discursive theoretical knowledge and toward compilation and abbreviation was reinforced. Not only did secular texts make a secondary claim on the resources of religious institutions, but debates such as the one about the female seed had limited interest in the absence of a sophisticated and diverse intellectual community. Thus the habits of condensation and compilation, developed during the Roman Empire at least in part to serve the educational needs and social pretensions of the literate secular elites, came to have other functions in the early Christian West, where the imperatives to preserve the remnants of ancient wisdom were mitigated by suspicion of its pagan origins and limits upon the occasions for displaying such knowledge for social advantage. It is therefore inappropriate to claim that it was the Romans who ruined science for the Latin West and that had the early Middle Ages inherited a more respectable scientific and medical legacy from Rome, the science and medicine of that period would have been much richer and truer to Greek traditions.[93]

Many of the forces and values which shaped Roman science, such as a preference for moral philosophy over natural philosophy, were shared by the intellectuals of the early Middle Ages. Still others, such as the appreciation of utility at the cost of theory, continued in new forms. The Roman intellectual preoccupation with the moral, the social, and the aesthetic had as its underpinnings not only certain strands of Greek thought but also the demands associated with the administration of local and imperial government and the needs of the classes which dominated the complex economic, political, and military systems. When these foundations crumbled, some of the values associated with them remained in some form or other, and the concern with right conduct and the good life was sustained by the development of Christianity in general and monasticism in particular. In this way, the older attitudes toward the study of nature and of the body took on a new meaning. It was not necessary to hold, as some radical Christians did, that the study of nature was pure vanity and thus a secondary concern; nor was it

93 Cf. Stahl, *Roman Science*, pp. 248–60.

necessary to condemn the flesh and thus minimize the significance of medical knowledge. The problems of economic and institutional survival, along with the development of doctrines of salvation, were sufficient to reinforce the relative indifference inherited from the Romans to the theories, debates, and systems that had been submerged in the transmission of Greek thought. Here the subject of sexuality, because of its early association with the Fall and its potentiality for sin, bore a special burden. Not that the Christians invented prudery. The pagan Celsus in his Latin medical encyclopedia had made a great show of modesty and announced his intention to follow the delicate practice of using Greek words for the genitals, the *partes obscenae*.[94] But the tone suited medieval Christian authors very well. For example, Isidore, archbishop of Seville in the early seventh century, calls semen *obscenus humor* and teaches that the word for "loins," *lumbus*, derives from the word for "lust," *libido*.[95] He reports that according to some, the word *femina*, "woman," comes from the Greek word for "fiery," because among humans and animals the female is more lustful than the male.[96]

In spite of the indecent associations of the words and what they signified, Isidore and other medieval authors did continue to preserve, to recompile, and to pass on the knowledge they had inherited about science and medicine in general and about reproduction, sex differences, and sexuality in particular. One reason for this persistence may be an unreflective reverence for and sense of duty toward the wisdom contained in the authoritative works of the past, but another reason was surely the adoption and adaptation of Roman notions of practicality by Christian authors. Roman practicality was, first and foremost, concrete. The achievements of Roman technology – for example, the engineering and administrative brilliance involved in some of the major public works projects of the empire – are justly celebrated. But there was also another aspect to Roman practicality, which both reinforced and was reinforced by the first. This was an attitude toward the world, reflected in Stoic philosophy and elsewhere, that human existence was at the center of nature and that nature existed to serve (or, at least, was only of interest insofar as it served) human purposes. Pliny's natural history reflected this outlook: almost all his entries on plants, animals, and minerals point out their medicinal or economic uses. Early medieval authors embraced and transformed this more general notion of utility. First, they Christianized it by developing classical teleology into a religious view: God has created everything for a purpose, and surely human salvation is central to God's purpose in the world. Genesis, as they understood it, authorized this anthropocentric view of Cre-

---

94 Celsus, *De medicina*, VI, xviii, 1; vol. 2, p. 268.
95 Isidorus Hispalensis, *Etymologiarum sive originum libri XX*, ed. W. M. Lindsay, 2 vols., Scriptorum classicorum bibliotheca Oxoniensis (Oxford: Oxford University Press, 1911), XI, i, 97, 98.
96 Ibid., ii, 24.

ation both in asserting that the human soul is made in God's image and in narrating the story in which God gives Adam dominion over the garden (nature) and empowers him to name the other creatures. Second, they made it not only an explicit but also a broad and prominent aspect of the study of nature and, to a lesser extent, of medicine.

This attitude toward nature provided a link between the emphasis on moral and social issues on the one hand and the notion of utility on the other. Medieval utility extended, therefore, beyond the realm of techniques for growing crops and remedies for curing illnesses into the realm of moral edification and human salvation. Whatever reservations early medieval compilers, copyists, or monastic and episcopal librarians might have had about the propriety or even about the applications of knowledge about sexuality and reproduction, they understood it to have a purpose. The information about nature and medicine contained in Isidore of Seville's *Etymologies* was to be useful, not so much in the sense that it would be applied to solve technical or ·medical problems (much less to explain the principles of the physical world) as in the sense that it would edify the reader or be used by teachers and spiritual leaders to promote rectitude and direct people's concerns toward their salvation. By repeating Pliny's warnings about the dangers of menstrual blood, Isidore gave later authors of treatises and sermons access to powerful material for their misogynistic warnings against the sexual lures of women.[97] Yet he stated firmly that since Scripture tells us woman was named immediately upon being created, the word *mulier* is applied to a person because of her femininity and not because she is sexually corrupt (i.e., not a virgin) – thus imparting a lesson about words, about the nature of women, and about the Fall all at the same time. Indeed, the integration of the study of words with the study of nature was an aspect of this medieval extension of utility.[98] Further examples of the expansion and Christianization of the "practical" through the study of words, nature, and spiritual matters abound in medieval versions of the Greek work known as *Physiologus* and in bestiaries.

These works contain descriptions of beasts, plants, and stones interpreted according to their moral and spiritual significance. For example, the beaver's genitals are useful in the mundane sense that they have (unspecified) medicinal powers, and he is therefore pursued by hunters. In a play on the word *castor* (beaver) which manifests the conviction that language, nature, and salvation are all bound up together, the beaver is said to castrate himself and toss his testicles to the hunter in order to save his life. Then, if pursued by another hunter, he lies on his back so the hunter will see he is without testicles and will go away. The story is useful on a higher level, because it teaches that if you cast off the temptation to sin, the devil will no longer

97 Ibid., i, 141.
98 Jacquart and Thomasset, *Sexuality and Medicine*, pp. 8-21.

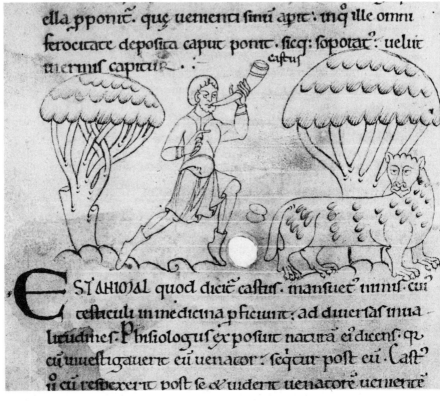

ella pponitc. que uemenca finti apic: inq ille omni
ferocitate depofita caput ponitc. ficq: fopotat': uelut
tueimif capitut.. .

E ST ahioial quod dicitc caftur. manfuet' innif cui
ceftıculi inmedıcına pficiunt; ad diuerfaf inua
litudinef. Pinfiologuf exposuit nacurā eī dicenf: qu
cū inuestigauerit cū uenacor: feqcur post eū. Caft²
ñ cū refpexerit post fe & uident uenacore uenientc

Figure 2. Beaver (Latin *castor*). The knowledge of nature was useful at several levels: medieval bestiaries not only passed on the information that the beaver's testicles (seen here between him and the hunter) had medicinal virtues but also taught that people can save themselves from the death of sin by cutting off their attachment to things of the flesh. (From a twelfth-century bestiary, Oxford, Bodleian, MS Laud. misc. 247, fol. 150v. Reproduced by permission of the Bodleian Library, Oxford.)

pursue you.[99] (See Figure 2.) Elephants are without sexual desire until the female picks some mandrake (which the *Physiologus* calls a "tree"), eats some, and gives some to her mate, after which the female conceives. (See Figure 6, p. 210.) They are, of course, compared to Eve and Adam, and the lessons of the Fall are invoked.[100] With time, compilers found more and

99 Francis J. Carmody, ed., "*Physiologus* latinus versio Y," University of California Publications in Classical Philology 12/7 (1941): XXXVI, pp. 128–9. Latin manuscripts of the *Physiologus* date from as early as the eighth century, and there is indirect evidence that translations existed earlier. Nikolaus Henkel, *Studien zum* Physiologus *im Mittelalter*, Hermaea: Germanistische Forschungen, n.s., 38 (Tübingen: Max Niemayer, 1976), pp. 21–8.
100 Carmody, "*Physiologus* versio Y," XX, pp. 117–19.

more useful lessons in these texts: the viper, whose story once stood for filial ingratitude and the failings of the Pharisees, later also acquires the lesson that women should put up with brutish husbands.[101]

The sense that knowledge of nature and the body was useful affected in turn the form it took, the genres that developed. The redefined and characteristically medieval practicality gave new meaning and new life to the information collected and passed down in encyclopedic works, handbooks, and little tractates on specific subjects. These writings, like the short works on obstetrics and gynecology, which continued to offer a more literal brand of practicality, reinforced the habits of excerpting, compiling, and condensing. Those who organized and executed the reproduction of medical and scientific knowledge made use of and produced variations upon the genres appropriate to these activities: lists of words and lists of recipes; instruction booklets on basic technical procedures, such as diagnosis by pulses and treatment by phlebotomy; isolated fragments squeezed into small blank spaces or the margins of manuscripts. The question-and-answer format, which served the double purposes of concision and pedagogy, found a secure place in literary production. And, finally, several other genres, although they were not as frequently reproduced in this period, presented themselves as legitimate modes of organizing knowledge because a few influential works produced at the threshold of the Middle Ages employed them. The commentary form, for example, which reemerged (renewed by translations from the Arabic) in natural philosophy and medicine in the twelfth century, had prototypes in the commentary of Chalcidius on Plato's *Timaeus* and the commentary of Macrobius on Cicero's *Dream of Scipio* and exerted a separate influence on the development of biblical exegesis.

Early medieval authors and readers of works on medicine and natural philosophy enjoyed considerable variety in the forms available to them, but those forms shared certain characteristics which influenced the contents and the dynamics of discourse on sexuality, sex difference, and reproduction. On the one hand, they seriously constrained the opportunities for either explanation or debate. The concise iteration of discrete parcels of information, although it invited applications – whether in medical practice or in sermons – did not provide literary space either for theoretical reflection, which might subsume discrete facts under an explanatory umbrella, or for the articulation and weighing of alternatives. On the other hand, this range of genres generally permitted – indeed encouraged – the preservation of diverse and even conflicting information and prescriptions and of facts and prescriptions originally based on diverse or conflicting assumptions. Later, as new genres developed which encouraged systematic explanation and the resolution of discrepancies, discussion and debate widened, but the toler-

101 Ibid., XII, p. 110; T. H. White, trans., *The Book of Beasts, Being a Translation from a Latin Bestiary of the Twelfth Century* (New York: G. Putnam's Sons, 1954), pp. 170–1.

ance for simultaneously entertaining seemingly incompatible facts and perspectives narrowed.

On the eve of the period of renewed translation and scholarly activity that gave rise to the elaboration of these new genres and introduced much fuller versions of Galenic medicine and Aristotelian science into the Latin West, the substantive diversity of information about reproduction and sex-related matters was striking: the opinions were neither elaborated nor systematized nor defended, yet they were various. The miscellaneous character of older sources made available in Latin and the eclecticism of many of the Roman authors who served as intermediaries provided rich choices, but because of the form early medieval works took, it is difficult if not impossible to tell where, if anywhere, they stand on specific questions. For example, the gynecological and obstetrical works found in one eighth- or ninth-century manuscript contain numerous recipes for inducing menstruation, often in the proximity of recipes for promoting conception. These might suggest a Hippocratic outlook on the connection between menstruation and gestation, as well, perhaps, as a Hippocratic pronatalism – the view that childbearing is healthy. But that speculation is difficult to sustain, for aids to conception might simply be attributable to the social demand for help with fertility problems, and the treatises also contain information on contraceptives.[102] There are recipes for bearing a boy and (fewer) recipes for bearing a girl: these and later works always implicitly place a higher value on sons, but in this case the recipes do not reflect the general ancient or specifically Hippocratic or Galenic associations of boys with right and girls with left. Similarly, there are recipes for suffumigation, a treatment effected by placing a source of specially constituted smoke or vapor below the vagina to influence the uterus. This might – but certainly does not necessarily – imply acceptance of the notion of a wandering womb.[103] The tracts contain no direct or indirect reference to the male (or female) semen, or indeed to the father's role at all. But this omission by no means implies adherence to a female-centered theory of reproduction; rather, it is a result of the way the subject is defined – in the manner of Soranus. Isidore of Seville, in his sections on the body and on medicine, offers slightly more expansive prose but a no more settled picture of reproduction and sexuality. We have already observed that he repeats wisdom that both denigrates and defends women; likewise he offers information that suggests now one view of male and female roles in reproduction, now another. For example, when he is introducing the concepts of body and flesh, he refers to "the seed of the male whence the bodies of animals

102 Egert, *Gynäkologische Fragmente*: for menstruation and conception, passim; for contraceptives, e.g., ibid., *Liber de muliebria*, 28 and 96b, pp. 37 and 44.
103 Egert, *Gynäkologische Fragmente*, passim.

and humans are conceived."[104] But when he is discussing embryology and comes to the resemblance of offspring to parents, he invokes a two-seed model.[105]

In short, the genres common to early medieval medical and scientific discussions of sex difference and reproduction reflected and reinforced a lack of concern with discursive science – with argument and explanation – and consequently made room for views based on divergent assumptions, or even simply contradictory opinions. As a result, when, starting in the late eleventh century, the Latin West began to seek out and contemplate a fuller version of ancient wisdom, it was receptive to several different sets of information about nature and, in particular, entertained both the Aristotelian and the Galenic versions of reproduction. Bits of both were, after all, already accepted, and there was no precedent for discomfort about the tensions between them. But, since the newly acquired knowledge included patterns of demonstration and argumentation, and the construction of consistent systems based on articulated general premises and was, in addition, accompanied by the results of thorough Arabic scrutiny, it contained both impetus and models for the development of new genres – forms of expression which celebrated the advantages of theory and system and which institutionalized the identification and resolution of inconsistencies. Both in the early Middle Ages, with the transmission of often fragmented and indirect elements of ancient knowledge, and in the later Middle Ages, with the transmission of systematic and often heavily glossed bodies of ancient knowledge, the Latin West adapted what it adopted, shaping the material as it assimilated it, revising and extending its form, and infusing it with significance specific to the Western context.

104 Isidorus, *Etymologiae*, XI, i, 15: "Crementum enim semen est masculi, unde animalium et hominum corpora concipiuntur."
105 Ibid., 145.

2

The emergence of issues and the ordering of opinions

From the late eleventh century on, several profound and massive changes in medieval learning made intellectual choices regarding views of sex difference and reproduction richer, clearer, and more difficult. The most significant of these changes were the simultaneous and related developments of new structures for the dissemination of ideas and a new body of texts. The rise of towns and the activities of ecclesiastical and secular courts, as well as some aspects of the older monastic traditions, gave rise to new occasions and forms for the discussion of sex difference and reproduction, culminating in the ascendancy of the universities and the scholastic medicine and natural philosophy which flourished there. At the same time, both encouraged by and lending impetus to the shifts in institutions of learning, scholars of the eleventh, twelfth, and thirteenth centuries undertook to translate vast quantities of material on natural philosophy and medicine from Greek and Arabic, bringing to the Latin West the works of Galen and Aristotle, whose opinions had been so long deflected, fragmented, and diluted during the preceding centuries, and also the works of the great Arabic writers, such as Avicenna and Averroes, who offered the West systematic and learned guides to the ancient sources.

The effects of this revolution in the institutions and substance of learning upon concepts of sex and reproduction were at once radical and limited. The effects were radical in the sense that the greater detail of information, the greater attention to theoretical arguments and consistency, and the greater precision and elaboration of ideas led to the recognition that the casual eclecticism of the earlier period could not withstand the challenge of new information and new standards of rigor. The sources featured in this chapter, Constantine the African's work *On Coitus*, Hildegard of Bingen's *Book of Compound Medicine*, and an excerpt of a treatise by William of Conches, represent the emergence of a broad-based, learned approach to a cluster of issues relating to sex, reproduction, and sex difference. Diverse in character, these works begin to construct coherent medical and philosophical frameworks within which the previously fragmentary materials could be understood. Thus, for example, they explored the respective roles of males and females in generation and the place of sexual pleasure in the economy of nature. The effects of the changes were limited, however, in the sense that they did not give rise to the dominance of a single theoretical model, but rather preserved much of the earlier spirit of synchretism and compromise.

By the late eleventh century, the learned community of western Europe possessed a significant amount of information and opinion about sex difference and reproduction. Derived, for the most part indirectly, from the writings of classical authors, this knowledge was miscellaneous and fragmented. A brief compilation on various general aspects of medicine ends with the assertion that semen arises in men out of the heat of the head and the phlegm in the kidneys – perhaps a crude echo of the Hippocratic and Galenic view that the semen originates in the brain and passes through the kidneys before taking on its final form in the testes. The text alludes to the classical qualities and humors (heat and phlegm) but associates the head, identified as cold by ancient authors, with heat.[1] Starting in the late eleventh century, the dilution and fragmentation of information and theories about reproduction underwent a gradual but radical reversal. Because of combined and mutually reinforcing interests in the recovery of classical texts and in the construction of systematic representations of nature, the Latin West extended and transformed its scientific and medical understanding of the sexes. Texts of the earlier period had occasionally manifested a specific interest in subjects relating to reproduction. For example, one manuscript of the same brief tract just referred to adds a separate section associating the conception of male children with menstrual blood, of female children with milk, and of twins with both. It gives signs for determining the sex of the fetus, including a classically derived left–right method: if the left breast swells more, the child will be a girl.[2] But this early medieval curiosity was sporadic, and its satisfaction was limited by the form and content of the sources available. By the twelfth century, a marked change was occurring both in the ambitiousness of the curiosity and in the means to satisfy it. The result was not simply more and more elaborate writing on many points of medicine and natural philosophy but also, by the end of the thirteenth century, a new consciousness of issues and problems related to these subjects and of disagreements and contradictions, which in turn gave rise to structured deliberations and discussions: is it the female semen or the menstrual blood (or both) that constitutes the female contribution to reproduction? Is

1 Sigerist, "Early Mediaeval Medical Texts," p. 88.
2 Ibid.

sexual pleasure for one or both of the sexes simply an incentive to reproduction or is it necessary for conception?

The emergence of debate on these and other subjects was a gradual and uneven process, fed by several different trends in the content and structure of medieval learning. The discussions took on their most elaborate and persistent form within the universities which took shape in the thirteenth century. But if university discourse on natural philosophy and medicine represented the epitome of these changes, the university was neither their first nor their only forum. Indeed, many of the new tendencies – the interest in systematic science, the development of new formats for discussing it, the elaboration of settings for teaching and learning, and the execution of translations – had roots in the same monastic tradition which in the earlier period had cherished and preserved (if also diluted and fragmented) the remnants of previously transmitted classical learning. And even as the universities came to the fore as the vanguard of scholarship, other institutions continued to foster and respond to the changes which were taking place.

Three examples will serve to illustrate the nature and variety of changes in the content and manner of thinking about the sexes in the period before the emergence of universities: the translations and treatises of an eleventh-century monk, Constantine the African, a medical tract by the twelfth-century abbess Hildegard of Bingen, and a fragmentary dialogue on subjects relating to reproduction probably copied in the early thirteenth century. Since these works are very different from one another in form and in content, they illustrate several distinct avenues of change. Constantine, although writing in a monastery, built on his cosmopolitan connections – his North African origins and his links with the city of Salerno – to make some of the first and most influential Latin translations of major Arabic medical works. Hildegard, operating in the most conservative environment of the three, illustrates the extent to which the monastic setting and monastic learning could adjust and evolve. The anonymous dialogue, reflecting rather than creating changes in sources of knowledge, was extracted from an early twelfth-century work and took a form which bridged the world of the monastery and the world of the university to express newly fashionable ideas. Diverse as these authors and their works are, they have in common that they have their roots in the older traditions and yet represent shifts in substance and approach which shaped late medieval ideas and institutions. All three manifest to a greater or lesser extent an appetite for more fully elaborated learning on subjects related to sex; all three attempt, albeit in very different ways, to give structure to discussions of these subjects; and all three lean away from the old forms of eclecticism, though each is in some sense eclectic. Finally, all are among the texts that gradually bring to light issues such as the role of female seed and the function of sexual pleasure that took their final form in the university-generated literature of the thirteenth and fourteenth centuries.

These three examples and the types of individuals and texts they represent do not fit into a linear narrative of scientific and medical progress. The kinds of intellectual activities they embody, whether translation into Latin, coordination of biblical and philosophical learning, or presentation of complex problems in accessible didactic form, all persisted side by side from the late eleventh or early twelfth century through the university-dominated thirteenth and fourteenth centuries. Constantine, the earliest, most complex, and most influential, presented to the Latin West a vast body of Arabic learning whose content and form profoundly affected the course of learned medicine; Hildegard, writing a century later but more tied to the older traditions, consolidated and integrated material from disparate sources; and the latest, the anonymous dialogue, although elementary in its presentation, took advantage of newly available ideas and shaped them into a focused set of questions.

CONSTANTINE THE AFRICAN: TEXTS AND READERS BEYOND THE MONASTERY

So momentous was the contribution of Constantine the African to medical learning that its implications were not yet fully played out by the end of the twelfth century, a century after his death. He presented the Latin world with a new set of texts on which to base the study of health and disease, and he communicated these texts beyond the cloister in which he worked to the town – the setting of the subsequent development of European thought. With access to the monastic tradition, he was nevertheless an outsider whose education and experience allowed him to see its shortcomings and lacunae; a member of a monastic community whose connections and influence went far beyond its walls.

Constantine was a converted Moslem from North Africa, and he clearly felt with some urgency the dearth of medical information and the poverty of medical understanding in the Latin world. As a monk at the Benedictine house at Monte Cassino in southern Italy, he imported, translated, and reshaped vast quantities of Arabic medicine over several decades toward the end of the eleventh century.[3] In doing so, he transferred to the West not only a strongly Galenic body of medical literature but also new ideas about the structuring of medical information and a new respect for the theoretical foundations of health care. Constantine supplied his Latin audience with little tracts on specific topics (sometimes excerpted from larger works), such as his treatises *On Coitus* and *On the Stomach*; he borrowed and abbreviated,

---

3 Constantine's life (about which little is known) and work (of which there is a great deal) await a full up-to-date treatment. See Michael McVaugh, "Constantine the African," in Charles Coulston Gillispie, ed., *The Dictionary of Scientific Biography*, 16 vols. (New York: Charles Scribner for American Council of Learned Societies, 1970–80), vol. 3, pp. 393–5.

sometimes mentioning and sometimes not mentioning his sources. He did his translating and composing (the two activities are not always distinguishable) at Monte Cassino, dedicated at least two works to its abbot, and collaborated with another Benedictine monk, Johannes Afflacius (like him, a converted Moslem). In these ways his work was tied to the monastic world, and although he enriched it considerably, he did not challenge it. It was thus monastic medicine, alive and active, that provided the setting for the initiation of a period of prodigious translations and intellectual growth in western Europe, not excluding new materials and new arguments concerning sexuality, sex difference, and reproduction.

But in other ways, Constantine's contributions were an important step in a process which conveyed medical and scientific knowledge out of the cloisters and into the courts, towns, and universities of Europe and which changed the character of medical and scientific knowledge, bringing into relief some of the tensions and contradictions concerning sex previously obscured by the form and content of monastic learning. In its substance (particularly in its attention to medical theory and natural philosophy), in its structure (particularly the organized and comprehensive character of his medical encyclopedia, the *Pantegni*, and his medical *vade mecum*, the *Viaticum*), and in its audience (including not only the monks of Monte Cassino but the bishop and the secular medical elite of the city of Salerno), the Constantinian corpus pointed outward to the shift in the character and locus of scientific and medical ideas that was to take place during the following centuries and that was to open them to interactions with broader religious, social, and cultural forces.

Both the consistency of Constantine's work with certain aspects of monastic medicine and the way in which it introduced some of these new elements – for example, persistently applied medical theory – are apparent in his little tract *On Coitus*. Like much monastic medicine, it is a short treatise on a specific cluster of topics. It is indirectly derived from ancient sources, whose authority it invokes from time to time. It contains a list of recipes of the sort often found in monastic and other early Latin manuscripts, in this case a series of fourteen recipes for increasing men's sexual desire, curing impotence, and related purposes. For example:

An electuary concocted by Isaac to prolong intercourse: 10 drams artemisia; 20 drams cleansed pine-nuts; 10 drams colewort, ragwort; 15 drams ginger; 7 drams anise; grind and rub for a very long time with butter and temper with honey. Give five drams to the patient on going to bed, then let him drink sirup or broth of parsnips; also, let his stomach and testicles be rubbed with oil of elder in which camomile is steeped.[4]

4 Paul Delany, "Constantinus Africanus' *De Coitu*: A Translation," *Chaucer Review* 4 (1969): 64. The translation given here is Delany's. Cf. Constantinus, *De coitu*, ch. 16, pp. 168, 170.

The clipped style, the mostly herbal and vegetable ingredients, the variety of forms the medicines take (potions, pills, ointments, vapors – only the last absent from this particular list), the accretion of a number of recipes presented without distinction for a single condition (from time to time one may be labeled "tested" or "really works"), and the (sometimes fabricated) citation of an authoritative source would all have been familiar in the early medieval monastic setting.[5]

If some things about Constantine's *On Coitus* fit neatly into traditions familiar in the monastery, many things about this work were new, starting with the subject matter: the production and nature of male semen, and male sexual and reproductive health and disorders. Of more obvious, if still oblique, relevance to celibate male communities than gynecological literature, these topics had not commanded much attention in the medical literature of the early Latin West. That Constantine decided to produce such a treatise attests at once to the vast quantity of medical information and opinion (on these subjects and others) to which he had access through Arabic writings, and at the same time to a sense of interest or need expressed by Constantine's southern Italian colleagues or perceived by Constantine himself. Without direct evidence there is no way to pinpoint the origins of this interest, though reasonable conjectures might include (in addition to those entertained in connection with the transmission of gynecological literature) the supposition that monks contending with such problems as celibacy or nocturnal emissions might have some immediate interest in some of these matters, and the supposition that the growing secular connections of the monastery – particularly with the medical community in Salerno – led it to look outward in its production of texts.

In addition to the new subject matter, some of the authorities Constantine cites are different. Though monastic medicine enhanced its legitimacy by acknowledging a real or imagined debt to Hippocrates, Galen, and others, Constantine added whole new sets of names to be reckoned with. These were physicians and scholars of the Islamic world, learned in ancient medicine (especially the works of Galen) and members of a cosmopolitan culture in which medical and scientific studies flourished. Isaac Israeli, mentioned in the set of recipes cited above, was a Jewish physician of the tenth century who wrote in Arabic and who was one of Constantine's main authorities. (See Figure 3.) Constantine introduced not only the names but also the ideas and the forms of expression of many Middle Eastern and North African authors to his Latin readers. In particular, the large-scale integration of medical and natural philosophical theory into medical writings was new to the West, and it necessarily took forms different from those of the early

5 Like whole works, specific recipes or opinions were sometimes pseudonymously attributed. Constantine may have seen this recipe attributed to Isaac Judeus, but Cartelle (Constantinus, *De coitu*, p. 169, n. 1) has not found it in any of Isaac's extant works.

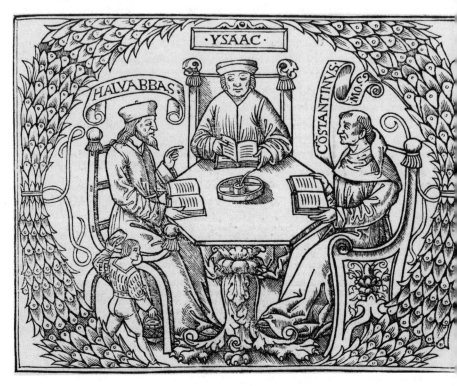

Figure 3. Constantine the African, Ali ibn Abbas ("Haly"), and Isaac Israeli. Constantine was and was seen as a transmitter of medical knowledge from outside Latin Christendom. In this early sixteenth-century woodcut, Constantine the monk sits with the authors of his major Arabic sources, a Moslem and a Jew. (Isaac, *Opera omnia* [Lyon, 1515], frontispiece. Photograph courtesy of the New York Academy of Medicine.)

compilations and recipe lists. In the treatise on intercourse Constantine presented the aphrodisiacs and other remedies only after proportionally lengthy discussions of the principles of generation and the origins of male health and pathology. He persistently invoked the classical idea of the four qualities in connection with reproduction, sex determination, diseases, and remedies, holding, for example, that a man's sexual appetite and reproductive potency depended on his particular complexion – his constitution with respect to the qualities hot, cold, moist, and dry. Furthermore, the explanations Constantine put forth in these remarks formed the basis for the prophylactic and therapeutic advice later in the work. Since, for example, he posited three things essential to intercourse (appetite, spirit, and humor), he saw the problems men might encounter – and the solutions to them – in terms of those principles.[6]

Constantine's general account of the reproductive process displays his inclination, derived from his Arabic sources, to sustain this consistency of explanatory principles and his desire to take advantage of the wealth of detailed information which those sources offered. Pursuing both consistency and detail was not without its difficulties, but Constantine was successful at placing the components of his picture in reasonable alignment: he did not expose and confront the tensions as later authors were to do. Coordinating as best he could the association of sexual arousal and semen with several different organs and several different paths, Constantine located the three essential elements at three different points of origin in accordance with Galenic notions of the division of labor among the major organs: appetite comes from the liver, windy spirit from the heart, and seminal humor from the brain. For procreation, two fluids must converge: first, the windy spirit, which, prompted by the appetite from the liver, arises in the heart and descends through vessels and the testicles into the penis, causing erection; and second, the seminal fluid, which passes from the brain through veins behind the ears into the spinal marrow, whence it descends through the kidneys into the testicles and penis. The male then ejaculates the semen into the female's deep hollow space, which closes to retain it.[7] Elsewhere Constantine consolidates even further, saying that when the senses stir the heart, two forms of the hot, dry spirit are produced: one descends directly, and the other passes to the brain, whence it descends to rejoin the first.[8] If Constantine succeeded in sustaining the association of the semen with heart, brain, marrow, liver, and kidneys (and in accommodating Hippocrates, Aristotle, and Galen) without falling into inconsistency, he failed to assimilate fully another version of the origin of semen – pangenesis. This theory, attacked by Aristotle, held that the semen is drawn from *all* parts of the body (thus potentially explaining the resemblance of child to parent), and it surfaced, appropriately attributed to Hippocrates, in Constantine's discussion of the ill effects of excessive copulation.[9] His work thus contains but does not confront what was to become grist for elaborate analyses when Aristotle's *Generation of Animals* was translated in the thirteenth century and when the format for sorting out differing theories was developed within the universities.

This description of the first stages of reproduction, taken from Constan-

6 See, e.g., ibid., ch. 13, pp. 142, 144.
7 Ibid., chs. 1 and 2, pp. 78–82.
8 Constantinus Africanus, *De humana natura vel de membris principalibus corporis humani*, in Albucasis, *Methodus menendi* . . . (Basel: Henricus Petrus, 1541), pp. 318–19.
9 Constantinus, *De coitu*, ch. 11, p. 132; ch. 1, p. 81 and n. 2. See also *Theorica*, III, 107, in idem, *Pantegni*, in Isaac [Israeli], *Opera omnia*, 2d foliation (Lyon: Andreas Turinus, 1515), fol. 25ra.

tine's tract *On Coitus*, suggests a view of the process in which the male makes the central contribution and the female serves as a receptacle. Perhaps because this particular work was aimed at explaining and curing men's sexual and reproductive disorders, its author, though borrowing from Hippocratic and Galenic medicine for the anatomy and physiology of seed production, gives an Aristotelian slant to the male and female roles, without suggesting the existence of any tension between the two perspectives. Constantine was in a position to recognize the lack of agreement about the female contribution. In his comprehensive work, the *Pantegni*, although he echoed Aristotelian rhetoric, saying that the sperm is to the menstrual blood as the craftsman is to the material, he referred to Hippocrates and Galen and specified that both male and female sperm are necessary for conception, since the female seed tempers the dangerously powerful male seed.[10] Indeed, he gave a well developed version of the Galenic parallels (and distinctions) between male and female in anatomy, production of sperm, and pathway of sperm to the point of conception.[11] At pains to put forward details about reproduction, Constantine risked undermining his attempts at systematic and consistent treatment, but he did manage to avoid a direct clash of theories within any individual work. Later, scholastic authors would address head on the exact sense in which female seed is "necessary" to generation.

Maternal influence after the moment of conception offers another example of the way in which Constantine's work smooths over potential conflicts and inconsistencies in an attempt to present a coherent picture and at the same time to incorporate disparate elements of his sources. Classical medicine had entertained two models of sex determination: one depending on the uterine environment and the other on the seed. In his tract *On Human Nature*, where Constantine subscribed to the existence of female testicles and sperm, he took the position that if the parents' sperms come together on the warm right side of the uterus, the child will be a boy; if on the cool left side, the child will be a girl; if in the middle, the child's sex will depend on the relative quantities of the two sperms.[12] He thus constructed a layered explanation in which each of the theories has a place. In *On Coitus*, the most male-oriented of his works, he added yet other causes: the dominance of the man's left or right testicle and the strength of the man's libido. But, seeking coherence and avoiding fragmentation, he placed them along with the uterine explanation within the framework of the four qualities, and particularly the hot–cool axis. Following the classical consensus, Constantine regarded

10 Constantinus, *Theorica*, III, 34, in idem, *Pantegni*, fol. 14ra. See also idem, *De humana natura*, p. 319.
11 Constantinus, *Theorica*, III, 34, in idem, *Pantegni*, fol. 13vb; and *De genitalibus membris* in Monica H. Green, "The *De genecia* Attributed to Constantine the African," *Speculum* 62 (1987): 314–15, 322–3. In demonstrating Constantine's authorship of the latter work, Green shows that it was substantially excerpted from the *Pantegni*.
12 Constantinus, *De humana natura*, p. 319.

heat as the cause of masculinity and cold as the cause of femininity. Because the parts on the right side (the right testicle and the right half of the womb) are close to the liver and therefore nourished by the pure blood which originates there, they are warmer than those on the left.[13] Similarly, heat explains the association of strong male libido with male offspring. Men whose testes are warm and moist (whether from general constitution, diet, or season) will have great sexual appetite and male offspring, because warmth produces both.[14]

In the end, although Constantine mentioned female testes and female sperm, declaring the latter to be necessary for procreation, their status and function remained unsettled, for the role he accorded to the female in the reproductive process was ill-defined, except where the influence of the uterine environment was concerned. There the principles of left and right and hot and cold extended to the female body, making the womb an active receptacle. Constantine's treatment of sex determination, like his treatment of the reproductive process in general, involved juggling a variety of perspectives. He kept them from disarray, accorded them a fluid and sometimes elusive relationship, and avoided setting them down side by side to examine their flaws or incompatibilities. In this respect, his approach represents a new, more systematic and deliberate eclecticism, preparing the way for but not yet engaging in the debates to come.

The concept of natural heat, which implicitly underlies at least some of Constantine's views on reproductive roles and sex determination, and the system of the four qualities in which it is embedded play a significant part in his ideas about sexual desire and pleasure as well. Sexual desire (which he usually calls *appetitus* or *libido*) along with the spirit and humor of which semen is composed, is one of the three things necessary for intercourse and therefore for procreation. Like semen, appetite depends on warmth: a man warmed by wine will have ample supplies of both; a man with warm testicles will be licentious as well as fertile.[15] According to Constantine, appetite arises from the liver, results from "windiness" (associated with the spiritous component of semen), and depends on the testicles. Eunuchs, who lack testicles, also lack libido.[16] Although appetite is not a sufficient condition for intercourse – there are those who desire it but are constitutionally unable to fulfill that desire[17] – it is nevertheless a necessary one. Constantine was therefore interested in ways to stimulate sexual appetite, and he offered specific recipes for that purpose, such as a concoction of mashed garden

13 Constantinus, *De coitu*, ch. 7, p. 106; idem, *De genitalibus membris* (Green "*De genecia*," pp. 319–20).
14 Constantinus, *De coitu*, ch. 5, pp. 96–8.
15 Ibid., pp. 196–8.
16 Ibid., ch. 12, pp. 138–40; ch. 6, pp. 102–4.
17 Ibid., ch. 12, p. 140.

roots, honey, egg yolks, and various herbs and seeds.[18] Conversely, since intercourse is not always appropriate or healthy, he offered recipes of a cooling sort – lentils prepared with lettuce seed, for instance – to extinguish desire.[19] Women's sexual appetite, however, received little attention from him. We know he believed women had sexual appetites, since at one point he included degree of libidinousness in a list of factors determining the size of a woman's *vulva* – a word used in the Middle Ages to refer variously to the vulva, the vagina, or a woman's sexual parts generally.[20] But although an allusion he made to the sensitivity of the mouth of the uterus might refer to desire (or to pleasure), and although in one version of the reproductive process he constructed parallels between female and male, Constantine wrote about neither the presence nor the failure nor the medicinal encouragement of women's libido.

If appetite is instrumental in intercourse, pleasure is both a motive and a consequence. In the prologue to *On Coitus* he says the Creator, who has instituted intercourse so that animal kinds may be perpetuated, has provided the organs necessary for procreation and has endowed them with such pleasure that all animals enjoy intercourse.[21] If there is a certain tension between this natural theology and the asceticism of monastic principles, a tension we will see manifested on the subject of sexual abstinence, Constantine nonetheless remained well within the bounds of orthodoxy on this point.[22] He may have been familiar with the formulation of Nemesius, the fourth-century Christian philosopher whose work on human nature was translated by Alfanus, archbishop of Salerno, a colleague of Constantine and former member of the Benedictine community at Monte Cassino. Nemesius held that desire for intercourse was natural but that unlike some appetites (such as the desire for food) which must be fulfilled for survival, this one can be denied, making virginity possible.[23] In any case, the invocation of divine intention and utility is in accord with monastic habits of thought.

Both the praise of God's provisions and the focus on animals may have been meant to soften the impact of the treatise's subject (men's sexual function and dysfunction), but elsewhere Constantine stated clearly that almost all humans like intercourse – not because it produces children, but "irratio-

---

18 Ibid., ch. 16, p. 182. See also ch. 13, p. 142; ch. 14, pp. 150–2; and ch. 17, pp. 180–2.
19 Ibid., ch. 15, pp. 154–6.
20 Constantinus, *De genitalibus membris* (Green "*De genecia*," p. 314).
21 Constantinus, *De coitu*, Prologue, p. 76.
22 See Monica H. Green, "Constantinus Africanus and the Conflict between Religion and Science," in G. R. Dunstan, ed., *The Human Embryo: Aristotle and the Arabic and European Traditions*, (Exeter: University of Exeter Press, 1990), pp. 47–69.
23 Nemesius Emesenus, *De natura hominis: Traduction de Burgundio de Pise*, ed. G. Verbeke and J. R. Moncho, Corpus Latinum commentariorum in Aristotelem Graecorum, suppl. 1 (Leiden: E. J. Brill, 1975), ch. XXIV, p. 108, and XVII, p. 97. This edition is of a slightly later translation.

nally," because it is a source of pleasure.[24] In spite of its place in the divine plan and its near universality, Constantine did not take a great interest in the operations of sexual pleasure (as distinguished from desire), for which he usually used some form of the word *delectatio*, and none of his recipes is aimed at enhancing it. In *On coitus*, which focuses on men, he associates sexual pleasure with the emission of male semen, but he does not establish any necessary connection between ejaculation and pleasure or between pleasure and conception, nor does he say whether nocturnal emissions involve pleasure.[25] Of women he says (in the *Pantegni*) only that the mouth of the uterus is sensitive to pleasure, but he also implies that the opening and closing of the uterus to receive and retain the seed is related to that sensitivity.[26] In keeping with his limited interest in the subject of pleasure, Constantine makes his most significant statement almost incidentally. After a series of chapters on the senses, he treats the general subject of pleasure and pain. By way of example, he mentions the expulsion of a potentially harmful accumulation of sperm, which results in more pleasure than pain. He adds, "Pleasure in intercourse is greater in women than in males, since males derive pleasure only from the expulsion of a superfluity. Women experience twofold pleasure: both by expelling their own sperm and by receiving the male's sperm, from the desire of their fervent *vulva*."[27]

Constantine's work only hints at what will, for various reasons, become subjects of extended discussion two centuries later – for example, the place of pleasure in conception and the comparison between male and female pleasure. What he did, however, for these subjects, for reproduction in general, and indeed for medicine as a whole was to translate and communicate information, theories, and a model for sustained discourse that were to be significant features of medicine and natural philosophy in the following centuries.

The concern, found in Constantine's works, with theoretical foundations and with explanations based upon them, in conjunction with the more general interest in philosophical discourse that developed in the late eleventh and twelfth centuries and that both fed and fed upon the translations of Greek and Arabic natural philosophy, was to give rise to a new standard of consistency in medical writing. Medical treatises and, in the thirteenth and fourteenth centuries, medical commentaries and disputations absorbed – at

---

24 Constantinus, *Theorica*, V, 107, in idem, *Pantegni*, fol. 25ra: "irrationabiliter."
25 Constantinus, *De coitu*, ch. 5, pp. 98–100. Weaker seed, nocturnal emissions (*pollutiones*), and the conception of daughters are all related to cool, moist testicles.
26 Constantinus, *Theorica*, III, 34, in idem, *Pantegni*, fol. 13vb.
27 Ibid., VI, 17, in idem, *Pantegni*, fol. 28rb: "Delectatio in coitu maior est in mulieribus quam in masculis, quia masculi delectantur tantum in expulsione superfluitatis. Mulieres dupliciter delectantur, et in suo spermate expellendo et masculi recipiendo ex vulve ardenti desiderio."

first loosely and implicitly, then strictly and self-consciously – standards of logic and demonstration drawn especially from Galen and Aristotle and reshaped by the Arabic and Latin traditions. In his treatise on intercourse Constantine carried the same principles of hot, cold, moist, and dry through his treatment of the varieties of testicles and semen, the production of male and female offspring, and the correction of disorders. His work has a striking coherence to it even though he did not, as authors did in the centuries to follow, construct syllogisms and refute opposing positions.

The prominence of theory in the writings of Constantine reflects the Galenic character of his Arabic sources (the East had preserved and developed the philosophical aspects of ancient medicine far more fully than the West) and the interests of his Western audiences, which were already manifesting an appetite for new, more discursive forms of inquiry. The treatise on intercourse has an expository style; ideas and information are connected thematically and logically, the repertoire of verbs goes well beyond the "take" and "apply" of remedy books, and the way information is presented differs from the miscellaneous character of compilations on particular subjects. One modern scholar complains that the author of an early twelfth-century anatomical text which borrows extensively from Constantine "frequently wandered from descriptive anatomy to elaborate discussions of humoral physiology and made repeated references to the teleological concepts of Galen. Apparently this master had fallen completely under Arabic influence."[28]

Constantine's influence spread slowly at first, becoming evident initially in medical works from Salerno in southern Italy, such as the anatomical text just mentioned. The eventual fusion of Constantine's work with the traditions of the Salernitan medical community illustrates one path by which medical and natural philosophical learning migrated from the monastery to the town, where it would ever after be centered.[29] Salerno was a cosmopolitan coastal town with a layered ethnic history, a location suited to intercultural contact, and a well established secular and ecclesiastical administrative center. Its reputation as a center of medical knowledge dated back to the

28 Morris H. Saffron, *Dictionary of Scientific Biography*, s.v. "Salernitan Anatomists." On the debt of the *Demonstratio anatomica* to Constantine, see G. W. Corner, *Anatomical Texts of the Earlier Middle Ages: A Study in the Transmission of Culture*, Carnegie Institute of Washington, Publication 364 (Washington: National Publishing, 1927), pp. 21–5.

29 The timing and extent of Constantine's influence have been much debated. The view that Constantine's work was the cause of the great flourishing of Salernitan medicine in the twelfth century is untenable, as is the position that Constantine's influence was negligible. See Schipperges, *Assimilation der arabischen Medizin*; Morris Harold Saffron, ed. and trans., *Maurus of Salerno: Twelfth-Century "Optimus Physicus" with His Commentary on the Prognostics of Hippocrates*, Transactions of the American Philosophical Society, n.s., 62/1 (Philadelphia: American Philosophical Society, 1972), intro., pp. 11–15; Lawn, *Salernitan Questions*; idem, ed., *The Prose Salernitan Questions Edited from a Bodleian Manuscript (Auct. F.3.10)*, Auctores Britannici Medii Aevi 5 (London: British Academy at Oxford University Press, 1979).

second half of the tenth century (a century before Constantine's time), when it was known particularly for its practitioners' empirical knowledge and practical success.[30]

The earliest medical writings that can be definitively linked to Salerno reflect this pragmatic bent, containing little of a theoretical or philosophical nature. The word "monkish" can be applied to these first works of bookish medicine,[31] many of which probably originated in the thriving and powerful Benedictine houses in Salerno and at Monte Cassino, a considerable distance away but with close ties to Salerno. Thus at the time of Constantine's translations and treatises, Salerno was home to a renowned group of practitioners (some of them monks), for whom medical learning, formerly undoubtedly communicated by apprenticeship, had begun to include written works containing recipes and compilations of the remnants of classical medicine. Constantine made his contribution in the context of a developing interest in fuller written treatments of the basic elements of medical practice (such as the analysis of urines and pulses) and a growing concern for understanding the theoretical foundations of medicine. At about the same time that Constantine was producing a body of medical texts derived from the Arabic versions of Greek medicine, others were translating texts, mainly from the Greek. These translations were gradually assembled by several generations of medical teachers into an introduction to the art of medicine, which came to be known as the *Articella*.[32] Compared with what Constantine transmitted of Greek and Arabic thought on sexuality, obstetrics, and gynecology, this collection, eventually including seven basic works, contained little that contributed significantly to the discussion of such subjects as the male and female contributions to reproduction. But one work in the group, Johannitius's general introduction to medicine, the *Isagoge*, contained a passage touching on the generative power of the sperm that caught

30 For the history of medicine at Salerno see Kristeller, "School of Salerno," esp. pp. 143–69, for the period discussed here. See also Karl Sudhoff, "Salerno, eine mittelalterlische Heil- und Lehrstelle am Tyrrhenischen Meere," *Archiv für Geschichte der Medizin* 21 (1929): 43–62; and, for more recent bibliography, Saffron, *Maurus of Salerno*.

31 Kristeller, "School of Salerno," pp. 147, 148. See also Augusto Beccaria, *I codici di medicina del periodo presalernitano (secoli IX, X e XI)*, Storia e letteratura 53 (Rome: Edizioni di Storia e Letteratura, 1956).

32 For the history of the *Articella* texts and the role played by them and the commentaries on them from the late eleventh to the early thirteenth century, see the summary provided by Paul Oskar Kristeller in *La Scuola Medica di Salerno secondo ricerche e scoperte recenti*, Quaderni del Centro studi e documentazione della Scuola Medica Salernitana 5 (Salerno: Centro studi e documentazione della Scuola Medica Salernitana, 1980). Much of the argument and evidence there is more fully presented and documented in his "Bartolomeo, Musandino, Mauro di Salerno e altri antichi commentatori dell'*Articella*, con un elenco di testi e di manoscritti," in *Studi sulla Scuola medica salernitana* (Naples: Instituto Italiano per gli Studi Filosofici, 1986), pp. 97–151, which is a translation, with additions and corrections, of "Bartholomaeus, Musandinus and Maurus of Salerno and Other Early Commentators of the *Articella* with a Tentative List of Texts and Manuscripts," *Italia medioevale e umanistica* 19 (1976): 57–87.

the attention of later commentators, and the collection as a whole played an important role in the development of late medieval medical thought and medical education.

The *Articella* and the Constantinian corpus differed significantly, the former deriving more directly from Greek texts and fitting more closely the practical orientation of early Salernitan medicine, and the latter deriving from Arabic texts and incorporating a significant body of theory and natural philosophy, but the two had much in common. Both were manifestations of a trend toward learned, written medicine, and both reflected an appetite for more detailed and comprehensive discussions of medical subjects than had been afforded by the fragments and compilations of earlier monastic medicine. Furthermore, although both point to the growing significance of secular medical learning, both had links with monasticism – two of the works included in the *Articella* can be traced to translators associated with the Benedictine monastery at Monte Cassino, perhaps even to Constantine himself and to his friend Alfanus, the abbot (who later became archbishop of Salerno).[33]

Not only do these two strands in the development of medical literature in southern Italy have much in common, but they also begin almost immediately to interact, so that by the end of the twelfth century, they are no longer really separable. Whereas it was once thought that the medical community of Salerno resisted the theorizing, academic tendencies of newly translated Arabic works, new evidence indicates that the monastic schools' bookish practice of writing commentaries on sacred and grammatical texts was applied by Salernitan medical teachers to one of the texts in the *Articella* as early as the second quarter of the twelfth century – and that one of the commentaries even cites Constantine.[34] Indeed, as Kristeller argues, we see in the context of the urban, secular teaching of medicine the precedent-setting application of the commentary form to medical and natural philosophical subjects.[35] Thus, in the course of the twelfth century, as interests shifted and new texts were both translated and created within the sphere of Salerno, accompanying changes in medical education began to become apparent. These are especially evident in the emergence of this new genre of text, the medical commentary, a product of a method of teaching in which a

33 Alfanus may have translated Hippocrates' *Aphorisms* from the Greek; Constantine may have translated Johannitius's *Isagoge* from the Arabic. The evidence for both attributions is circumstantial. Kristeller, "Bartolomeo, Musandino e Mauro," pp. 109–11. It is less likely that Constantine is responsible for the *Articella*'s versions of Hippocrates' *Aphorisms* or *Prognostics*. Kristeller, *La Scuola Medica di Salerno*, p. 12.
34 Kristeller, "Bartolomeo, Musandino, Mauro," p. 143; idem, *La Scuola Medica di Salerno*, p. 10.
35 Paul Oskar Kristeller, "Beitrag der Schule von Salerno zur Entwicklung der scholastischen Wissenschaft im 12. Jahrhundert: Kurze Mitteilung über handschriftliche Funde," in Josef Koch, ed., *Artes liberales von antiker Bildung zur Wissenschaft des Mittelalters*, Studien und Texte zur Geistesgeschichte des Mittelalters 5 (Leiden: E. J. Brill, 1959), pp. 84–90.

master presents an authoritative text to a group of students by reading and expounding upon it. In Salerno the format was a part of the formalization of medical learning which would culminate with the creation of a corporate body of medical masters and eventually of a full-blown university, with examinations and licensing procedures. Although medical commentaries appeared before the full influence of the newly translated texts was felt, their popularity and their form were no doubt influenced by familiarity with the fact that the Arabs and indeed Galen himself had made use of the commentary for research and instruction. This method of teaching and this genre of text became increasingly favored not only in Salerno but in other towns, such as Bologna, Paris, and Oxford, where students gathered geographically and institutionally apart from the older ecclesiastical centers of learning, in what were eventually to become the corporations of faculty or students known as universities. Commentaries will therefore be among the most important sources for the analysis of later medieval ideas on sexuality, sex difference, and reproduction.

The practical and theoretical traditions interacted. If practice-oriented works of the *Articella*, such as Hippocrates' *Aphorisms* and *Prognostics*, were brought into the intellectual mainstream by the addition of commentaries, the often more abstract material of the Constantinian corpus found its way, by the end of the twelfth century, into a large body of question-and-answer texts closely tied to practical medical education and known as the Salernitan Questions.[36] The presentation of a series of questions and answers had precedents in classical literature, the most relevant of which for our subject are the Latin version of Soranus's *Gynecology*, the pseudo-Aristotelian collections of questions known as *Problems*, and Seneca's *Natural Questions*. But the association of this form with Salernitan medicine is clearly more than a neoclassical affectation. Although oral traditions are difficult to trace, it is reasonable to assume that pragmatic medical education in Salerno included, in conjunction with apprenticeship, the rote learning of certain basic terms and facts. If this is the case, the early, oral answers to the questions were certainly much shorter than those that have come down to us in writing and probably contained far fewer allusions to general medical explanations in terms of theoretical concepts such as qualities and pores. Indeed the later history of this genre suggests that the same questions might once have had quite different answers.[37] By around 1200, the period of the earliest written example to come down to us, the collections of opinions associated with Salerno included comments on various sexual subjects, many of which are

36　Brian Lawn has pioneered the study of these texts, beginning with *Salernitan Questions*. He offered additions, especially concerning the relation of the Salernitan Questions to the work of William of Conches, David of Dinant, and John Blund, in the Italian version, *I Quesiti Salernitani: Introduzione alla storia della letteratura problematica medica e scientifica nel Medio Evo e nel Rinascimento*, trans. Alessandro Spagnuolo ([Salerno]: Di Mauro, 1969).

37　Lawn, *Prose Salernitan Questions*, especially the comparative tables.

closely linked to those contained in *On Human Generation*, discussed later. By that time, both the questions and the answers had been influenced by the works of Constantine (particularly with regard to semen, coitus, and related topics) and by the learned medical masters of late twelfth-century Salerno, for example, Urso of Calabria, who wrote commentaries on the *Articella* and independent treatises reflecting a deep interest in the principles and explanatory power of natural philosophy. By that time, too, the whole array of medical learning, from oral to written, from practical to theoretical, from question-and-answer to commentary and treatise, was firmly established in the secular, urban environment of Salerno and had begun to take hold in other towns.

In order to explore the effects of the greater influence of ecclesiastical institutions and theological ideas, in order to illustrate the continuing liveliness of the monastic traditions, and in order to reach a point of convergence between southern and northern learning in the form of question-and-answer literature on sexual subjects, we turn now to the north and back to the cloister.

HILDEGARD OF BINGEN: EXTENSION AND INTEGRATION

When she composed her medical works during the middle of the twelfth century, Hildegard of Bingen was abbess of a convent in the Rhine Valley.[38] Though extraordinary for the scope and force of her writings and idiosyncratic in the manner and matter of her medical and natural philosophical expression, Hildegard provides an illustration of the way in which the old forms of monastic thought adapted in the face of the new learning without being radically transformed. Her comments on reproduction and sex difference range beyond the medical compendia, gynecological tracts, and compilations of remedies of early monastic medicine and beyond the concerns of the natural philosophers of her time. But her approach remains eclectic and unsystematic. She adopts neither the organized and comprehensive format of Constantine the African's *Pantegni*, which set an example for medicine beyond the cloister, nor the influential strategies being developed by contem-

---

38 On Hildegard and her scientific and medical views see Hans Liebeschütz, *Das allegorische Weltbild der heiligen Hildegard von Bingen*, Studien der Bibliothek Warburg 16 (Leipzig and Berlin: B. G. Teubner, 1930); Charles Singer, "The Scientific Views and Visions of Saint Hildegard," in *Studies in the History and Method of Science*, 2d ed. (London: William Dawson, 1955), vol. 1, pp. 1–55; Heinrich Schipperges, trans. and intro., *Hildegard von Bingen, Heilkunde: Das Buch von dem Grund und Wesen und der Heilung der Krankheiten* (Salzburg: Otto Müller, 1957); Bernhard W. Scholz, "Hildegard von Bingen on the Nature of Women," *American Benedictine Review* 31 (1980): 361–83; Peter Dronke, "Problemata Hildegardiana," *Mittellateinisches Jahrbuch* 16 (1981): 97–131; idem, *Women Writers of the Middle Ages: A Critical Study of Texts from Perpetua (†203) to Marguerite Porete (†1310)* (Cambridge: Cambridge University Press, 1984), pp. 144–201.

porary philosophers and theologians like Peter Abelard and Peter Lombard to sort out and evaluate differences among authorities.

Hildegard's situation and temperament inclined her to seek vivid and forceful representations of matters related to sexuality and at the same time to place them within an acceptably conservative context. A visionary mystic whose cosmic imagery was dramatic and detailed, she was also a firm administrator and influential figure within the Church. She was intellectually omniverous, apparently taking in information from all manner of learned and popular sources, but she may have acquired much of it second-hand, since she was without regular access to a community of scholars or even to an important library. She did not often name, indeed she may not even have always known, the sources from which some of her statements were ultimately derived.[39] Like many of her contemporaries, her purpose in writing about nature and health was to set down, and sometimes to interpret, what was known, not to advance knowledge or to enter into exchanges intended to resolve inconsistencies. The book on medical simples attributed to Hildegard is a massive conventional compilation of remedies.[40] Her *Book of Compound Medicine* is shorter and more complicated, starting with a loose scientific exegesis of the account of the Creation and incorporating various principles of anatomy, physiology, and psychology, as well as addressing many disorders and their cures.[41] In some respects, including the extent to which it treats matters of sexuality and sex difference, the work is idiosyncratic, marked by Hildegard's extraordinary personality and position as a woman writer, but in other respects it reflects the traditions and the environment of the cloister.

Hildegard's treatise opens with an exposition of the early chapters of Genesis. Works of this kind proliferated in the monasteries and cathedral schools of the twelfth century: they used the increasingly refined methods of biblical exegesis, which was an aspect of renewed and reformed religion and theology, and at the same time – because the story of Creation enumerates so many aspects and occupants of the natural world – they provided an occasion to explore questions of natural philosophy that intrigued many twelfth-century intellectuals. Hildegard's version of Creation is brief, crude, and fitfully organized, but it gives her the opportunity to write about meteo-

---

39 Although Charles Singer saw evidence Hildegard had read modern works ("Scientific Views and Visions"), subsequent studies are more agnostic about her direct access to such sources (Liebeschütz, *Das allegorische Weltbild*, esp. pp. 8 and 99–103) or deny it altogether (Schipperges, *Hildegard von Bingen, Heilkunde*, pp. 42–5). The most careful recent study is Dronke, "Problemata Hildegardiana," pp. 107–17, which suggests specific, sometimes probably indirect, connections with classical philosophical and medical sources.

40 Hildegard, *Liber simplicis medicinae* [also known as *Physica*], ed. C. Daremberg, in *Opera omnia*, ed. Friedrich Anton Reuss, *Patrologia Latina* 197 (1853), cols. 1117–353.

41 Hildegard, *Causae et curae* [also known as *Liber compositae medicinae*], ed. Paul Kaiser, Bibliotheca scriptorum Graecorum et Romanorum Teubneriana (Leipzig: B. G. Teubner, 1903).

rology, astrology, and tides, and in two ways it provides a framework for her subsequent discussions of diseases and remedies.[42] First, it presents the story of human Creation and the Fall, not just as pious window dressing but as the explanatory basis for phenomena ranging from the physiological differences between women and men to the occurrence of menstruation. Thus the names of Adam and Eve occur in the later books of the treatise, when Hildegard introduces a section on moods with Adam's postlapsarian melancholy[43] and when she accounts for sexual attraction.[44] (Her use of early passages in Genesis to illuminate the origins of sex differences is explored in Chapter 4.) Second, her version of Creation allows her to set out some basic principles of the natural world, such as the relationship between the human body and the four elements, which serve later in the sections on diseases and their cures. For example, when she prescribes a bath and an unguent made of several herbs and menstrual blood as a remedy for the sort of leprosy which arises from excessive libido, she explains the recipe by the relationship of hot and cold in the ingredients, as well as by the specific operation of each.[45]

Partly, perhaps, because of the loose organization of the work (virtually no topic is treated in a thorough and compact manner), and partly because of a lack of precedent, Hildegard set aside no specific section of the *Book of Compound Medicine* for consideration of sex difference or reproduction. The subjects come up early in the work in response to biblical cues; later there is a section on physiognomic types which incorporates aspects of male and female sexuality; then, among the cures, there is a series of items on gynecology and obstetrics; and in a final, astrological chapter separate patterns are distinguished for women and men.[46] But unlike many of her predecessors and contemporaries who were writing similarly wide-ranging works encompassing numerous aspects of natural philosophy or medicine, Hildegard undertakes a significant exploration of the nature of female and male.

Her interest in reproduction surfaces early in the work, when she is surveying inanimate Creation: the elements, meteorological effects, the waters of the earth. In a section on the heavenly bodies she pauses in her discussion of the moon to warn that we ignore its influence at our peril. The example she chooses is the effect of the moon's phases on the conception of

---

42 Hildegard gives a much fuller interpretation of parts of Genesis in her *Book of Divine Works: Liber divinorum operum simplicis hominis* [also known as *De operatione dei*], ed. Joannes Dominicus Mansi, in *Opera omnia*, ed. F. A. de Reuss, *Patrologia Latina* 197 (1853), cols. 739–1038. On the organization of this work, see Liebeschütz, *Das allegorische Weltbild*, p. 130, n. 1; Schipperges, *Hildegard von Bingen, Heilkunde*, intro., pp. 41–2. Schipperges devises new divisions and titles for his translation.

43 Hildegard, *Causae et curae*, bk. II, pp. 145–6.

44 Ibid., pp. 136–7.

45 Ibid., bk. IV, pp. 212–13.

46 The authenticity of the last book (bk. V of the Kaiser edition) has been questioned: Schipperges, *Hildegard von Bingen, Heilkunde*, intro., p. 42.

children. The choice is unexceptional, given the strong association of astrology with nativities even before the influx of Arabic texts leads to the full development of that science. But Hildegard goes on to digress on other factors affecting offspring. A man should have a beard before he approaches a woman, and the woman should be mature, not a girl. Furthermore, a man who is a glutton and a drunk will become leprous and twisted, and one in whom lust and bodily excess lead to uncontrolled desire will lose his seed. A man who is restrained in his consumption of food and drink and who pours forth his seed appropriately will beget proper offspring.[47] This digression illustrates the way in which Hildegard takes advantage of an opportunity to mention human generation. It also provides an example of her practice of speaking about sex and reproduction in a vocabulary drawn from moral discourse. This habit of speech stems partly, no doubt, from her unflagging piety but also from her monastic environment and education, which lent a biblical cast to the diction of her medical as well as her visionary writing. She does not seem to have been fully familiar with the vocabulary of anatomy and pathology that was beginning to take hold in the twelfth century as a result of translations such as those produced by Constantine. Hildegard's shifting rhetoric struck a delicate balance between the humility of simple and religious intonations and the authority of learning.[48] Words such as the vague and biblical "loins" (*lumbi*) abound. Yet even in the first book of the treatise, closely tied to the early chapters of Genesis, she adeptly invoked the language of elements and qualities which, although available in traditional works such as Isidore of Seville's, was also a staple of modern natural philosophy as it was taking shape in the works of clerics who wrote and taught in cathedral towns and who, like Hildegard, used the Creation as a point of departure.

More remarkable than Hildegard's tendency to moralize nature is her tendency to naturalize Creation, an inclination which clearly reflects the changes in the intellectual climate that were occurring in the twelfth century. These changes were not linear, nor did they go undebated or unopposed, but they represented a significant field of contention for intellectuals of the decades before Hildegard composed her *Book of Compound Medicine*, sometime around midcentury. In addition to providing the occasion for encyclopedic introductions to large bodies of knowledge, both the biblical story of the Creation and the account of the coming-to-be of the world found in the Latin version of Plato's *Timaeus* (the latter encased in a Neoplatonic commentary) gave those who sought it the opportunity to explore specific natural philosophical theories and their implications. In a mythic work influenced by the *Timaeus*, for example, Bernard Silvester,

47 Hildegard, *Causae et curae*, bk. I, p. 18.
48 Joan Cadden, "Wissenschaft, Sprache und Macht im Werk Hildegards von Bingen," *Feministische Studien* 9 (1991): 69–79.

one of the new breed of urban intellectuals, closed with an account of
reproduction, which he represented as a process battling against the disintegration of nature into the primordial substance from which it had emerged.
Two genies (perhaps the male and female principles) fight for the cause:

Invincible, with the weapons of generation they do battle with death: they restore
nature and perpetuate the species. They do not allow the mortal to die, nor what is
falling to have fallen, nor humanity to have perished from its stem. The penis wages
war against Lachesis and, skillful, reties the threads cut by the hand of the Fates.[49]

In a didactic work of natural philosophy which refers frequently to Scripture and the Church Fathers, William of Conches, likewise a teacher in the
urban schools of northern France, rejected a literal interpretation of the story
that Eve was made from Adam's rib, in favor of the notion that she, like
him, was created from a special clay in which the four elements were perfectly balanced – or, in her case, *almost* perfectly balanced.[50] The authors of
such works, insofar as their identities and lives are known to us, seem to
have been members either of monastic communities or of cathedral chapters. Hildegard may be numbered among them, in the sense that she also
took on the task of exploring and reformulating the relationship between a
spiritual or moral interpretation of the world and a rational or natural interpretation. (Hildegard's visionary works, which have been mined by scholars for their cosmological content represent another approach to the same
problem.)[51] But whereas many of them show signs of being aware of each
other's work and sometimes even of having traveled to each other's schools,
Hildegard does not seem to be part of a network of scholars possessing an
explicit awareness of occupying a common intellectual terrain.[52]

Like William of Conches, when Hildegard came to the creation of Adam
and Eve, she gave it a physiological gloss. She has been speaking of the four
elements (earth, water, air, and fire) of which the created world is composed
(indeed, she has introduced human Creation with a lengthy discussion of the
four humors as well). Finally, she sums up by saying that there are four and

---

49 Bernardus Silvestris, *Cosmographia*, ed. Peter Dronke, Textus minores in usum academicum
   53 (Leiden: E. J. Brill, 1978), bk. II, ch. 14, ll. 161–5: "Cum morte invicti pugnant,
   genialibus armis: / Naturam reparant, perpetuantque genus. / Non mortale mori, non quod
   cadit esse caducum, / Non a stirpe hominem deperiisse sinunt. / Militat adversus Lachesim
   sollersque renodat / Mentula Parcarum fila resecta manu." See Winthrop Wetherbee, trans.,
   The Cosmographia *of Bernardus Sylvestris* (New York: Columbia University Press, 1973), p.
   164, n. 108; and Brian Stock, *Myth and Science in the Twelfth Century: A Study of Bernard
   Silvester* (Princeton, N.J.: Princeton University Press, 1972), pp. 216–18.
50 Guilelmus de Conchis, *Philosophia*, ed. and trans. (into German) Gregor Maurach with
   Heidemarie Telle (Pretoria: University of South Africa, 1980), bk. I, ch. 13, §43–5, pp.
   38–40.
51 Singer, "Scientific Views and Visions."
52 The links among these authors did not imply agreement on the interpretation of nature, so
   Hildegard does not stand outside some specific "school" of thought. See Stock, *Myth and
   Science*, esp. pp. 237–73.

only four elements and that the superior, celestial beings are of fire and air, whereas the inferior, terrestrial ones are of water and clay. Having thus substituted the biblical "clay" (*limus*) for the natural philosophical "earth" (*terra*), Hildegard is ready to address human creation. God makes Adam's external members of clay and water and gives them the fiery and airy spirit of life. This spirit becomes a constituent of blood, which is composed of all the elements. He then shapes the internal organs separately and infuses them – especially the marrow and the veins – with the spirit of life, which is like a worm writhing in its home or sap in a tree. Although she soon calls this spirit (*spiraculum*) a soul (*anima*), she has reduced it to physiological stature, once again using a shift in vocabulary to create a tenuous link between the scriptural and scientific readings.[53]

And Eve? She was indeed formed from Adam's side. But Hildegard's reading looks no less to the physical aspect of the story than the version of William of Conches. Made from the strongest elements, especially the robust earth, Adam is strong and hard. Made from his flesh and marrow, Eve is softer and weaker – and since she is not burdened by the weight of earth, her mind is sharper and loftier.[54] (The qualities of mind, *acuta* and *aerea*, are susceptible of more derogatory translation, and it is possible the ambiguity was intentional.) As the scriptural version of the story has natural implications, so the physical version has theological repercussions. We are fortunate that Eve transgressed first, because, Adam being stronger, his fault would have been irremediable. But we are unfortunate in that each generation is farther and farther from the original clay, and thus, it is weaker and weaker – presumably in both the physical and the moral sense.[55] The consequences of differential creation – Adam by the transformation of earth, Eve without transformation from his flesh – are at the foundation of much of what Hildegard has to say about sex differences. They play a role similar to that of the hot–cold contrast in classical theory, determining, among other things, the nature of the female and male reproductive contributions. Later in the work, when she is discussing diseases and their remedies, she occasionally refers back to these properties without, however, alluding to their origins: the flesh of the male peacock is efficacious in the treatment of dropsy because of its strength,[56] but the parts of female birds are used in a cure for the effects of a fall because females are more taciturn.[57] Hildegard's

---

53 Hildegard, *Causae et curae*, bk. II, pp. 41–2. A little later she retells the infusion of the soul (*anima*) in more traditional terms (bk. II, p. 45).

54 Ibid., pp. 46–7; idem, *Liber divinorum operum*, pt. III, vis. vii, ch. 3, col. 963.

55 Hildegard, *Causae et curae*, bk. II, p. 47. Discussions about the order of the Fall and its significance date back at least to Augustine: e.g., *De civitate dei*, Corpus Christianorum, Series Latina, 47–8; Aurelii Augustini opera 14 (Turnhout: Brepols, 1955), bk. XIV, ch. xi, vol. 2, pp. 432–3.

56 Hildegard, *Causae et curae*, bk. IV, p. 208.

57 Ibid., pp. 206–7.

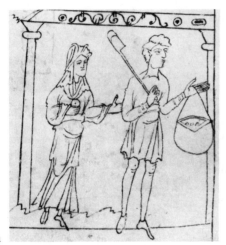

a

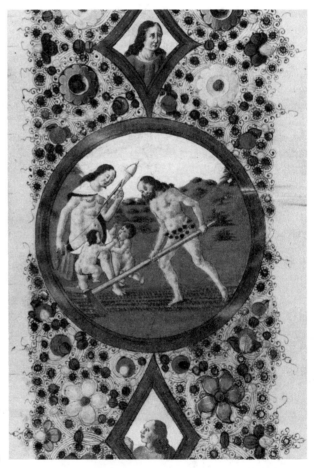

b

naturalistic interpretation of Creation thus has implications for the construction of ideas about masculine and feminine natures.

The Fall likewise has multifarious implications. Hildegard placed the social consequences of the Fall in a relatively cheerful light, emphasizing not the sweat of toil and the pain of childbirth but rather the division of labor based on the different modes of creation: man, earth-born and strong, brings forth fruit from the earth; woman, made without essential transformation, engages in the artificial work of the manual crafts and bears infants in her womb. (See Figure 4.) She linked the bearing of children, both carrying and generating them, with woman's airy substance, perhaps suggesting spaciousness, perhaps malleability.[58] The Fall's physiological consequence, however, is grave: the disturbance of the perfect balance of humans found in the prelapsarian state. Once Adam (no mention of Eve in this context) has eaten the apple, things go awry – most immediately because he has accepted serpent-approved food, which produces a case of melancholy, presumably because serpents have a cold, dry nature. In general the Fall is the source of elemental disarray, which produces humoral superfluities and thereby all manner of physical and emotional ailments.[59] Once this principle is established, however, Hildegard seldom invokes the sin of Adam when discussing diseases and cures, the main exception being a section that emphasizes afflictions of the mind and spirit.[60]

Hildegard's versions of the Creation and the Fall carry over into what she says about the male and female contributions to reproduction and about the nature and function of sexual pleasure. Several passages dealing with procreation reveal Hildegard's sense of the part played by the two parents in the production of offspring. She holds that as a result of human transgression the purity of the blood has been undermined, necessitating

---

58 Ibid., bk. II, p. 59: ". . . infantem in utero portat et eum generat."
59 Ibid., pp. 36–9. The omission of Eve's sin from Hildegard's phrasing is probably a reflection of contemporary rhetorical convention.
60 Ibid., pp. 143–8.

Figure 4. Adam and Eve at work. In their depictions of the original work of women and men, medieval artists added to the tasks mandated in Genesis. (*a*) In this early eleventh-century manuscript, Eve is holding the whorl of a spindle for spinning thread, and Adam carries not only the spade of an agricultural worker but also the bag of a herder. (Elsewhere in the manuscript, Eve is shown giving birth to Abel.) (Oxford, Bodleian, Junius 11, fol. 45r. Reproduced by permission of the Bodleian Library, Oxford.) (*b*) In this midfifteenth-century manuscript, perhaps reflecting the preoccupation with fertility after the plague and new images of the family, Eve is spinning and caring for Cain and Abel, while Adam is hoeing. (Origin, *Homiliae,* Modena, Biblioteca Etense, MS lat. 458 [= alpha.M.1.4], fol. 1r. Reproduced by permission of the Biblioteca Etense.)

the emission of seed, which takes place in the heat of lust.[61] She does not entertain the question of whether procreation would have occurred in Paradise, but it is certainly her conviction that it would not have occurred *in this way*. It is pleasure (*delectatio*) deriving from the serpent and the forbidden fruit that gives rise to a new person, for it is pleasure which agitates a man's blood, Hildegard tells us, thus at one stroke accounting for the beginning of the reproductive process and introducing the doctrine of original sin. The stormy, overabundant four elements within his body overwhelm the four faculties that constitute his judgment and "produce from the blood a poisonous foam, which is the seed [*semen*]." On this point, men and women differ:

For in the transgression of Adam, the strength of man in his genital member is turned into poisonous foam, and the blood of woman is turned into a contrary effusion. For his blood has seed from the strength and true nature of man, since from earth he was made flesh. But her blood, since it is weak and subtle from the true nature of woman, does not have seed but only emits a subtle and small foam. For she is not [constituted] in two ways, as man is, of earth and flesh, but only taken from the flesh of man, and thus she is weak and fragile and is the vessel of man.[62]

A woman's blood, like a man's, does become agitated (Hildegard sometimes names the cause as *amor*, a word absent from her discussion of male arousal), and she emits something like foam, but it is more blood-colored than white. As she says later, "The foam of seed from her is more rarified than that emitted by the man – small and so scanty, [it is] to the man's foam as a scrap of bread to his whole [loaf]."[63]

For Hildegard, then, the male produced semen and the female did not, or at least not a significant seed. Because of her derivative nature, woman has neither the proper force nor the proper substance to make the white foam which either is or contains the seed. To the extent that she regarded the seed as an exclusively male contribution, Hildegard's position agreed with Aristotle's, but the reasons she gave were very different from his, which emphasized form and heat. In addition, she did not place female nature in a particularly negative light. If the male's emission is the standard to which the female's is compared, it is also his which arises from storm and superfluity,

61 Ibid., p. 33.
62 Ibid., p. 60: "Et haec omnia de nimietate superfluitatis quasi tempestatem faciunt et de sanguine venenosam spumam, quod semen est, educunt. . . . Nam in transgressione Adae fortitudo viri in genitali membro versus est in venenosam spumam, atque mulieris sanguis versus est in contrariam effusionem. De forti enim et de recta natura viri sanguis eius semen habet, quia de terra caro factus est. Sed de recta natura mulieris sanguis eius, quia debilis et tenuis est, semen non habet, sed tantum tenuem et parvam spumam emittit, quoniam de duobus modis terrae et carnis non est, ut vir, sed tantum de carne viri sumpta est; et ideo debilis et fragilis est et vas viri est."
63 Ibid., p. 76: ". . . spuma seminis ab ea rarius quam a viro eicitur et modica et tantae exiguitatis ad spumam viri ut frustum panis ad integritatem eius."

and his which is called poisonous.[64] Furthermore, as the process of procreation continues, the female contribution takes on more significance.

Hildegard imposed a certain symmetry on the process of conception. It is a consequence of her reasoning about human Creation. The biblical representation of man and woman as "one flesh" cannot refer to Eve's having been made from Adam, since, Hildegard had insisted, that process is precisely what made their flesh different. For her it referred to the act of copulation, during which the man's and woman's flesh are drawn into each other.[65] In addition, when the man's semen is ejaculated into the woman, it is cold.[66] The woman's quasi foam joins to itself the man's seed, which it warms and comforts and makes into a blooded creature. Contrary to the classical consensus, it is the mother's heat which causes the substance to coalesce and to grow into a thing with blood. Hildegard described this process both in terms of the foods derived from the mother's body and, more impersonally, in terms of the effects of the four elements, whose matter and qualities shape and temper the stuff of the "seed," now the beginning of a person. The female role here goes well beyond simply extending a predetermined or preexisting form; it involves giving the fetus shape and definition. Even the foods derived from the mother do more than just sustain the conceptus – they change it.

It is easier to identify what the female contribution does than to say what it is. That its origin is parallel to the origin of semen – sexual excitation – suggests that it is a secretion associated with intercourse. That it is connected with blood both in its appearance and in its effects suggests that it is (or is linked to) menstrual blood. (Lack of clarity about the female fluid or fluids involved in procreation was a persistent problem – and eventually an issue – in late medieval discussions of reproductive roles.) In contrast, although it is not difficult to identify the substance Hildegard referred to as a man's foam, she was less specific about how it operates in the course of conception. It is cool and white and needs both the heat and the blood from the mother to become a fetus.

Given Hildegard's interest in qualities, elements, and humors, her reversal of the usual hot–cold dichotomy is striking evidence of the freedom afforded her by the limitations and fragmentation of medical and natural philosophical knowledge that persisted in monastic sources and perhaps in the limited library of the convent, even as the intellectual scene in the large

64 Ibid., pp. 59–60. The storm of elements is associated with humanity (*homo*), not man (*vir*), but it culminates in the production of semen, which is attributed specifically to *vir*.
65 Ibid., pp. 67–8. See also idem, *Scivias*, ed. Adelgundis Führkötter with Angela Carlevaris, Corpus Christianorum, Continuatio mediaevalis 43-43A (Turnholt: Brepols, 1978), pt. II, vis. v, ch. 25, p. 196. Hildegard does not seem to mean that the man takes the woman's substance into his body, but rather that as the woman draws in the man's seed, the seed (an extension of the man's "flesh") takes in some of the woman's emission.
66 In the same passage, Hildegard says once that the man's blood sends the cold foam to the woman and once that it becomes cold after ejaculation: *Causae et curae*, bk. II, p. 60.

monastic and cathedral schools and in the towns was undergoing vast changes. Hildegard is consistent in her attribution of hot and cold: the earth from which man comes is a cold element; semen's poisonous qualities are also associated with cold; and when Hildegard included menstrual blood in a remedy for the venereal form of leprosy, she explained that the other ingredients are tempered by its heat.[67] She did not, however, systematically invoke heat as an active principle. In particular, Hildegard had other ideas for treating the question of the determination of a fetus's sex (which classical authors had agreed depended in one way or another upon heat and cold) and its general disposition.

The strength of the man's semen determines the sex of the child; the feelings of the parents toward each other determine its temperament.[68] Hildegard's view of sex determination is based, once again, on the implications of the two-phase Creation. Strong seed produces a male, for man is formed from clay, a stronger material than the flesh from which woman was formed. Strength of seed comes into play in the Hippocratic account of sex difference, but there the issue is which of two seeds will prevail; it enters into the Aristotelian account, but there it must contend with the passively resistant matter provided by the female. Hildegard has constructed her own theory based on a single (male) seed with more or less power, but without either an active Hippocratic or a passive Aristotelian counterpart. The assignment of this role to the male seed underscores in three ways the primacy of the male in Hildegard's thinking. First, it is the father who has the sole power to determine the sex of the child. Second, "strong" is matched with a male outcome, "weak" with a female outcome. (Later we shall see that in characterizing the feminine and masculine, Hildegard blunted these value implications of sex differences by representing them as distinctions rather than dichotomies.) Finally, though less clearly, there is the suggestion, consonant with cultural assumptions, that sons are better than daughters.

Sex is not, however, the only dimension of the offspring shaped by the conditions of conception. Hildegard diluted the prominence (though not the monopoly) of the father in sex determination by interlacing with it the matter of the child's character, influenced equally from the maternal and paternal sides by the love the parents bear for each other at the time of conception. The way she combined the determination of sex and temperament can be summarized as follows:

1. If the paternal seed is strong and parents love each other properly, they will produce a virtuous son.
2. If the paternal seed is strong and the man loves the woman properly, but she does not love him, they will produce a son who is weak and not virtuous.

67 Ibid., bk. IV, pp. 212–13.
68 Ibid., bk. II, p. 35–6.

3. If the paternal seed is thin and the parents love each other properly, they will produce a virtuous daughter.[69]
4. If the paternal seed is thin and either of the parents does not love the other, they will produce a daughter.
5. If the paternal seed is strong and neither parent loves the other, they will produce a bitter boy.
6. If the paternal seed is thin and neither parent loves the other, they will produce a bitter daughter.[70]

There are certain asymmetries in this account, but it effectively accords equal influence to the two parents' feelings. (The exact nature of these feelings is not easy to determine. The language Hildegard used, *rectus amor caritatis*, implies a righteous affection without lust. Perhaps she was alluding to the parents' properly chaste sexual inclinations. Several times, however, she adds "at that moment," suggesting that this exalted feeling is potentially transitory.) Hildegard is not perfectly consistent on the origin of character traits, suggesting elsewhere, when illustrating the bodily effects of the Fall, that weak seed or the seed of a man who is ill may affect the health and disposition of the child.[71]

A woman's body in general and her uterus in particular, as well as the fluid or fluids she emits, influence the outcome of the reproductive act. When Hildegard offered treatments for sterility, she was concerned with the seed of the man and with the womb of the woman.[72] And to the passage in which she enumerated the permutations of the father's determination of sex and both parents' determination of character, she appended a brief comment about appearance: "The heat of women who have a plump nature overcomes the seed of the man, so that the infant's face takes shape mostly in their likeness. But women who are by nature thin usually generate a child in the likeness of the father."[73] Since plump was healthier than thin, the former case could not be regarded as unnatural or unhealthy. Thus Hildegard had once again deflected attention from the centrality of the male contribution. This was all she had to say about the vast problem of family resemblance, which ancient authors, particularly Aristotle, had struggled with and which later scholastics were to debate.

Although she did allude to the power of heat in this treatment of inherited

---

69 Hildegard uses the word *tenuis* (thin, weak, subtle) here and in connection with the quality of woman's body as it was created from man's.
70 Hildegard has simplified and moralized the notion of innate temperament here; what she says later about men and women of different temperaments is more complicated and more tied to classical physiological notions: ibid., pp. 70–6 and 87–9.
71 Ibid., p. 33.
72 Ibid., bk. III, pp. 182–3.
73 Ibid., bk. II, p. 36: "Calor autem mulierum, quae pinguem naturam habent, semen viri superat, ita quod infans secundum similitudinem earum multotiens in facie formatur. Sed mulieres, quae macres in natura sua sunt, infantem ad similitudinem patris in facies multotiens generant."

appearance, Hildegard did not try to suggest any single explanatory principle which would tie together the three sorts of parental influence: sex determination, character formation, and physical resemblance. If not systematic,
her picture of reproductive roles is, nevertheless, not confusing. Women and
men have distinct natures. Although they are not in any sense opposites,
they are essentially different, a circumstance which has many physiological
implications. The lack of opposition is played out in the language Hildegard
used to name the differences. Although she frequently called man "strong"
(*fortis*), she did not usually describe woman simply as "weak" (*debilis*), as
Aristotelians were to do, but rather chose words that have less negative
connotations, for example, "soft" (*mollis*) and "fragile" (*fragilis*).[74] The
man's strength seems to accord him a dominant role in reproduction: he
alone produces seed, and he effects the critical determination of the child's
sex. But in fact, beyond this one power, the man does not have a dominant
influence. Indeed, the vaguely defined female effusion and the mother's
marital affection, body type, and uterus taken together play an equal or
leading role in other aspects of reproduction.

These scattered comments on the female and male contributions to reproduction bear the stamp of the monastic environment in which Hildegard
was raised and in which she wrote. Although the Rhineland was a commer-
cially, politically, and culturally busy place during Hildegard's lifetime, and
although she did travel very widely for a supposedly cloistered nun, she
does not seem to have had access to a great monastic library or scholarly
community of the kind that had been assembled at some of the larger male
institutions, such as those at Chartres or Paris. In that respect, Hildegard's
intellectual formation is probably more typical of women and men inhabit-
ing twelfth-century cloisters than that of urban teachers like William of
Conches and Bernard Sylvester or of her contemporaries at the great monasteries of St. Victor and Clairvaux. Her natural philosophy and theoretical
medicine were fragmented. She dealt with questions about reproduction in
a variety of contexts, from the Creation to the remedies for venereal disease.
Her treatment of them echoes with notions accumulated indirectly from
classical traditions: the origin of the male seed, the fetal determination of sex
as an exercise of power, and the effects of the qualities, elements, and
humors in generation, health, and disease. She was consciously calling upon
the resources of the abridged, compiled, reshuffled, unreconciled, but rich
and authoritative traditions of the ancients as they reached her through the
textual traditions and education of Western Christendom. But her interest in
natural philosophy and theoretical medicine was persistent as well, and in
this respect her intellectual inclinations may reflect the rising passion for
such matters. Even in the later books of the treatise, which contain long

74 Ibid., pp. 46, 47.

series of ailments and cures, Hildegard paused frequently to give the cause of a disease or the reason for a recipe. Pork should not, for example, be given to a patient suffering symptoms from a fall, for it will too easily excite the libido.[75] The conservative character of her sources and format was thus tempered with a spirit of curiosity and independence, just as her fundamental notion of male strength was tempered by the range of ways in which she saw the female influencing reproduction.

The place Hildegard gave to Genesis in the early sections of the treatise is another sign of the monastic character of her learning. The long expositions of aspects of Creation are linked both to the monastic method of exegesis – the exposition of sacred texts – and to the moralizing agendas of widely assimilated works like the *Physiologus* and Isidore of Seville's *Etymologies*. She was imaginative in her arrangement and elaboration of some specific points, such as the unhealthy snake-borne food, but to the extent that her work focused on the understanding of Scripture, her enterprise was an essentially conventional one. Yet the work as a whole is not structured to deliver a religious or moral message. One of the richest of her explanatory principles – the difference in composition of male and female flesh – is closely tied to a specific biblical passage, but much of those parts of the book that deal with human nature and the natural order is written in the language of the secular sciences. Likewise, although there are allusions to the Fall of Adam in the later, medical sections, they are scattered and unelaborated. In other works of Hildegard's, such as the book of visions, *Scivias*, the balance of natural science and moral or theological concerns is weighted toward the latter. In the *Book of Compound Medicine*, however, Hildegard's goals and language give primacy to the examination of nature and, most specifically, to the human body. Thus on the matter of the mutual illumination of Scripture and nature, Hildegard once again fits within monastic traditions, while at the same time mirroring the changes occurring in those traditions, especially the increasing appetite for the intellectual exploration of natural phenomena.

The same delicate balance of tradition and innovation is present in Hildegard's treatment of sexual desire and pleasure. If anything, the available texts on medicine and natural philosophy dealt less with these matters than with the reproductive roles of the sexes, and the religious and moral traditions dealt with them more. Yet Hildegard, often employing language more associated with sermons than with science, nevertheless put forward an unusually elaborate and naturalistic view of sexuality. Like her comments on the reproductive process, what she had to say about desire and pleasure is scattered throughout the work, with the most extensive passages occurring in its first two, more general, books.

---

75 Ibid., bk. IV, p. 207.

Hildegard used a diverse vocabulary to denote pleasure and desire, and she described sexual arousal in several different ways. She said that the male has veins running from his liver and his stomach to his loins, and that the wind of pleasure arises from the marrow and falls into the loins, setting the taste for pleasure in motion in the blood.[76] In the female, the wind of pleasure arises from the marrow and falls into the womb, which is attached to the umbilicus, setting her blood in motion toward pleasure.[77] In variations on this account, Hildegard did not seem concerned with consistency or precision, saying at one point, for example, that the wind of desire rises out of the marrow, passes through the chest, touches the brain, pierces the heart and liver, and falls into the genitals.[78] The path of sexual feeling is clearly related to the path of the semen, but she did not trouble to seal the connection. She also referred at various times to the blood, the brain, and the marrow as the origin of this movement. The three are closely linked. The marrow (*medulla*) – the same stuff found in the bones – is a spiritous substance associated with feeling, linked to the brain and heart, and affecting the blood; it bears the heat which Hildegard associated with arousal.[79] But Hildegard did not pursue these relationships systematically.

Like her general descriptions of arousal, Hildegard's vocabulary has flexibility and range. She most often used the word *delectatio* to suggest not only pleasure or delight but also a desire or appetite for them. Thus she employed the word to denote sexual excitation without necessarily implying the fulfillment of desire. She spoke, for example, of "those who desire to satisfy their appetite [*delectationem*]"[80] and warned that a person (apparently of either sex) who is aroused (*in delectatione*) up to the point of emitting foam, but then retains it, may get sick.[81] Although *delectatio* can cause problems, the word does not necessarily have a negative connotation for Hildegard, whereas *libido* (lust) invariably makes trouble. Both men and women are susceptible to it, and it can lead both sexes into adultery, though, for reasons that will become clear shortly, Hildegard used the word more frequently in connection with men.[82] On the other end of the scale, the word *amor* (love) occurs in connection with both sexes' desire for intercourse and connotes moderation. Hildegard used another word for "love," *dilectio*, in the introduction to a lengthy section on such matters as nocturnal emissions and the ages of sexual maturity and fertility. This *dilectio* is the result of the creation of woman from man. She compared it to fire, and even before the Fall, it

76 Ibid., bk. II, p. 69.
77 Ibid., p. 76.
78 Ibid., p. 142. This account refers to men. A similar but not identical path is described for women on p. 104. See also p. 142, on both sexes.
79 Ibid., p. 140.
80 Ibid., p. 142.
81 Ibid., bk. IV, p. 192.
82 Ibid., bk. II, p. 68.

already had some connection with desire. Following the Fall, it was transformed into a mutual feeling like "the trembling of a threshing floor which is struck with many blows and heats up, when the grain is shaken out on it" – and, in this postlapsarian form, takes the name *delectatio*.[83] A variety of other words are involved in the characterization of desire and pleasure, but none so persistently as those suggesting heat, fire, and burning (especially *calor*, *ignis*, and various forms of *ardeo*).

Both heat and wind are essential features of desire and pleasure. Hildegard used the notion of heat to good effect in her rich metaphorical language, as when she said that a man's *delectatio* is like a fire which alternately flares up and dies down; a woman's is like the sun, gentle and productive of fruit.[84] At other times heat and fire bear their more technical meanings derived from their place in the scientific system of qualities and elements. In old age, for example, the natural process of cooling eventually leads to a decline in the "heat of pleasure" (though a man or woman of robust constitution may enjoy sexual pleasure until the seventieth or eightieth year); and to extinguish a person's desire and lust, one employs herbs with cooling properties.[85]

Like heat, which has both metaphorical and technical senses in Hildegard's treatise, wind is both a physiological component of and a source of imagery about sexual desire and pleasure. The notion of wind is most concretely expressed in her description of male arousal, for it is this wind arising from the marrow which enters the testicles. They act as bellows to inflate the penis, causing erection. But Hildegard also entertained a more general notion of the winds of desire, which are calmer, she claimed, in women, because the place into which they descend is more spacious. Thus, whereas a man may be wracked by the storm of lust (*tempestas libidinis*), a woman experiences only the much more manageable wind of pleasure (*ventus delectationis*) and is capable of greater self-control.[86] The relationship of heat and wind in the physiology of desire is clarified by Hildegard's comparison of different types of men. One group's sexuality is more fiery than windy. These men are easily aroused, find restraint almost impossible, and become sick if they do not have intercourse with women. Another group's is more windy than fiery. In these men the wind tempers the heat of the fire, so they are able to abstain from or to perform honorably the offices of love.[87]

In this last example, Hildegard's natural philosophical tendencies have edged out her literary inclinations: wind's cool quality, not its disruptive

---

83 Ibid., pp. 136–40; p. 137: ". . . in similitudine horrei aerae, quae multis ictibus percutitur et ad calorem perducitur, cum grana in eo excutiuntur."

84 Ibid., pp. 70, 76.

85 Ibid., bk. II, p. 139; bk. IV, p. 194.

86 Ibid., bk. II, p. 76.

87 Ibid., pp. 70–2. See Joan Cadden, "It Takes All Kinds: Sexuality and Gender Differences in Hildegard of Bingen's *Book of Compound Medicine*," *Traditio* 40 (1984): 161–4.

potential, comes to the fore. But the physiology of desire, like its anatomy and vocabulary, is unsettled in Hildegard's descriptions, shifting from one set of terms and associations to another. Although she clearly regarded sexual impulses and behaviors as interesting subjects, she did not see them in terms of problems to be solved, issues to be resolved, or phenomena to be explained by a consistent theory. Once again, in this respect, she represents the tradition in which she was educated and the environment in which she lived. Yet her comments do suggest certain general perspectives on desire and pleasure. She did seem to presume some connection between them and fertility, both in men and in women, and she was concerned with their possible ill effects – medical and moral: delectation is a good thing in that it serves procreation; it is a bad thing in that it opens the door to physical and spiritual dangers.

Every person after Adam and Eve originates from sexual desire or pleasure (*delectatio*),[88] for the disorder of the humors after the Fall opened the way for the "storm of begetting."[89] Hildegard often associated sexual appetite and pleasure with reproduction and called the impulse which arises from the marrow "the wind of the most agreeable love of begetting."[90] Not only does male desire play an essential role by causing the descent of the seed and the erection of the penis, but it is "with the will of love" that the woman's blood receives the seed and as a result of her desire that her uterus draws it in and closes to retain it.[91] Hildegard's observations about infertility underscore the link between *delectatio* and reproduction. Impotent men have little libido, their desire is insufficient to produce an erection, and they do not have appropriate seed.[92] Certain women who are healthier without men have no (or fleeting) pleasure of the flesh and are usually sterile.[93] Hildegard may even have been suggesting indirectly that a woman must have an orgasm to conceive, for she asserts that even after *delectatio* (that ambiguous experience), the woman may not release seed because the veins of her womb are clogged.[94]

If procreation depends on sexual arousal, it does not necessarily follow that sexual arousal implies procreation. For example, young people (boys of fifteen or sixteen, girls from twelve to fifteen or sixteen) have a taste for sexual pleasure and produce the associated foam, but neither the delectation nor the foam is mature or fertile.[95] Indeed, in several different contexts, Hildegard takes up the subject of nonreproductive sex. Apparently referring to both

88 Hildegard, *Causae et curae*, bk. II, p. 60.
89 Ibid., bk. I, p. 18: ". . . tempestas geniturae. . . ."
90 Ibid., bk. II, p. 140: ". . . ventum suavissimi amoris geniturae producit."
91 Ibid., p. 67: ". . . cum voluntate amoris. . . ." See also p. 104.
92 Ibid., 75.
93 Ibid., p. 89.
94 Ibid., pp. 76–7.
95 Ibid., pp. 138–9.

women and men, she enumerates the different conditions under which a person's marrow may give rise to sexual excitement. Although the nature of the emissions varies according to the conditions, *delectatio* is involved in each case. A person aroused by thoughts sometimes emits foam even when the genitals are not touched at all; touch alone may lead to the emission of foam; and contact with another person – or other living thing – may give rise to an emission. Nocturnal emissions may occur either without visions or dreams, in which case pleasure is apparently not involved, or with visions, in which case the heat characteristic of waking pleasure is present.[96] Much of what Hildegard had to say about this range of sexual experiences is matter of fact and surprisingly nonjudgmental. Like the sexual activities of the immature, acts other than heterosexual intercourse do not produce healthy seed or lead to procreation, but they are not unequivocally represented as harmful or sinful per se. Excesses of food and drink, idle thoughts, and the intervention of the devil may incite unhealthy or blameworthy desire,[97] but it is more immoderation than desire or pleasure that is the root of the ensuing ills. And although there is a moral tone to much of what Hildegard says (she says at one point that it is unnatural and shameful for a man to ejaculate except with a woman),[98] in this work she focuses on the *physical* manifestations of immoderation. The offspring of adulterous unions and of men who cannot control their stormy libidos will be defective in body and behavior.[99] Hildegard's language here is much more restrained than in her visionary work, *Scivias*, where she describes the diabolical conditions – including the mother's great ardor – under which the Antichrist was conceived.[100]

Immoderate pleasure and desire can be physically harmful both if indulged and if restrained. After mentioning that men and women can have sexual pleasure until they are very old, Hildegard warned that those who discharge their seed in lust risk blindness, whereas those who do so moderately will not be harmed, and she later gives a recipe to cure men and women whose inordinate libido has led to eye trouble.[101] On the other hand, proper sexual emissions resulting from proper *delectatio* can have a positive effect, especially as a means of purging the blood. Without proper release, symptoms ranging from madness to ulcerations may arise. Unfortunately, the overlibidinous, with their agitated blood and their insufficiently cooked seed, emit foam too weak to constitute proper purgation.[102]

Hildegard and other authors working in a monastic setting at the time when western Europe was beginning to receive newly translated medical

96 Ibid., pp. 137–8.
97 Ibid., p. 140.
98 Ibid., pp. 137–8.
99 Ibid., bk. I, p. 18; bk. II, pp. 68 and 71.
100 Hildegard, *Scivias*, pt. III, vis. xi, ch. 25, pp. 589–90.
101 Hildegard, *Causae et curae*, bk. II, pp. 139–40; bk. IV, pp. 192–4.
102 Ibid., bk. II, pp. 73 and 160–1.

and scientific classics from the Greek and Islamic worlds preserved elements of the monastic style of thought and expression while responding to the wealth of ideas circulating widely by the end of the twelfth century. These are not the ancestors of modern medicine. Like the monasteries and convents themselves, the medical learning that stayed within the cloister eventually lost status and influence. But in the late Middle Ages medical and natural philosophical writing continued to flourish in these settings, reflecting and adapting to, if eventually no longer shaping, the newer and more influential academic and secular contours of European medicine and science. Furthermore, in this setting, as in settings outside the cloister, Western thinkers engaged in a struggle to understand and accommodate diverse theories and information about sex, sex difference, and reproduction with each other and with the evolving Christian doctrines on the subject. Finally, clerics from the monasteries and the cathedral schools, many of whom spent significant parts of their lives in cloisters, paved the way for the institutions and the curriculum of universities, especially in northern Europe. Among them were scholars like Peter Abelard, who gathered students around himself in Paris and other towns, and Peter Lombard, whose theological *summa, The Sentences,* lay at the foundation of much university theology. Their lives, their teaching, and their writing formed bridges between the learning of the cloister and the learning of the university.

QUESTIONS AND ANSWERS ON HUMAN GENERATION

Hildegard reflected rather than influenced the growth of natural philosophy and theoretical medicine, whereas Constantine had begun to build bridges between clerical learning and the wider world. From the early twelfth century on, northern European texts, some of them directly or indirectly influenced by Constantine, began in form and content to reveal new trends in scientific and medical learning. Among these are three groups of related texts which expand on topics relating to sexuality and reproduction: the works of William of Conches, written in the second quarter of the twelfth century; a number of mostly English manuscripts dating from the turn of the thirteenth century on and containing question–and–answer literature influenced by Constantine and the Salernitan traditions; and a set of manuscripts containing a didactic dialogue that apparently took on its specific form around 1200. The material on sexual and reproductive matters in the question–and–answer literature, known as the Salernitan questions, relied heavily on the same work of William's from which the more fluid dialogue between master and student was excerpted.

Like Constantine's general work of medicine, the *Pantegni,* William of Conches's general work of natural philosophy, *On the Philosophy of the*

World, contains a few chapters on sexuality and reproduction.[103] These chapters, both in the subjects covered and in the explanatory principles invoked, reflect a strong Salernitan influence. More specifically, they suggest a familiarity with the work of Constantine and with the format and particulars of the Salernitan question literature.[104] William did not, however, as Constantine did, isolate and expand that material into a separate treatise. Having written about sperm and menstruation, about age, time, and complexion in relation to coitus, and about conception and infertility, and having mentioned the beliefs that women, though cooler than men, have stronger libidos and that women do not contract leprosy (*lepra*) from intercourse with lepers, he declares coyly that he will not say much about these matters, lest he offend monks who might read his work.[105] William revised *On the Philosophy of the World* a number of times, and a later version, known as the *Dragmaticon* and written when William was in the service of a secular prince, puts forth the views and the tone borrowed by later compilers.[106]

As Constantine had found it appropriate to produce a separate tract on intercourse, so an anonymous twelfth-century reader of William's work saw fit to borrow and modify the sections made up of an exchange between a philosopher and his interlocutor on sex and generation. This dialogue is reproduced more or less intact in at least four surviving manuscripts dating from the late twelfth through the fourteenth century. It appears twice as a short freestanding set of questions and twice at the head of a longer text that highlights the dialogue form and goes on to treat the main organs of the body, growth, respiration, sleep, hair, baldness, and the senses.[107] It is also closely

103 Chs. 8–14 in bk. IV of Guilelmus de Conchis, *Philosophia*, deal with reproduction, sexuality, and obstetrics.
104 See Lawn, *Quesiti Salernitani*, pp. 70–8 and n. G, pp. 236–8, on William's relation to the Salernitan Questions; see the apparatus to his *Prose Salernitan Questions*, for William's apparent reliance on Constantine.
105 Guilelmus de Conchis, *Philosophia*, bk. IV, ch. 14, pp. 97–8.
106 Guilelmus de Conchis, *Dialogus de substantiis physicis* [= *Dragmaticon*] (Strasburg: Iosias Rihelius, 1567; repr., Frankfurt-am-Main: Minerva, 1967), esp. bk. VI. For a summary of what is known of William's life and the problematic chronology of his work, see Guillaume de Conches, *Glosae super Platonem*, ed. Eduoard Jeauneau, Textes philosophiques du Moyen Age 13 (Paris: Librairie Philosophique J. Vrin, 1965), pp. 11–16.
107 Lawn at first saw the correspondence between William's chapters and the prose Salernitan questions as evidence that William had borrowed from and abbreviated a Salernitan prototype (*Salernitan Questions*, pp. 53–4). As a result of the research he did to edit the prose questions, he later concluded that the compiler of the prose questions in his manuscript B must have been borrowing from William – perhaps from a lost early version of the *Dragmaticon* (*Quesiti Salernitani*, nota aggiunta G, pp. 236–8). Of the freestanding texts devoted mainly to sex and generation, the longer, dialogue form appears to have been constructed by adding the shorter, nondialogue version summaries of opinions on other subjects drawn from old sources, such as the works of Boethius, and new sources, such as Aristotle's *Parva naturalia*, available in Latin toward the end of the twelfth century. But it is also possible that the shorter was lifted from the longer, since the practices of both excerpting and compiling that were developed in the early Middle Ages persisted in later centuries.

related to the opening elements of a long series of more formal questions and answers published by Brian Lawn as *The Prose Salernitan Questions*.[108] The dialogue form, which William used in his *Dragmaticon*, gives a more dynamic tone to the text, making a bridge between the older Salernitan question-and-answer format and the later scholastic format.[109] The chapters of William of Conches thus become both beneficiaries of and contributors to the Salernitan tradition broadly construed, and both their origins and their fate illustrate the extent to which northern European intellectuals, operating in a very different context from the Salernitan teachers and writers, embraced the form and some of the content of the new Italian medical learning.[110] Though these comments on sexuality and generation were originally embedded in William's works of the first half of the twelfth century, they acquired a life of their own in their later form as prominent components of widely distributed question-and-answer literature. There, even in the cases where the sexual and reproductive questions form only the first fraction of a larger collection of questions on various aspects of the natural world, the works are misleadingly but significantly labeled "The Secrets of Women," and "Philosophy or Disputation on Human Generation."[111] For convenience, I use the title *On Human Generation* to refer to the group of questions copied separately from William's *Dragmaticon,* on the one hand, and from the *Prose Salernitan Questions,* on the other. Whereas Brian Lawn had taken the prominence of this sort of question in one manuscript as a sign that its English compiler was "unusually preoccupied with sexual matters and gynecology," the discovery of additional manu-

---

108 The manuscripts are Oxford, Bodleian, MS Auct. F.3.10, fols. 118r–161v, edited by Lawn in *Prose Salernitan Questions*, in which the questions on sex and generation are at the head of a much larger body of questions; Cambridge, Trinity, MS O.2.5, fols. 75ra–85vb, and Paris, Bibliothèque Nationale, MS lat. 14809, fols. 298v–312v, in both of which the questions on sex and generation are at the head of a different and less extended collection of questions; and Paris, Bibliothèque Nationale, MS lat. nouv. acq. 693, fols. 183r–184v, and Zurich, Zentralbibliothek, MS Car. C. 172, fols. 3v–6v, both of which contain the questions on sex and generation as a short independent work.

109 Seneca's *Natural Questions* and Plato's *Timaeus* provided models for the dialogue form, which was especially popular in the twelfth century; e.g., Adelardus, *Die Questiones Naturales des Adelardus von Bath,* ed. Martin Müller, Beiträge zur Geschichte der Philosophie und Theologie des Mittelalters 31/2 (Münster: Aschendorff, 1934); and Richard C. Dales, ed. and trans., *Marius on the Elements,* Publications of the Center for Medieval and Renaissance Studies, UCLA, 10 (Berkeley and Los Angeles: University of California Press, 1976). See Haskins, *Studies in the History of Mediaeval Science*, pp. 20–42.

110 That the tradition was appropriated by northern Europeans is apparent from William's familiarity with it, from the presence of Salernitan material in the works of other twelfth-century authors, from the fact that the manuscripts of the sex-related question sets seem to have originated mainly in the north, and from the strong evidence that the anonymous compiler of Lawn's manuscript B was English. See Lawn, *Salernitan Questions,* chs. 2 and 4.

111 In Cambridge University, Trinity, MS O.2.5, the work has the heading "Secreta mulierum maior" written in a hand different from the copyist's; in Bibliothèque Nationale, MS lat. 14809, the copyist has closed with "Explicit philosophia sive disputatio de generatione humana."

scripts which are not simply copies of that one suggests that interest in the subjects was not idiosyncratic but broadly based.[112]

How, then, does this group of question-and-answer texts approach matters of sexuality and reproduction? Following William of Conches, and like Constantine before him, the longer versions of this work open with an apologia, in this case explaining why, though the soul is superior to the body, we should consider the body first. Like Constantine's initial reference to the Creator and William's fear of offending monks, this question constitutes a nod toward ecclesiastical sensibilities. But, whereas William declined to address certain questions in his *On the Philosophy of the World*, there is no self-censorship here. The text goes on to justify its approach on epistemological grounds: it is the body which first presents itself to our consciousness (*cognitio*).[113] Later, having discussed prostitution, rape, and venereal disease, one version, written in the form of a dialogue between master and student, has the student say, "I do not dare ask any more about intercourse, since it is not a respectable subject." To which the master replies, invoking the name of Hippocrates, that "nothing natural is shameful."[114] Having thus established the respectability of the subject, the longer versions continue (and the shorter version, having skipped the formalities, begins): "Sperm, then, is the seed of humanity."[115] The biblical beginning, which Hildegard had carefully placed at the center of her introduction to procreation and which William had treated elsewhere, is nowhere to be seen as the naturalism of the question-and-answer tradition comes to the fore.[116]

Drawing upon the Hippocratic notion of pangenesis, which was in turn supported by a widely circulated pseudo-Galenic text, *On Human Generation* represents sperm as a very pure derivative of all the body's members.[117] In

112 Lawn, *Prose Salernitan Questions*, p. xvii. The four additional manuscripts appear to be derived from a version of the questions that originated before the Bodleian manuscript, because they are closer to William's version and lack passages that Lawn has plausibly hypothesized were the additions of an anonymous English master, such as the example of the five masters (pp. xv–xvi).

113 Cambridge University, Trinity, MS O.2.5, fol. 75va; and Bibliothèque Nationale, MS lat. 14809, fol. 298v. Lawn, *Prose Salernitan Questions*, B, 2 and 3, are preceded by an even more extensive prologue with much fuller theological references.

114 "Discipulus: De coitu quia materia adeo non honesta est, amplius non querere audeo. . . . Philosophus: Nihil naturale est turpe." Bibliothèque Nationale, MS lat. 14809, fol. 300r; Cambridge University, Trinity, MS O.2.5, fol. 76va. Here and hereafter I have chosen the clearest readings without noting variants, except where the sense might be substantially affected. On coy and genuine protestations of respectability, see Joan Cadden, "Medieval Scientific and Medical Views of Sexuality: Questions of Propriety," *Medievalia et Humanistica*, n.s., 14 (1986): 157–71.

115 Cambridge University, Trinity, MS O.2.5, fol. 75ra; Bibliothèque Nationale, MS lat. 14809, fol. 298v; Bibliothèque Nationale, MS lat. nouv. acq. 693, fol. 183r: "Sperma igitur est hominis semen." The *Prose Salernitan Questions*, however, have a lengthy preamble in which not only Christ but also Truth, Justice, and Mercy figure (Lawn, B, 1).

116 Guilelmus de Conchis, *Dragmaticon*, bk. III, p. 77.

117 The *De spermate*, or *Liber de xii portis*, begins, "The sperm of man descends from every humor of the body. . ." ("Sperma hominis descendit ex omni humore corporis. . ."):

answer to the student's vague challenge that this is hard to believe, the master presents two different kinds of explanation: one abstract and theoretical, the other concrete and empirical. First, similars are born of similars – in other words, in order for generation to produce human flesh and bone and other parts, it must draw upon flesh and bone and other parts. Second, we have evidence that the process occurs in this way from the fact that if a father has a chronic disease such as gout, the child will have it too. In a challenge that rings more of a university disputation than of a rote-learning session, the student asks how it is possible, then, that when a man lacking a limb has intercourse with a woman, the resulting child is not missing the same limb. The answer, like the example of inherited disease, seems to imply that only the father produces formative seed, for rather than solving the difficulty by saying that the deficit is made up by the mother's seed, the philosopher of the dialogue answers simply that nature flees imperfection and creates the missing limb by borrowing the components of other parts – bones, flesh, nerves, and so on.[118] The impression that only the man's sperm is at issue is confirmed by a statement (echoing Constantine) that there are three things necessary for intercourse: the semen itself; heat, which refines the semen; and spirit, which erects the penis and expels the semen.[119]

Complementing this view of the male role is some later discussion of the uterus as a receptacle for semen. It is like an upside-down vase. (See Figure 5, p. 179.) In some respects, the operations of the uterus, insofar as it has any, are mechanical, not formative. The mouth of the uterus can open and close to admit and retain the semen, and its interior is hairy to keep the seed from slipping out. Thus prostitutes usually do not get pregnant, for frequent intercourse causes their wombs to close up, preventing the semen's entry, or else it causes the hairs to wear down, making their wombs as slippery as marble. In addition, the environment of the uterus must be of a hospitable complexion, for seed can be destroyed by dryness or by harmful fluids. And finally, it must have sufficient retentive power to hold the fetus through the period of gestation.[120]

In spite of these indications that only male seed is actually formative, the

Oxford, Bodleian, MS Ashmol. 1471, fols. 68r–71v; Vera Tavone Passalacqua, trans. and comm., *Microtegni seu De spermate* (Rome: Instituto di Storia della Medizina dell'Università di Roma, 1959), p. 48.

118 Cambridge University, Trinity, MS O.2.5, fol. 75ra–b; Bibliothèque Nationale, MS lat. nouv. acq. 693, fol. 183r; Bibliothèque Nationale, MS lat. 14809, fols. 298v–299r; Lawn, *Prose Salernitan Questions*, B, 4–5.

119 Cambridge University, Trinity, MS O.2.5, fol. 75rb; Bibliothèque Nationale, MS lat. nouv. acq. 693, fol. 183r. Cf. Lawn, *Prose Salernitan Questions*, B, 6; Constantine, *De coitu*, ch. 1, p. 80; and idem, *Viaticum*, in Isaac [Israeli] *Opera omnia*, 2d foliation (Lyon: Andreas Turinus, 1515), VI, i, fol. 164ra.

120 Cambridge University, Trinity, MS O.2.5, fol. 76ra–rb; Bibliothèque Nationale, MS lat. nouv. acq. 693, fol. 183v; Bibliothèque Nationale, MS lat. 14809, fol. 299r; cf. Lawn, *Prose Salernitan Questions*, B, 10 and 13. On the Constantinian origins of the notion of uterine villosity, see Jacquart and Thomasset, *Sexuality and Medicine*, pp. 25–6.

view of conception projected by these texts suggests otherwise. First of all, the role of the uterus goes beyond holding the fetus. Not surprisingly these question-and-answer texts reiterate the classical notion that the relative heat of the right side of the womb produces male children, and the left produces females. (Fetuses not all the way over to one side or the other will be manly females or womanly males.)[121] They also invoke the notion of the seven-celled uterus, a late ancient anatomical conceit which developed and retained some influence because, among other things, it suggested a way of explaining multiple births, reflected observations of animal anatomy, and resonated with a numerological outlook.[122] Although the cells of the uterus were usually represented simply as compartments, here the womb "has seven cells of the human figure, stamped in the manner of coins," implying that each compartment can mold a fetus, imparting a specific form to it.[123] The allusion to the left–right principle is the only explanation offered for sex determination in this set of questions, an explanation which the seven-cell picture traditionally supports. (The three cells on the left housed females; the three on the right, males; and the one in between, hermaphrodites.) With respect to the female role in procreation, however, both that theory and the notion of the uterine cells as stamps are greatly outweighed by a separate discussion of the necessity of female seed and its relation to female pleasure.

The roles of pleasure and seed in conception converge most prominently in a sequence of four linked questions, beginning with, "Since whores have intercourse very frequently, how is it that they rarely conceive?"[124] Accepting the presumed fact that prostitutes are infertile (a perception that may result from the effects of infection, malnutrition, or contraceptive practices, or that may arise from cultural associations of barrenness with immodest behavior), the philosopher answers:

Conception cannot be effected from one seed. A woman will not conceive unless the sperms of the man and the woman come together. Prostitutes, therefore, who

121 Cambridge University, Trinity, MS O.2.5, fol. 77ra; Bibliothèque Nationale, MS lat. nouv. acq. 693, fol. 184r; Bibliothèque Nationale, MS lat. 14809, fol. 300r; cf. Lawn, *Prose Salernitan Questions*, B, 24.

122 Fridolf Kudlein, "The Seven Cells of the Uterus: The Doctrine and Its Roots," *Bulletin of the History of Medicine* 49 (1965): 415–23; Robert Reisert, *Der siebenkammerige Uterus: Studien zur mittelalterlichen Wirkungsgeschichte und Entfaltung eines embryologischen Gebär-muttermodells*, Würzburger medizinhistorische Forschungen 39 (Pattensen: Horst Wellm, 1986).

123 Bibliothèque Nationale, MS lat. nouv. acq. 693, fol. 183v; Bibliothèque Nationale, MS lat. 14809, fol. 299v: "7 habens cellulas humane figure ad modum monete impressas." Cambridge University, Trinity, MS O.2.5, fol. 76ra, reads "humidas et frigidas" for "humane figure." Cf. Lawn, *Prose Salernitan Questions*, B, 12.

124 Bibliothèque Nationale, MS lat. nouv. acq. 693, fol. 183v; Cambridge University, Trinity, MS O.2.5, fol. 75vb; Bibliothèque Nationale, MS lat. 14809, fol. 299r: "Cum prostitute meretrices frequentissime coeant, unde est quod raro concipiunt?" Cf. Lawn, *Prose Salernitan Questions*, B, 10.

have intercourse only for money, have no pleasure, and neither generate nor emit anything.[125]

Two points are immediately clear from this passage. First, female seed or sperm, as well as male, is required for conception to occur. Second, in women at least, the production of seed depends upon the experience of pleasure (*delectatio*). (Of male pleasure we learn that it is generated when the semen flows through the sensitive penis.)[126]

How does this explanation of prostitutes' sterility – that they do not experience pleasure in intercourse – relate to the explanations mentioned earlier – that their wombs are closed or slippery? The answer illustrates the transitional character of the group of works to which *On Human Generation* belongs. No longer do they heedlessly accumulate disparate material, but neither do they yet systematically confront and resolve different perspectives. The question-and-answer format was initially nondiscursive: the questions were not always grouped topically, and the answers were not always consistent with each other. The new information available in the twelfth century allowed compilers of question sets like *On Human Generation* or the *Prose Salernitan Questions* to collect multiple answers to a single question, as when the philosopher explains why childhood, although warm and moist, is not an age appropriate to conception, first because the pores are not large enough to permit the passage of semen, and second because childhood is warm and moist not in essence but only in its relation to birth.[127] *On Human Generation*, however, goes beyond the traditional accretion of independent answers to recognize the complexity of the questions and the potential tensions between the answers. After the master has explained that prostitutes are sterile because they do not experience pleasure and the associated emission of necessary seed, the pupil (a younger, less worldly man?) objects that, on the contrary, prostitutes can be seen racked by love, yet, in spite of pleasure, rarely conceive. In response to this objection, the master offers the alternative explanation (more anatomical and less theoretical, it may be the earlier of the two answers): their wombs are either closed up or too slippery. The exchange by no means approximates the complexity of scholastic disputations which were soon to dominate the exchanges of the intellectual elite, but it reflects a clear recognition of problems to be resolved concerning the relationship between pleasure and conception.

125 Cambridge University, Trinity, MS O.2.5, fol. 75vb; Bibliothèque Nationale, MS lat. nouv. acq. 693, fol. 183v; Bibliothèque Nationale, MS lat. 14809, fol. 300.: "Conceptio ex uno semine fieri non potest. Nisi non conveniunt viri et mulieris spermata non concipit mulier. Prostitute igitur que solo precio coeunt nullam delectationem habent nec aliud gignunt nec emittunt." Cf. Lawn, *Prose Salernitan Questions*, B, 10.
126 Cambridge University, Trinity, MS O.2.5, fol. 75rb; Bibliothèque Nationale MS lat. nouv. acq. 693, fol. 183v; cf. Lawn, *Prose Salernitan Questions*, B, 6.
127 Cambridge University, Trinity, MS O.2.5, fol. 75vb; Bibliothèque Nationale, MS lat. nouv. acq. 693, fol. 183v. See Lawn, *Prose Salernitan Questions*, pp. xiv–xv.

The next question and answer pursues and develops the issue further, shifting the scene from the sexual responses and reproductive status of prostitutes to those of rape victims:

I recall you said just now that a woman cannot conceive without [emitting] seed, which is not plausible. For we see women who have been raped, protesting and crying, and who have suffered violence even at that moment [of intercourse who] have conceived. Hence it appears these women have had no pleasure at that time, and without pleasure, seed cannot be emitted.[128]

In the previous question, the juxtaposition of two assumptions about prostitutes suggested an awareness of discrepancies of the sort ignored in early compilations and even in the more coherent works of Constantine and Hildegard. Here, theory (the necessity of female semen) and fact (the pregnancies of rape victims) confront each other directly and vividly. Lurking behind the casually phrased challenge is a logically constructed one. If a woman must experience pleasure to emit seed, and seed is necessary for conception, then there is no conception without pleasure. But in rape there appears to be conception without pleasure. In order to sustain the conviction that female seed is necessary, the response must either concede that emission can occur without pleasure or reject the assertion that in cases of rape there can be conception without pleasure. The response offered by the philosopher in *On Human Generation* is repeated by later authors as well.[129] Conception can indeed occur as the result of rape, but not without the woman's pleasure (and the seed resulting therefrom):

If in the beginning the act displeases the women raped, yet in the end it pleases [them] because of the weakness of the flesh. For there are two wills in humans, namely, the rational and the natural, which we often see fighting within us. [What] is displeasing to reason is pleasing to the flesh. And if, therefore, there is not the rational will in the raped women, there is nevertheless [the will] of carnal pleasure.[130]

---

128 Cambridge University, Trinity, MS O.2.5, fol. 76ra: "Ad memoriam venit mihi quod nuper dixisti quod sine semine mulier concipi non potest quod non est verisimile. Videmus enim raptas reclamantes et plorantes etiam in isto tempore passas violenciam concepisse. Unde apparet illas nullam habuisse delectationem, sed sine delectatione non potest sperma emittit." Bibliothèque Nationale, MS lat. nouv. acq. 693, fol. 183v, starts the question at "Videmus." Cf. Lawn, *Prose Salernitan Questions*, B, 11.

129 See Jacquart and Thomasset, *Sexuality and Medicine*, p. 64. Cf. David of Dinant, who, although writing before the full translation of *Generation of Animals*, anticipates later scholastic opinion by dissociating female pleasure from conception on the authority of Aristotle: Marian Kurdziałek, "Anatomische und embryologische Aeusserungen Davids von Dinant," *Sudhoffs Archiv für Geschichte der Medizin und der Naturwissenschaften* 45 (1961): 10–11.

130 Cambridge University, Trinity, MS O.2.5, fol. 76ra–rb; Bibliothèque Nationale, MS lat. nouv. acq. 693, fol. 183v: "Et si raptis in principio displiceat opus, cum in fine ex fragilitate carnis placet. Item in homine sunt due voluntates, scilicet rationativa et naturalis, quas sepe in nobis repugnare videmus. Displicet rationi et placet carni. Et si igitur in rapta non est voluntas rationis, est tamen delectationis carnis." Cf. Lawn, *Prose Salernitan Questions*, B, 11, which reads ". . . displicet enim rationi quod placet carni. . . ."

There are really two answers here. The first, a modern pornographic commonplace, is that women move from revulsion to pleasure in the course of a rape and therefore do emit semen in the end. Although the carnal weakness which causes the change is not associated exclusively with women, the answer does emphasize women's weakness. The second answer, more sophisticated and abstract, invokes the human condition in general: that our reason and our flesh are often at war with one another. The relationship between protest and pleasure is not a temporal one but rather one of categories: a woman can withhold rational consent, even though, on the carnal level, she may experience pleasure and thus emit seed. Since both hinge on carnal acquiescence, there may seem little to choose between the two explanations. However, especially from the twelfth century on, medieval law and theology accord great importance to intention and consent, and the steadfastness of the higher, rational human will is far more important than the weakness of the lower, animal nature.[131] Thus, in the course of making explicit issues concerning the reproductive role of the female sperm, the text implicitly poses problems about female sexuality. Is a prostitute's sterility a consequence of her willingness to engage in sex for money? Does a rape victim's pregnancy occur in spite of her withholding consent by an exercise of rationality? Or do both experience pleasure, because it is women's nature to do so?

The problem remains unspoken and unanswered. The text veers away from the digression to return to the point: how can one doubt the existence of female sperm, when children often resemble their mothers and inherit their mothers' infirmities? And to press the point even further, there is yet another question on conception. Paired with the question about the fecundity of rape victims, it asks why women "who have intercourse only with their husbands and with great pleasure often do not conceive."[132] Pleasure and the consequent emission of seed may be necessary for conception, but they are not sufficient. Once again, the response contains two types of explanation. The first concerns the properties of the uterus, which may be too fat, too dry, too soft, or lack sufficient retentive power. The second concerns the two sperms, male and female, one or both of which may be too hot, too cold, too moist, or too dry, each excess producing specific impediments to conception.

Several aspects of this sequence of questions and answers on pleasure, semen, and conception are remarkable. First, the existence and importance of a female seed are not merely alluded to, mentioned, or even asserted, but

131 Because of Augustine's influence, an interest in the will permeates many aspects of medieval culture. In connection with natural philosophy and psychology it figures prominently in the work of Nemesius, for example.

132 Cambridge University, Trinity, MS O.2.5, fol. 76rb; Bibliothèque Nationale, MS lat. nouv. acq. 693, fol. 183v: "Que cum solis maritis coeunt cum magna delectatione videmus frequenter non concipere." Cf. Lawn, *Prose Salernitan Questions*, B, 13.

actively and persistently argued for. Not since antiquity had the case for a female semen been so fully presented in the West. But with the exception of the brief reference to children's resemblance to their mothers and the inheritance of maternal infirmities, the dialogue gives no account of the exact contribution of the female seed or its relation to the male seed. Other questions in the text deal with such obstetrical and embryological topics as the nourishment of the fetus and the term of gestation, but they do not elaborate upon the specific roles or influence of maternal or paternal seed. Thus *On Human Generation*, William of Conches's *Dragmaticon*, and the *Prose Salernitan Questions* disseminated a two-seed version of reproduction without providing it with the specificity and evidence it would need to survive in a scholastic environment of disputation and Aristotelian influence. A second remarkable aspect of this group of texts is that notwithstanding the lack of detail about the female seed's effects, they defend the principle in a manner far more structured and far more thorough than earlier texts. And finally, they give more prominence to the subject of pleasure – and female pleasure in particular – than any of the earlier works dealing with reproduction, including ancient scientific and medical writings.

Unlike Constantine's terse general explanation for the existence of pleasure – that it encourages an act which perpetuates the species – this sequence of questions placed the issue of pleasure mainly within the functional context of reproduction. But the perspective on pleasure in *On Human Generation* extends still further. Two additional questions in the text expand the subject in relation to the female libido. The first compares women's sexual appetite with men's; the second compares it with that of female animals. In the first case the matter under discussion is the relation of intercourse to complexion, the mixture of qualities that constitutes an individual's physiological makeup. A question about the complexion best suited to intercourse leads to the conclusion that a warm and moist constitution most favors the act. (The answer does not contain anything like Constantine and Hildegard's reflections on the constitutional basis of sexual types, although one compiler adds such material, naming contemporary individuals as examples of the types. For instance, Hugh of Mapenor, later bishop of Hereford, is said to have little sexual appetite and great sexual potency.)[133] Once again, *On Human Generation* pursues the implications of a basic tenet: "Since woman is naturally cold and moist, how is it that she is more heated in libido than man?"[134] Woman's libidinousness, like her coldness, is taken for granted; the problem is how to reconcile her cool complexion with her sexual heat. One answer is

133 Lawn, *Prose Salernitan Questions*, B, 8, and introduction, pp. xv–xvi.
134 Cambridge University, Trinity, MS O.2.5, fol. 75va; Bibliothèque Nationale, MS lat. nouv. acq. 693, fol. 183v: "Cum igitur mulier sit naturaliter frigida et humida, unde est quod ferventior est viro in libidine?" Cf. Lawn, *Prose Salernitan Questions*, B, 7. The question of relative libido is discussed at length in Chapter 3.

that woman is like wet wood, which is hard to get burning, but which, once it is ignited, burns hotter and longer. A second answer is that since (contrary to Hildegard's view) the womb is cold and the semen is warm, the womb rejoices when it receives the semen. (Another analogy, that of snakes seeking a warm place, eerily illuminates this point.) And the conclusion, apparently borrowed from Constantine, is that "woman's pleasure in intercourse is double: from the emission of her own seed and from the reception of another's seed. But man's pleasure is simple, from emission alone."[135] Like the passages which use prostitutes and raped women as examples, this discussion (which, in passing, reconfirms the presence of female semen) takes the question of desire and pleasure beyond the functional, though the occasion and rhetoric are scientific. Indeed, it draws into the sphere of natural philosophy socially and morally based ideas of female sexuality.

The second question on desire and pleasure that goes beyond the mechanics of procreation occurs later, between a group of questions dealing with menstruation and a group dealing with embryology. "Once conception has occurred, other animals refrain from intercourse. Women have intercourse more gladly at that time."[136] Why? Once again, the premise is that women have great, and in this case functionless, desire. The main answer, however, like one of the answers to the question about rape, refers not to the specifically feminine but rather to human nature in general. Unlike animals, who only have a sense of the present, we have in addition memory of the past and expectations about the future. "And so it is that a woman, remembering past pleasure, desires the same."[137] This conclusion, which links desire to the higher human faculties, was not popular later, probably because Aristotelian psychology accorded animals the faculties of memory and fantasy. It is also in a sense inconsistent with the answer on rape, which portrayed the experience of pleasure as arising from the animal, or lower, nature of woman, while her mind or will was clear of it. But the two answers share the view that desire and pleasure have a psychological as well as a physical dimension.

This set of questions, clustered together by an anonymous twelfth-century compiler, many borrowed from William of Conches and closely

---

135 Cambridge University, Trinity, MS O.2.5, fol. 75va; Bibliothèque Nationale, MS lat. nouv. acq. 693, fol. 183v: "Duplex est igitur delectatio mulieris cohitus, in emissione proprii seminis et in receptione alterius seminis. Viri autem simplex delectatio est in sola emissione." Cf. Lawn, *Prose Salernitan Questions*, B, 7; and Constantinus Africanus, *Theorica*, VI, xvii, in idem, *Pantegni*, fol. 28.

136 Cambridge University, Trinity, MS O.2.5, fol. 76vb; Bibliothèque Nationale, MS lat. nouv. acq. 693, fol. 184r: "Facta conceptione cetera animalia cessant a coitu. Mulieres tunc libentius coiunt. . . ." Cf. Lawn, *Prose Salernitan Questions*, B, 23.

137 Cambridge University, Trinity, MS O.2.5, fol. 77ra; Bibliothèque Nationale, MS lat. nouv. acq. 693, fol. 184r: "Unde est quod mulier reminiscens preterite delectationis similem desiderat." Cf. Lawn, *Prose Salernitan Questions*, B, 23. Another reason given is that the fetus increases her warmth.

related to a set of prose Salernitan questions, does not constitute a comprehensive treatment of reproduction or sexuality. Some issues of interest to contemporaries, such as sex determination and the male libido, are barely mentioned in *On Human Generation*, while others are given full and emphatic treatment. The strong presumption of the existence and essential role of female semen is reiterated at several points. Although the arguments neither contain any claims about the exact function of that substance nor compare it with the male semen, they constitute a firm and consistent statement of the case for a female reproductive contribution beyond fetal nutrition and the uterine environment. Unlike Constantine, who, in spite of his active interest in men's desire and pleasure, ignored women's, and unlike Hildegard, who, though she carefully characterized women's sexual arousal and compared it with men's, did not discuss its purpose, these questions and answers insist on the existence and the reproductive significance of female pleasure.

The naturalistic answers, sometimes several for a single question, did not preclude a concern for some of the moral issues which Hildegard addressed and which had been found earlier in the work of Isidore of Seville and others. The very inclusion of sustained allusions to prostitution and rape suggests the suspect and dangerous nature of sexuality. They must have stood out starkly even against the background of questions concerning such a delicate subject as intercourse. And at the same time, misogynistic assumptions punctuate the discussions of women in sexual contexts: they are more libidinous than either men or animals, and they experience sexual pleasure even when raped. (It will be noted that the rapist does not figure in the analysis.) Yet *On Human Generation* maintains a strained ambiguity toward the ominous side of sexuality in general and female sexuality in particular. Introduced as limiting cases in connection with contested issues, these subjects are mostly addressed obliquely. The inquiry as a whole is rendered at least nominally respectable by the maxim that nothing natural is shameful, and women's sexual appetite is neither denied nor condemned directly. Some of the answers do at least partly explain it, leaving in place the negative suppositions but setting them in a positive light: the higher human faculties explain women's response to rape and their continued interest in sex after conception. To add to the ambiguity, the accretion of distinct answers to a single question leaves matters unresolved: do women who are raped experience pleasure at a certain moment or on a certain level? These ambiguities, however, are less the result of internal inconsistencies or reticence about the subject than they are of the work's perspective. Hildegard raised and addressed issues of behavior and feelings from a moral and often scriptural perspective and attempted to coordinate them with medical and philosophical naturalism. *On Human Generation*, although sensitive to questions of propriety, is not attempting to synthesize the ethical and natural aspects of sexual response or function. Behavior and experience here figure as examples of physiology and, more prominently, psychology – as subjects of natural philosophy. In this respect, the text is in the naturalistic tradition of Constantine and his Arabic sources. But Constantine, insofar as he commented on the links between physical and mental states where sex was concerned, was content to put them in terms of complexion and temperament: he did not venture into the more philosophical realms of will and reason.[138] The latter were subjects associated not with the emergent theoretical medicine characteristic of Salerno but rather with the philosophical anthropology which had begun to emerge in the works of authors like William of Conches, steeped in the learning of northern ecclesiastical centers.

In form as in content, the little set of questions about reproduction shows signs of interactions and transitions occurring by the end of the twelfth century, when it was first extracted from the works of William of Conches and others. At its roots, the question-and-answer pattern to which *On Human Generation* adheres was a catechistic vehicle for imparting condensed facts and doctrines. Terse, dogmatic, and bearing no necessary connections to one another, though often clustered by general subject, these questions and answers reflected the condensed and fragmented character of early medieval learning, as well as something about the methods of medical education, which was probably not very text oriented.[139] However, like the contemporary collections of Salernitan questions, the questions and answers in *On Human Generation* show a number of changes in this traditional genre. First, the accretion of multiple answers to a single question, a process consistent with the habits of monastic learning, is visible at a number of points. The pairing of concrete anatomical or physiological answers with more abstract natural philosophical ones suggests that the practice of providing multiple answers evolved along with the tenor of medical and natural philosophical inquiry. Second, this text goes beyond the simple question-and-answer pattern by following up answers with objections and doubts, which occasion elaboration or modification of the initial answer. Thus it transforms the sense of the word "question" from the pretext for a statement to the demand for an argument, and in doing so it illustrates the impact of the expansive intellectual mood and the more generous texts and educational practices of the period; that is, it reflects the moment of the inception of universities. The fascination with dialectic that had infected the northern schools and the application of commentaries to medical texts that had flourished in the south influenced the formerly simple format of question and answer. One

138 See Mary Frances Wack, "The *Liber de heros morbo* of Johannes Afflacius and Its Implications for Medieval Love Conventions," *Speculum* 62 (1987): 324–44.
139 In addition to Lawn, *Prose Salernitan Questions*, see Talbot, "Medical Education in the Middle Ages."

result was that reproduction and sexuality, like many other subjects at this time, became the objects of investigations, not just of comments.

Indeed, in its shorter form (i.e., the version in which all the questions and answers concern human sexuality and procreation), *On Human Generation* suggests a special interest in exploring those subjects. Even in its longer form, where questions about the senses and other subjects follow, as in the related *Prose Salernitan Questions*, the prominent position of the questions on generation and pleasure at the front of the work gives them special weight. The long form of the text represents yet another trend and suggests something about the diversity and interaction of genres in the twelfth and thirteenth centuries: it is written as a dialogue. Apparently borrowed from William of Conches, along with much of the substance, this humanistic form had gained popularity in the twelfth century. Unlike the terser form, which points toward the development of more formal settings of scientific discourse and, in particular, toward the universities, the dialogue invokes a more intimate exchange within the less elaborately institutionalized monastic or cathedral or medical schools, or even in the households of noble patrons.[140] The differences between the dialogue and question-and-answer forms are not great – they consist, for the most part, of the presence or absence of the word *discipulus* before the questions and *philosophus* before the answers – but they have separate and distinct associations.

In many respects, then, this set of questions on generation is at a crossroads. It is indebted to intellectual developments in southern and northern Europe; it draws on medicine and natural philosophy; it has moral as well as naturalistic vibrations; it has links to simple question and answer, to dialectic, and to dialogue; it might address audiences in ecclesiastical schools, university towns, or courts. It occurs in manuscripts both in the company of works on medicine, astronomy, and physiognomy and in the company of biblical commentary and works on charity and penance, indicating that the boundaries between different types of learning were not barriers to interaction and that their audiences were diverse. Not a product of a university environment, *On Human Generation* was copied well into the university period. Thus, while the works of university masters turned such subjects as female semen, sex determination, and pleasure into occasions for intricate, abstract, and clever disputations, the need persisted for shorter, simpler guides of the sort which the earlier medical, monastic, and cathedral schools

---

140 William addressed the *Dragmaticon* to Geoffrey of Anjou and presented it in the form of a dialogue between himself and his patron. Of the long form of the text in question, one manuscript (Cambridge University, Trinity, MS O.2.5) is a dialogue between Philosopher (*philosophus*, sometimes abbreviated "P") and Disciple (*discipulus*, sometimes abbreviated "D"); the other (Bibliothèque Nationale, MS lat. 14809) gives only "P" and "D," except that in a single instance *Dux* (duke) introduces a question. This manuscript also drops the dialogue labels after the initial section on generation.

had produced. These up-to-date but nevertheless elementary compositions found their way into their usual places in monastic libraries and no doubt also into the hands of those pursuing or directing propaedeutic studies, especially in university towns.[141]

That a little work on reproduction should be so situated suggests that its subject was among those that engaged the interest of a significant portion of the European intellectual elite. Although it would be unreasonable to claim that at a time of such an explosion of intellectual curiosity, human generation held a privileged place in the constellation of scientific and medical concerns, it is reasonable to assert that the subject had established itself as serious and intriguing.

A convergence in learned medieval thinking about the sexes occurred in the period from the late eleventh to the early thirteenth century, but it was more a convergence of concern and of scholarly activity than it was a convergence of opinion. Constantine wrote in the late eleventh century from a medical perspective, Hildegard wrote in the middle to late twelfth century in a traditional monastic environment, and William of Conches and the compilers of *On Human Generation*, who built on his work, wrote from the perspective of natural philosophy in the late twelfth and early thirteenth centuries, but all posed and addressed questions about sex and reproduction that involved highlighting and clarifying the natures and functions of males and females. Although the goals and forms of their works differed significantly, each made a place for sexual and reproductive issues. Among the questions which began to crystallize during this period were two which contributed materially both to subsequent discussions in the context of scholastic medicine and philosophy, treated in the next chapter, and to the concepts and vocabulary by which medicine and natural philosophy participated in the construction and representation of gender, treated in Part II. These were, first, the respective contributions of the male and the female to the conception of a fetus and the formation of offspring and, second, the relationship of male and female sexual pleasure to reproduction.

These differently educated, positioned, and oriented writers had helped to reflect and promote a broadly based interest in these matters among the Latin-literate intellectual elite, but they did not reflect any consensus on specific assertions or theories, or even on the appropriate emphases. Con-

---

141 An instructive case study of such dissemination is Michael Johnson, "Science and Discipline: The Ethos of Sex Education in a Fourteenth-Century Classroom," in Helen Rodnite Lemay, ed., *Homo Carnalis: The Carnal Aspect of Medieval Human Life*, Center for Medieval and Early Renaissance Studies, Acta, 14, for 1987 (Binghamton, N.Y.: State University of New York, 1990), pp. 157–72.

stantine was especially interested in male sexual function; Hildegard was more concerned with the process and implications of procreation; and *On Human Generation* attended particularly to females in its attempts to clarify the principles of reproduction. Constantine sometimes ignored and sometimes asserted the importance of the female seed; Hildegard gave it hardly any attention but introduced female influence in other forms; and *On Human Generation* took its existence and function most seriously, favoring its significance for conception. None of the texts examined the nature of the "female seed" or the meaning of the term: that task was left to the later university scholars. Constantine gave sexual pleasure a brief justification (made much of by later authors) and treated it only tangentially as it figured in men's ability to have intercourse; Hildegard brought out the uses and dangers of desire and pleasure, distinguishing between the sexes in this respect; and *On Human Generation* linked pleasure closely to a woman's ability to conceive, exploiting both its philosophical and its prurient possibilities.

The lack of settled opinion reflects not only the different backgrounds and intentions of the authors but also the rich and open possibilities of medicine and natural philosophy during a period of rapid growth and change. It has implications both for the subsequent development of scholastic opinions and for the interactions of medical and natural philosophical ideas of sex difference with social and religious understandings. With respect to the development of university disputations on female seed and on male and female pleasure, the absence of a set of dogmas or received opinions did not simply leave later scholars free to create their own formulations; instead, along with the ancient texts which were translated into Latin in the twelfth and thirteenth centuries, the variety of ideas provided the basis and the raw materials for complicated and unsettled exchanges. More important, with respect to the relationship of medicine and natural philosophy, on the one hand, and the social and cultural environment, on the other, the diversity within the former as well as the complexity of the latter precluded either a comfortable complicity or a contentious confrontation of social and scientific views of sex difference. Rather, as the chapters on gender, sterility, and abstinence demonstrate, there was divergence and convergence, coexistence and negotiation, tension and accommodation.

The importance of the early medieval transmission and of the emergence of issues in the period just treated lies not only in their contributions to the more sophisticated and specialized work of later scholars but also in their connections with institutions and audiences. Even in a later Latin culture dominated by university learning, more people knew the name of Constantine the African than knew the name of the prolific and sophisticated medical professor Bernard of Gordon, and more people learned about the natural world through direct or indirect access to encyclopedias that resembled the work of William of Conches or Hildegard of Bingen than learned about it through access to the writings of the prolific and sophisticated philosopher and theologian Albertus Magnus. The articulation of scholastic questions about seed and pleasure does not, then, displace the earlier traditions just examined; rather, it adds a dimension and an impetus to them.

3

Academic questions: Female and male in scholastic medicine and natural philosophy

OLD WINE AND NEW BOTTLES: TRANSLATED TEXTS AND SCHOLASTIC METHODS

The rich and idiosyncratic presentations of sex differences in the period from the late eleventh to the early thirteenth century emerged in a variety of contexts and connected with a variety of concerns. Although their authors drew upon earlier texts and traditions, they did not refer to any agreed-upon set of authorities; and although some writers considered matters of reproduction and sexuality in a thorough and structured manner, they embraced no common method of investigation. As a result, the scattered topics of discussion – the components of male sexual potency, the relative tempestuousness of male and female sexuality, the possibility of conception resulting from rape – lent themselves to often colorful modes of expression. During the thirteenth and fourteenth centuries, the shift of intellectual activities to universities and to the literary forms developed in connection with university instruction at once enriched and impoverished medieval conversations about reproduction and sexuality and the ways in which they reflected ideas about sex difference. On the one hand, the careful and sophisticated study of texts by Greek and Arabic authorities focused and deepened the treatment of matters relating to female and male natures and functions; on the other hand, the gravitation of scholarship toward subjects defined by those texts and the development of highly structured rules for the presentation of opinions placed some constraints both upon subject matter and upon the language and forms within which it was discussed. In addition, the increased convention and formality pose special problems for deciphering within the works of the intellectual elite reflections of larger social and cultural understandings of female and male.

The question of the reproductive contributions of the female and the male, the manner in which a fetus comes to be either female or male, and the character and quantity of female and male sexual pleasure were among the issues which commanded the attention of thirteenth- and fourteenth-century academics. Each of these subjects was grounded in the interests of earlier medieval writers and each was enriched by the new influx of Greek and Arabic learning, although in different ways and to different degrees. Classical authors had directly addressed the roles of males and females in procreation and the causes of male and female offspring, but not the relationship between male and female pleasure. In the hands of scholastic authors, therefore, the first two topics were the subject of fuller and more authoritatively grounded debate, whereas the last allowed more room for the expression of medieval ideas less bound to classical precedents. On the surface, the answers arrived at by late medieval physicians and natural philosophers suggest a simple pattern of concepts about sex difference: the father's seed is the active and formative principle both in reproduction and in sex determination, and the man experiences more significant pleasure in intercourse. But beneath the surface, in the array of specific arguments, in the interplay of philosophical and medical opinion, and in the use and transcendence of sources, scholastic discussions present a complex and multivalent view of the specific issues and project a richer and more ambiguous picture of sex differences.

Sources and translations

The questions that emerged concerning reproduction and sexuality during the period from Constantine's translations to the turn of the thirteenth century became more focused, more precise, and more contentious with the translation and deployment of additional texts and with the rise of the universities. In particular, the translations of Avicenna's *Canon of Medicine* and Aristotle's *Generation of Animals* provided a massive infusion of information and reasoning, while the creation of formalized approaches to authoritative texts provided a method and forum for the careful analysis of the facts and logic involved. The new material and new approach did not so much change academic opinion about the role of male and female semen or the nature of male and female pleasure as they delineated the problems and multiplied and elaborated the terms in which they were addressed. The results at once highlighted the difficulty of establishing consistent answers that accounted for ordinary experience and at the same time revealed the recurring hope of resolving paradoxes and dispelling doubts. If female and male both have fully active sperm, why does nature require such duplication? If not, why do some children resemble the father and others the mother? If women's sexual pleasure is associated with an emission, what is it and what role does it play? If not, what is the purpose of women's pleasure?

In one sense, the full Latin translations of Avicenna's medical encyclopedia from Arabic and of Aristotle's treatises on living creatures, first from

Arabic versions and then from Greek, offered no surprises to European students of medicine and science. The ideas of Aristotle and Galen, Avicenna's main source, had filtered into the Latin tradition through late ancient intermediaries and had been preserved, sometimes with and sometimes without attributions, in the period of condensation and compilation. The Constantinian translations had added immeasurably to European access to Galenic ideas, and the translation of some of Aristotle's works on other subjects had made the Aristotelian approach to nature familiar to European intellectuals interested in natural philosophy and medicine. But in another sense, the availability of Avicenna's *Canon* and Aristotle's writings on animals made a great deal of difference. Their massive and thorough character, if finding some precedent in Constantine's major works, were on a scale and at an analytical level hitherto unfamiliar to those studying medicine or the natural philosophy of living things.

The *Canon of Medicine*, written in Arabic by Avicenna (Abu Ali al-Husain ibn 'Abdallah ibn Sina) at the beginning of the eleventh century, is a detailed survey of medical learning, both theoretical and practical. Avicenna, who had studied many classical and Arabic medical works, drew heavily on Galen, but his work is by no means a compilation; rather, it is a synthesis, incorporating as well Platonic philosophy, Aristotelian natural philosophy, and the cumulative wisdom of Hellenistic, Persian, and Arabic authors, all presented according to Avicenna's own vision of the field. Gerard of Cremona, translator of many medical and scientific works from Arabic, rendered the *Canon* into Latin sometime during the second half of the twelfth century – an awe-inspiring achievement, for the text (as printed in the sixteenth century) is more than a thousand pages long.[1] By the end of the first quarter of the thirteenth century its influence began to be felt; by midcentury it was widely known in European medical faculties; and by the end of the century parts of it had become crucial elements of the medical curriculum. Beyond the university, the *Canon* found a place in monastic libraries and was used by authors of general works on natural philosophy.[2]

Sexual and reproductive subjects crop up here and there throughout the *Canon*. In the anatomical section of the first book, for example, there is a short chapter on muscles in the penis, attributing to them a role in opening up the pores for the semen and causing erection.[3] But the main discussion

---

1 Avicenna, *Liber canonis* (Venice: Pagininis, 1507; repr., Hildesheim: Georg Olms, 1964).
2 See Nancy G. Siraisi, *Avicenna in Renaissance Italy: The Canon and Medical Teaching in Italian Universities after 1500* (Princeton: Princeton University Press, 1987), esp. pp. 44–56; and Danielle Jacquart, "La réception du *Canon* d'Avicenne: Comparaison entre Montpellier et Paris au XIIIᵉ et XIVᵉ siècles," in *Histoire de l'école médicale de Montpellier*, vol. 2 of *Actes du 110ᵉ Congrès national des sociétés savantes, Montpellier, 1985: Section d'histoire des sciences et des techniques* (Paris: Ministère de l'Education Nationale, Comité des Travaux Historiques et Scientifiques, 1985), pp. 69–77.
3 Avicenna, *Liber canonis*, bk. I, fen i, doctr. 5, summ. 2, ch. 25, fol. 17vb.

occurs in the third book, which treats diseases of specific parts of the body. Its two major divisions on men's and women's generative parts contain a great deal of specific information about various sores and abscesses affecting the testicles, the penis, and the uterus, as well as a range of gynecological and obstetrical problems, from removing a dead fetus to correcting menstrual retention.[4] Avicenna introduces the discussion of male disorders with a general treatment of the purpose of intercourse and the causes of erection and sperm; and he opens the discussion of female disorders with an account of conception and the growth of the fetus. The latter section was frequently alluded to in late medieval treatments of male and female reproductive contributions and was the subject of several commentaries which will be discussed later.

Avicenna's work was influential not only because it consolidated a vast amount of information on all the major subdivisions of theoretical and practical medicine but also because it was, and was perceived as, a vehicle for the transmission of ancient learning. The presence of Avicenna's work in the university curriculum and in the libraries of monasteries and medical practitioners complemented and reinforced the value of the Hippocratic and Galenic canon – itself continually being extended by additional translations. With respect to reproduction, sexuality, and sex difference, the Greek influence remained largely indirect, however. Hippocrates' *On the Nature of the Fetus*, translated in the midthirteenth century, was the subject of only one commentary in the fourteenth;[5] Galen's monumental *On the Use of Parts*, which contains ample relevant material and was available in Latin in abbreviated form from the late twelfth century, did not play a direct role in the main conversations about reproductive roles, sex determination, and sexual pleasure in the natural philosophy or medicine of the late Middle Ages.[6] Indirectly, however, the spirits of Galen and, to a lesser extent, the Hippocratic writers hovered over the scholastic debates. For Avicenna not only transmitted some of their ideas but also named them as authorities and called attention to significant divergences among Hippocrates, Galen, and Aristotle. Differences between Galen and Aristotle or, as they were sometimes construed, between medical and philosophical authorities were highlighted in scholastic debates about the biological natures and roles of males and females.

Consciousness of these differences and of their implications for general theories of nature and life was heightened dramatically by the translation

4 Book III, fen xx and xxi, contain the central body of Avicenna's views concerning reproduction.
5 Kibre, *Hippocrates Latinus*, XI, pp. 189–91.
6 See May's Introduction in Galen, *On the Usefulness of the Parts of the Body*, pp. 5–6. A full translation of *On the Use of Parts* from the Greek dates from 1317. On the narrow influence of the twelfth-century abbreviation translated from the Arabic, see Roger French, "*De juvamentis membrorum* and the Reception of Galenic Physiological Anatomy," *Isis* 70 (1979): 96–109.

and assimilation of Aristotle's major works on animals – *History of Animals,
Parts of Animals, Generation of Animals* – first from Arabic in the early thirteenth century by Michael Scot, who also translated Avicenna's compendium on animals, and then from Greek just after midcentury by William of
Moerbeke. These works, usually grouped together under the title *On Animals*, found a secure if not central position in the curricula of the universities'
arts faculties.[7] Like Avicenna's *Canon*, Aristotle's *On Animals* is a work of
enormous size and scope. It contains many passages relevant to sex difference, not the least of which is the extensive treatment of the reproductive
division of labor contained in the books on generation. Like Avicenna,
Aristotle encouraged reflection on the issues and implications of reproductive theories not only by laying out his own arguments but also by summa-
rizing and refuting his Hippocratic and pre-Socratic predecessors at a number of points, thus confirming for medieval readers what the *Canon* had
already suggested: that the subject of sex difference as embodied in questions about reproductive contributions and sex determination was a rich
field for inquiry and debate.

Medieval interest in elaborating and resolving questions which reflected
in one way or another on the definitions of female and male natures and
functions was thus encouraged by newly recovered classical precedents, as
well as by the traditions developed in the context of monastic learning
before the impact of the new translations. In particular, lines of battle had
been drawn in antiquity over the existence and role of a female seed and
over the relation of the male seed to the form and substance of the offspring.
Whether the female produced anything which could properly be called
semen (and therefore properly parallel male semen), and if so what exactly it
was and how far the parallel extended, were questions already explicit in the
works of the ancient Greeks and their Arabic interpreters. Medieval authors
laid hold of and even exaggerated the differing opinions of their authorities,
reshaping and giving urgency to the problem of male and female reproductive contributions.

But medieval interests were not defined solely by ancient precedents.
University lecturers on medicine and natural philosophy had some freedom
to choose topics for discussion according to their interests.[8] They and those
who borrowed and reworked their scholarship pressed beyond the center of
ancient concerns. Often taking their cues from their medieval predecessors,

---

7 The contents of what was called *De animalibus* included two additional works in the Greco-
Latin version. See *De generatione animalium translatio Guillelmi de Moerbeka*, vol. XVII 2 of
Aristoteles Latinus, ed. H. J. Lulofs, Union académique internationale, Corpus philosophorum Medii Aevi (Bruges and Paris: Desclée de Brouwer, 1966), Praefatio, pp. ix–xiii.
8 Scholars' freedom was especially exercised in the choice of quodlibetal questions, but as
Nanci Siraisi points out in connection with commentaries such as those on Avicenna's
chapter "On the Generation of the Embryo," they might also decide to lecture or write on
specific sections of authoritative texts (*Avicenna in Renaissance Italy*, pp. 60–1).

they isolated and developed two sets of questions which had not been of special concern in antiquity. The first, the determination of the fetus's sex, had arisen in ancient texts as an element in discussions of other subjects, notably the origin of the semen and the possibility of maternal influence. In scholastic philosophy and medicine, the determination of sex acquired status as a scientific problem in its own right. The second, the nature and function of female and male sexual desire and pleasure, has even less basis in the texts of the newly translated authorities, although Aristotle mentioned it briefly in his refutation of a formative role for the female. It too commands the attention of thirteenth- and fourteenth-century academics.

Compared with the attention accorded Aristotle's logical works or Hippocrates' *Aphorisms*, late medieval interest in Aristotle's *On Animals* and even Avicenna's *Canon* was not great, if we can take numbers of manuscripts and the existence of works about the texts as indicative of their prominence. Furthermore, the curricula of the arts and medical faculties were far from preoccupied with sex. Yet the subject does have a certain persistence and, perhaps more important, a certain ubiquitousness. As we shall see, questions about reproductive contributions, sex determination, and pleasure crop up not only in commentaries on the *Canon* and *On Animals* but also in texts concerned with theology and ethics. Signs that consideration of these subjects was broad and active also appear in widely disseminated texts which are not direct products of the university environment but which have incorporated the discussions. Members of religious orders sent to universities to take a degree in arts and then perhaps continue in theology returned to their orders to teach and write; students from the arts and medical faculties found positions or set up practices in courts and municipalities.[9] The appropriation of academic ideas concerning sex difference indicates that interest was active, not just pro forma, and also suggests the pathways these ideas followed into a broader social and cultural milieu.

Dissemination: Institutions and forms of scholasticism

The dissemination of the ideas contained in newly translated texts occurred in part through the well-established institutions and genres of learned discourse. But the information and opinions of Aristotle, Avicenna, and others was most fully and enthusiastically received and presented in the newer forms developed within the context of university teaching. Enriched by the early contributions of the learned humanistic traditions and the talented personnel of the monasteries, the secular urban schools at Salerno and else-

9 On the dissemination of university learning, see Palémon Glorieux, *La littérature quodlibétique de 1260–1320*, Bibliothèque thomiste 5 and 21, Section historique 18 (Le Saulchoir, Kain: Revue des Sciences Philosophiques et Théologiques, 1925; Paris: Librairie Philosophique J. Vrin, 1935), vol. 2, pp. 19–28.

where in Italy were the source of the Italian universities of the following centuries. Because these schools remained largely independent of ecclesiastical control and because they were not dominated by (indeed often did not have) faculties of theology, the study of medicine, natural philosophy, and indeed philosophy in general found room for expression and development in the medical faculty. As a result, many later participants in the debates about such subjects as female seed were, as we shall see, teachers of scholastic medicine in southern Europe. In northern Europe, on the other hand, although the universities were not the direct descendents of the monasteries, they did owe more to ecclesiastical institutions, personnel, and authorities. Thus, although in both northern and southern Europe from the thirteenth century onward the study of natural philosophy had a significant place in the faculties of arts, in northern Europe, where clerical influence is more pervasive and where the greatest prestige was attached to the study of theology, it was not only teachers of natural philosophy and medicine but also theologians who carried on the discussion of subjects like nocturnal emissions.[10]

Thus the teachers and writers who contributed to university discussions on sex difference constituted an international collection of men variously trained and pursuing diverse careers, many of whom were, nevertheless, aware of each other's work. In the 1240s Peter of Spain, whose father had been a physician, and Albertus Magnus, an older Dominican scholar and teacher who had studied briefly in Padua, both arrived to study and then lecture at the university of Paris – Peter in the arts faculty, Albertus in theology. Each went on to a distinguished career in the Church, Albertus becoming head of the Dominican order in Germany, then bishop of Regensburg, and Peter becoming bishop of Braga in Portugal, then a cardinal, and finally dying as Pope John XXI. Yet both continued to pursue their scholarly interests. Peter, who taught briefly at the nascent university in Siena, wrote extensively on Aristotelian logic and natural philosophy, including a major work on animals. In addition, he wrote commentaries on a number of standard medical texts and composed two general works on medicine. Albertus Magnus, who managed to give series of lectures on scientific subjects at the school of advanced theological studies that he had started at Cologne for the Dominicans, produced a prodigious array of works on all aspects of

10 The standard history of the development of medieval universities is Hastings Rashdall, *The Universities of Europe in the Middle Ages*, new ed. by F. M. Powicke and A. B. Emden, 3 vols. (Oxford: Clarendon Press, 1936). More recent studies include Gordon Leff, *Paris and Oxford Universities in the Thirteenth and Fourteenth Centuries: An Institutional and Intellectual History* (New York: John Wiley and Sons, 1968; repr., Huntington, N.Y.: Robert E. Krieger, 1975); and Nancy Siraisi, *Arts and Sciences at Padua: The Studium of Padua before 1350*, Studies and Texts 25 (Toronto: Pontifical Institute of Mediaeval Studies, 1973). Siraisi and Pearl Kibre summarize the development of northern and southern universities with special reference to the teaching of science in "The Institutional Setting: The University," in David C. Lindberg, ed., *Science in the Middle Ages*, Chicago History of Science and Medicine (Chicago: University of Chicago Press, 1978), pp. 120–44.

natural philosophy. Giles of Rome, another churchman, who studied and taught theology at Paris toward the end of the thirteenth century, wrote not only on standard subjects of Aristotelian science but also on the medical subject of embryology.

Perhaps the paradigm for the links between north and south, natural philosophy and medicine, and ancient and medieval learning was Peter of Abano, whose career as a university teacher began in Paris in the late thirteenth century and ended in Padua in the early fourteenth. He taught and wrote on both philosophy and medicine (including astrology), and he translated a number of ancient works from Greek into Latin. His most influential work, the *Conciliator*, collected the opinions of ancient scientific and medical authorities on a wide variety of topics and sought to explain the differences among them. By the time Peter of Abano arrived, northern Italy had two thriving and structured centers of learning, Padua, where Peter settled, and Bologna, where in the second half of the thirteenth century Taddeo Alderotti, a prominent medical practitioner and widely read scholar, had helped to shape the curriculum and the institution. Taddeo taught logic and medicine and wrote extensively on medical classics such as Hippocrates' *Aphorisms*. He had a number of prominent and productive students, one of whom, Dino of Florence, taught and practiced medicine in Florence, Siena, Padua, and Bologna in the early decades of the fourteenth century. Northern Italy continued to be in the vanguard of scholarship in medicine and in the branches of natural philosophy which served it, so that at the end of the fourteenth century, when a physician named Jacopo of Forlì, who taught medicine, logic, and philosophy during his career at Padua and Bologna, took up the subject of the generation of the embryo, he had a considerable tradition to draw on and cited the work of Giles of Rome, Dino of Florence, and others.[11] Along with many others, including philosophers from the university at Oxford and medical writers from the university at Montpellier in southern France, these individuals were shaped by and contributed to the new universities of Europe. In the process, they applied new methods of teaching and writing to subjects like generation, sterility, physiological constitutions, and sexual pleasures, which conveyed ideas about females and males.

Like the new institutions, the new modes of expression which they nurtured had precedents in the period before the emergence of university scholasticism. Monastic scholars had engaged in the exegesis of sacred texts, and medical authors in Salerno had glossed the group of medical classics which came to be known as the *Articella*. Medical authors knew that Galen had written commentaries on works of Hippocrates, and natural philosophers

11 Information on these individuals may be found in *The Dictionary of Scientific Biography*; and Lynn Thorndike, *A History of Magic and Experimental Science*, 8 vols. (New York: Macmillan and Columbia University Press, 1923–58). On Taddeo and Dino, see Nancy G. Siraisi, *Taddeo Alderotti and His Pupils: Two Generations of Italian Medical Learning* (Princeton: Princeton University Press, 1981), pp. 27–42 and 55–64.

were familiar with the late ancient commentary of Chalcidius upon Plato's *Timaeus*. In addition, the dialogue format, as well as the works of theologians from Augustine in the fifth century to Peter Lombard in the twelfth, suggested the pedagogical model of question and answer.[12] Finally, the didactic formats of the Salernitan medical questions and *On Human Generation* and of the pseudo-Aristotelian work known as the *Problems* influenced the form and content of the emerging genres.[13]

As teachers at the monastic and cathedral schools and free-lance teachers in urban centers gathered around them an increasingly numerous and cosmopolitan group of students, and as the timetable of the academic year and the curriculum took shape, the practice of reading and explicating an authoritative text took on a regular if flexible form known as the *lectio*. The text to be taught was divided into sections upon which the lecturer expounded in order. The place of a particular text in the curriculum and the status of the lecturer influenced the character of the exposition, which could range from cursory literal explication to freewheeling discussion including references to other works and lengthy digressions. These practices in turn shaped the literary form known as the "commentary," which became a widely used vehicle for teaching and research. Albertus Magnus's work on Aristotle's *On Animals*, written when he was bishop of Regensburg, is a massive example of the most expansive sort of commentary. To his summary and interpretations of Aristotle's views (heavily influenced by Avicenna's work on *On Animals*, which Michael Scot had also translated), Albertus added lengthy digressions, such as the six-chapter tract entitled "On the Dispute of Galen and Aristotle Concerning the Principles of Generation," and a medically oriented discussion of the causes of infertility. This sort of disengagement from the dominance of the authoritative text evolved further into the practice of posing and expounding problems related to but not necessarily fully treated or resolved in the text. University masters and other teachers thus presented to their students and sometimes committed to writing sets of *questiones* on a required text.

In addition to the day-to-day business of the university, which revolved around the public interpretation of authorized texts, faculty and students participated in and observed public disputations at specified times in the year and at specified stages of their education and certification. *Questiones* on a set

12 Viola Coloman, "Manières personnelles et impersonnelles d'aborder un problème: Saint Augustin et le XIIᵉ siècle. Contribution à l'histoire de la *quaestio*," in *Les genres littéraires dans les sources théologiques et philosophiques médiévales: Définition, critique et exploitation: Actes du Colloque international de Louvain-la-Neuve, 25–27 mai 1981*, Publications de l'Institut d'études médiévales, 2d series: Textes, études, congrès 5 (Louvain-la-Neuve: Institut d'études médiévales de l'Université Catholique de Louvain, 1982), pp. 11–30.
13 Danielle Jacquart, "La question disputée dans les facultés de médecine," in Bernardo C. Bazàn, John W. Wippel, Gérard Fransen, and Danielle Jacquart, *Les questions disputées et les questions quodlibétiques dans les facultés de théologie, de droit et de médecine*, Typologie des sources du Moyen Age occidental 44–45 (Turnhout: Brepols, 1985), pp. 281–315.

text or problems on any subject (called "quodlibetal questions") formed the basis for highly structured disputations. The format varied but usually included arguments pro and con, review of authorities on the subject (especially the author from whose work the question emerged), a determination or conclusion, and responses to the contrary arguments.[14]

When Albertus Magnus was teaching at Cologne, for example, he addressed the question whether generation by intercourse is the greatest pleasure. First he argued that it is not: (1) because the separation of compatibles causes sadness, and semen is highly compatible with the body which produces it; (2) because serving oneself is a greater source of pleasure than serving someone else, and unlike eating, which is for oneself, generation is for someone else; and (3) because pleasure is based on the senses, and whereas in nutrition two senses (touch and taste) are involved, in intercourse only one (touch) is involved. Then, because this set of questions is centered on an Aristotelian text, he enumerated Aristotle's reasons why generation by coitus is indeed the greatest of pleasures: (1) because everything takes pleasure in its proper operation, and between nutrition and generation, generation is the higher operation, being for the sake of the species, not just for the sake of the individual, and is therefore the source of a greater pleasure; (2) because pleasure is caused by the conjunction of compatibles, and semen, being refined from the same nutriment that constitutes the members, causes great pleasure as it passes through them in the process of intercourse; and (3) because the expulsion of a superfluity is pleasurable, and semen is a useful residue of superfluous nutriment. Finally, making his position clear without a separately labeled "determination," Albertus answered the first set of arguments: (1) if semen were nutriment about to be converted to a specific part, intercourse would cause the sadness of separation, but in fact it passes through the nervous parts, which do not need it; (2) the distinction should not be between serving oneself and serving someone else but between serving the particular (individual) and serving the general (species), the latter being superior; and (3) nutrition may have pleasure from more senses, but intercourse has more pleasure from touch, since what is being touched is more similar and more compatible than food.[15]

14 B. C. Bazàn, "La *quaestio disputata*" and J. F. Wippel, "The Quodlibetal Question as a Distinctive Literary Genre" both in *Les genres littéraires dans les sources théologiques et philosophiques médiévales: Définition, critique et exploitation: Actes du Colloque international de Louvain-la-Neuve, 25–27 mai 1981*, Publications de l'Institut d'études médiévales, 2d series: Textes, études, congrès 5 (Louvain-la-Neuve: Institut d'études médiévales de l'Université Catholique de Louvain, 1982), pp. 31–50 and 67–84 respectively; and Bernardo C. Bazàn, John W. Wippel, Gérard Fransen, and Danielle Jacquart, *Les questions disputées et les questions quodlibétiques dans les facultés de théologie, de droit et de médecine*, Typologie des sources du Moyen Age occidental 44–5 (Turnhout: Brepols, 1985).

15 Albertus Magnus, *Quaestiones super* De animalibus, ed. Ephrem Filthault, in *Opera omnia*, vol. 12, ed. Bernhard Geyer (Münster: Aschendorff, 1955), bk. V, q. 3, pp. 154–5. This work is referred to below as *Quaestiones de animalibus* and is to be distinguished from Albertus's more extensive commentary referred to as *De animalibus*.

Renaissance humanists maligned these exercises as empty formalisms, and they are the basis of the modern complaint that medieval theology or philosophy was concerned with determining how many angels could dance on the head of a pin. Although audiences of students and faculty certainly prized virtuosity in disputations, undertaken in some measure to demonstrate the participants' debating skills and logical prowess, and although the outcomes of some conventional questions were never in doubt, both the choice of the questions and the contents of the answers are revealing. An early fourteenth-century theologian asking whether the seed which organized the fetus was itself the potential of soul was approaching serious problems about the nature and unity of the soul and about the process of ensoulment.[16] The question another theologian from around 1300 was called upon to explore, while likewise possessing its serious dimensions, was no doubt also a crowd-pleaser: whether a man sins more by having intercourse with a prostitute than with a respectable woman.[17] Not only do the questions suggest what interested medieval academics (or at least what they took to be standard issues), but also the answers reflect their assumptions and the body of knowledge and opinion with which they expected each other to be familiar. As lectures gave rise to the literary forms of commentary and *questiones*, disputations gave rise to a genre of texts known as *questiones disputate*. Some, like Albertus's set containing the questions on maximum pleasure, were more or less faithful reports recorded by scholars who heard the oral debate;[18] others, like Jacopo of Forlì's on Avicenna, were more polished revisions by the author himself.[19]

Although the development of commentaries and questions as formal structures for the investigation of scientific and medical issues occurred within the universities, those forms and the specific subjects to which they were applied spilled out into wider literate circles, as Albertus Magnus's career suggests. Not only were the more conventional compilations and encyclopedias, now inflected with scholastic awareness of conflicting authorities and contemporary debates, available beyond the universities, but the pedagogical practices and related literary forms had currency outside the university curriculum.[20] For example, a work called *The Secrets of Women*, which included a wealth of Aristotelian and other material relating to sexuality, reproduction, gynecology, and obstetrics, was falsely attributed to the

---

16 Gui Terreni (de Perpignan), in Glorieux, *Littérature quodlibétique*, vol. 1, p. 173.

17 Nicholas Bar, in ibid., vol. 2, p. 138.

18 There is some uncertainty surrounding the nature and authorship of this set of questions, but see Ephrem Filthaut, Prolegomena, in Albertus Magnus, *Quaestiones de animalibus*, pp. xliii–xlv.

19 Jacobus Forliviensis, *Expositio supra capitulum* De generatione embrionis *cum questionibus eiusdem*, in Bassanius Politus, comp., *De generatione embrionis* (Venice: Bonetus Locatellus, 1502), fols. 2ra–17va. Wippel, "Quodlibetal Question," pp. 78–81.

20 Glorieux, *Littérature quodlibétique*, pp. 22–8; see also Ludger Meier, "Les disputes quodlibétiques en dehors des universités," *Revue d'histoire ecclésiastique* 53 (1958): 401–42.

learned Albertus Magnus, subjected to commentaries (though it never had an official place in a university curriculum), reproduced in more than seventy manuscripts, and, by the fifteenth century, was available in German and French translations.[21] *The Secrets of Women* illustrates the authenticity of late medieval curiosity within and beyond universities about sexuality and sex difference, as well as the ambiguity of university-style formality, which lent cool legitimacy to topics fraught with danger.[22]

The development of standard forms of presentation and rules of argument did not prevent thirteenth- and fourteenth-century scholastic writers from entertaining some of the wide range of questions which caught the attention of Constantine, Hildegard, and the compilers of the questions and dialogues on generation. Thomas Aquinas, like Hildegard of Bingen a century before him, reflected on the natures and functions of males and females in the context of divine Creation; medical professors writing about sterility invoked some of the same problems and solutions as Constantine; and *The Secrets of Women* passed on some of the misogynist lore that had been contained in the Salernitan literature, such as the assertion that a menstruating woman causes mirrors to become cloudy. But the introduction of newly translated authorities, the formalization of higher learning, and the increased communications among intellectual communities (facilitated by a surge in travel and in the production of manuscripts) helped to focus the attention of thirteenth- and fourteenth-century writers on specific issues.

Of the questions and problems relating to reproduction and sexuality addressed by authors of this period, those which reveal most about notions of sex difference concern the reproductive contributions of females and males, the causes of sex determination of the fetus, and the nature and function of sexual pleasure. The first of these, reproductive roles, gets at the very reason sex differences exist, and thus sets forth the definitions and functions of female and male. At the same time, it connects sex difference with principles which transcend the process of generation or even of biological function in general, touching on the metaphysics of form and matter and

---

21 [Ps.-]Albertus Magnus, *De secretis mulierum*, in *De secretis mulierum item De virtutibus herbarum lapidum et animalium* (Amsterdam: Iodocus Ianstonius, 1643). See Helen Rodnite Lemay, *Women's Secrets: A Translation of Pseudo-Albertus Magnus' De secretis mulierum with Commentaries*, SUNY Series in Medieval Studies (Albany: State University of New York Press, 1992). On the history, variations, and authorship of this work, see Lynn Thorndike, "Further Consideration of the *Experimenta, Speculum astronomiae* and *De secretis mulierum* ascribed to Albertus Magnus," *Speculum* 30 (1955): 413–43; Ernest Wickersheimer, "Henri de Saxe et le *De secretis mulierum*," *3ᵉ Congrès de l'histoire de l'art de Guérir, Londres, 17–22 juillet, 1922* (Antwerp, 1923), pp. 253–8; Brigitte Kusche, "Zur *Secreta mulierum* – Forschung," *Janus* 62 (1975): 102–23; Christoph Ferckel, "Die *Secreta mulierum* und ihr Verfasser," *Sudhoffs Archiv für Geschichte der Medizin und der Naturwissenschaften* 38 (1954): 267–74. On manuscripts and translations, see Margaret Rose Schleissner, "Pseudo-Albertus Magnus: *Secreta mulierum cum commento*, Deutsch: Critical Text and Commentary" (Ph.D. diss., Princeton University, 1987), pp. 6–9, 42–50, and appendix B.
22 See Schleissner, "*Secreta mulierum*," pp. 35–41.

the physics of the transmission of motion. From the point of view of the parents, the second set of questions, concerning the production of female or male offspring, is in part a special case of the problem of reproductive roles – the influence of father and mother upon the sex of the offspring. But the problem of sex determination led medieval authors to more diverse and complex causes, which in turn illuminate their effects – the essential features of sexual differentiation. In addition, the issue of sex determination had what might be called a practical side: it invited discussion of manipulations of the causes in order to influence the sex of the child. Finally, the third group of questions, those about pleasure, is haunted both by specific problems in natural philosophy (e.g., is the desire for sexual pleasure a result of having or needing heat?) and by more general moral and social concerns.

SEMINAL IDEAS: FEMALE AND MALE GENERATIVE CONTRIBUTIONS

Aristotle versus Galen?

Framed in terms of the competing opinions of authorities, especially as they were understood from the newly translated works of Aristotle and Avicenna, and treated according to the practices of scholastic argument, questions surrounding the existence and function of a female semen took on a clarity, specificity, and urgency foreign to earlier medieval treatments of reproduction and to the accommodating style of encyclopedists. Because of the explicit and heated character of the exchanges, modern scholars have recognized their significance for our understanding of medieval views about sex difference. They tend, however, to minimize the seriousness of the medieval discussions by simplifying the Aristotelian and Galenic views, by exaggerating the difference between them, and by assuming the effective dominance of an Aristotelian and misogynistic outlook, according to which either females had no seed or else anything labeled a female "semen" or "sperm" had neither moving nor forming influence upon the offspring. Some hold that this view was displaced in the Renaissance by a more flexible or feminist perspective derived either from Galen or from Soranus and others.[23] Medieval and Renaissance authors themselves sometimes repre-

---

23 M. Anthony Hewson, in *Giles of Rome and the Medieval Theory of Conception: A Study of the De formatione corporis humani in utero*, University of London Historical Studies 38 (London: Athelone Press, University of London, 1975), follows his subject, Giles of Rome, in minimizing the force of the Galenic position. (See review by Michael McVaugh, *Speculum* 52 (1977): 987–9.) Anne-Liese Thomasen, in "*Historia Animalium* contra *Gynaecia* in der Literatur des Mittelalters," *Clio medica* 15 (1980): 5–23, emphasizes the harmful effects of Aristotelian minimization of the female reproductive role upon concerns for women's health, and the positive effects of the Renaissance revival of the Soranus–Muscio tradition. Ian Mclean, in *The Renaissance Notion of Woman: A Study in the Fortunes of Scholasticism and Medical Science in European Intellectual Life*, Cambridge Monographs on the History of

sented the lines of disagreement as clearly drawn. In the seventeenth century, William Harvey, who wished to be associated with neither faction, represented the positions of Aristotelians and Galenists as virtually incommensurable, the former stated in metaphysical terms of active and passive, the latter in physiological terms:

> Nature has not, on account of the distinction into male and female, established it as a law that the one, as agent, should confer form, the other, as passive, supply matter, as Aristotle apprehended; nor yet that during intercourse each should contribute a seminal fluid, by the mixture of which a conception or ovum should be produced, as physicians commonly suppose.[24]

But if a seventeenth-century author had reasons to caricature the positions in order to enhance the force of his purportedly novel formulation, medieval authors' treatments of the subject are often subtle and complex and are seldom unambiguously tied to a single ancient authority. Indeed, as other scholars have pointed out, the cross-fertilization of medicine and natural philosophy in the scholastic environment allowed for far more diversity, compromise, and ambiguity than the simpler models suggest.[25] For example, Aristotle's *On Animals*, which contained his theory of generation, was one of only two nonmedical works on which lectures could be given at the university of Paris medical faculty, and the Paduan medical author and teacher Peter of Abano regarded it as required preparatory reading for medical students.[26]

   The oldest, most persistent way of representing scholastic debates about the existence and nature of the female seed in particular and the reproductive roles of females and males in general was indeed in terms of the conflicting opinions of two great authorities, Aristotle and Galen. "Aristotle and Galen were opposed to each other on this question," as Jacopo of Forlì bluntly put it in his question on Avicenna labeled "Whether the woman's semen actively enters into the formation of the fetus."[27] Although the reiteration of this

Medicine (Cambridge: Cambridge University Press, 1980), does not represent Aristotelian and Galenic views as diametrically opposed nor does he portray Galenism as essentially feminist, but he does see a Renaissance shift toward the Galenic perspective as good for women (e.g., pp. 37–8).

24 William Harvey, *Anatomical Exercises on the Generation of Animals*, in *Works*, trans. Robert Willis (London: Sydenham Society, 1847), pp. 300–1.

25 See, e.g., Jacquart and Thomasset, *Sexuality and Medicine*; and Nancy G. Siraisi, *Taddeo*, pp. 195–202.

26 Ernest Wickersheimer, *Commentaires de la faculté de médecine de l'université de Paris (1395–1516)*, Collection de documents inédits sur l'histoire de France (Paris: Imprimerie Nationale, 1915), Introduction, p. xxiv; Nancy G. Siraisi, "The Medical Learning of Albertus Magnus," in James A. Weisheipl, ed., *Albertus Magnus and the Sciences: Commemorative Essays, 1980*, Studies and Texts 49 (Toronto: Pontifical Institute of Mediaeval Studies, 1980), p. 380, n. 2.

27 Jacobus Forliviensis, *De generatione embrionis*, q. 4, fols. 15rb–vb: "Notandum quod de ista questione sibi invicem repugnantes fuerunt Aristoteles et Galenus" (fol. 15va).

opposition underscores the consciousness of the problems of antiquity and the habit of drawing the elements of both questions and answers from established authorities, it is subjected to a range of emphases and approaches.

A well known fourth-century Greek source, translated into Latin in the eleventh and then again in the twelfth century, briefly summarized the conflict and, in doing so, hinted at concerns which later medieval authors were to develop, but which Harvey preferred either to set aside or to treat from a different perspective:

> Women have all the same parts as men, but inside not outside. But then Aristotle and Democritus wish to connect nothing of women's semen to the generation of children; for they regard what is emitted by women more as sweat of [her reproductive] part than as a seed. Galen, refuting Aristotle, says women surely emit sperm and the mixture of the two produces a fetus (hence I have said that coitus is a mixing). But he does not say it is a perfect seed like that of a man, but rather undigested and more humid than it. Such seed of the woman as exists serves as food for the man's seed.[28]

In few words this text of Nemesius brings forth two important elements of the problem confronted by scholastic authors: first, that Aristotle and Galen disagree about the existence of a female seed with a reproductive role (a disagreement connected with the interpretation of male–female parallels), and second, that Galen's position does not create a clear dichotomy between a one-seed system and a system with two equivalent seeds, but rather raises a new set of questions about the *different* natures and functions of female and male semens. Scholastic authors had their work cut out for them, given the broad credibility of the two authorities and the complexity of the question, in which are embedded a whole set of difficult problems (How do children come to resemble their fathers? their mothers? Has nature made two seeds to serve one purpose? or one seed for no purpose? or similar structures for different purposes?).

Scholastic questions of generation and conception

How did those writing in the thirteenth- and fourteenth-century university environment approach this set of problems? The questions they posed to be answered in the course of a disputation or a series of lectures indicate what they came to view as the critical issues. Whether commenting on medical texts, such as the Hippocratic *On the Nature of the Embryo* and Avicenna's

---

28 Nemesius, *De natura hominis*, ch. 24, p. 109: "Sed et mulieres omnes easdem cum viris habent particulas, sed intus et non extra. Igitur Aristoteles quidem et Democritus nil volunt conferre mulieris semen ad generationem filiorum; quod emittitur enim a mulieribus sudorem particulae magis quam germen esse volunt; Galenus vero reprehendens Aristotelem, sperma quidem emittere mulieres ait et mixtionem utrorumque facere fetum (ideoque coitum mixtionem dici), non tamen perfectum germen esse dicit ut quod est viri, sed adhuc indigestum et humidius; tale autem existens mulieris germen cibus fit viri germini. . . ."

chapter "On the Generation of the Embryo," or on works of natural philosophy, such as Aristotle's *Generation of Animals* and the pseudo-Albertus *Secrets of Women*, thirteenth- and fourteenth-century authors framed their questions about the reproductive contributions of females and males in similar
ways: Do women produce sperm (or semen)? If so, does it play a necessary
role in reproduction?[29]

The challenge to late medieval scholars went well beyond the problem
of resolving conflicts among distant authorities: on these subjects as on
many others the *questiones* reflect exchange among moderns. One work on
Avicenna's chapter "On the Generation of the Embryo" refers to the opinions of Dino del Garbo and Gentile da Foligno. In its question "Whether
the sperm of the woman may have active power in the generation of the
fetus," it summarizes and takes exception to Giles of Rome's opinions.[30]
Not only did these questions become more explicit and persistent than
they had been in the works of writers like Constantine and Hildegard, but
they also became consistently asymmetrical: they focused on the abilities
and disabilities of females, not on the mutual interactions of male and
female elements. Although the answers to these questions almost invariably involve the roles of both sexes, what is at issue is females, and
particularly women. There are exceptions. The quodlibetal question posed
by Raymond Rigaut (neither a philosopher nor a physician but a theologian) has the unusual phrasing "Whether two seeds – namely, that of the
father and that of the mother – must converge for the generation of progeny."[31] And some authors were interested in the much less prominent and
less frequently posed question aimed at clarifying the role of the male
semen: does the sperm of the male enter into the substance of the fetus?[32]
But far more lecture time and far more manuscript pages were devoted to
the capacities and incapacities of females: does woman have sperm, and is
it necessary for generation?

29 Nancy Siraisi lists numerous instances of such questions in Italian medical literature (*Taddeo*,
   pp. 338–40); these and related questions are at the center of Hewson's analysis in *Giles of
   Rome*, esp. pp. 67–146. The questions of Albertus Magnus and others are treated below.
30 Dinus de Florentia, *Expositio supra capitulo* De generatione embrionis *cum questionibus
   eiusdem*, in Bassanius Politus, comp., *De generatione embrionis* (Venice: Bonetus Locatellus,
   1502), fol. 31ra: "An sperma mulieris habeat virtutem activam in generatione fetus et an
   etiam pro materia illius possit subiici." See Hewson, *Giles of Rome*. Siraisi points out that
   the attribution of this work to Dino is probably false (*Taddeo*, p. 200, n. 142).
31 "Utrum ad prolis generationem necessario concurrant duo semina, patris scilicet, et ma-
   tris." Cited in Ferdinand Marie Delorme, "Quodlibets et questions disputées de Raymond
   Rigaut, maître franciscain de Paris, d'après le Ms. 96 de la Bibl. Comm. de Todi," in Albert
   Lang, Joseph Lechner, and Michael Schmaus, eds., *Aus der Geisteswelt des Mittelalters:
   Studien und Texte Martin Grabmann . . . gewidmet*, Beiträge zur Geschichte der Philosophie
   und Theologie des Mittelalters, suppl. 3 (Münster: Aschendorff, 1935), vol. 2, p. 831.
32 Among the authors surveyed by Siraisi, only one, Dino del Garbo, poses this question
   (*Taddeo*, p. 339).

Do women produce something which might properly be called a "seed" or "sperm"? Medieval answers range from "no, but . . ." to "yes, but. . . ." They reflect the conflict between what were understood to be the philosophical (Aristotelian) and medical (Galenic) opinions and a pervasive unwillingness to choose sides unequivocally. In spite of his expressing different views elsewhere, in his set of *questiones* on Aristotle's *On Animals*, Albertus Magnus makes the strongest case for the Aristotelian position that women do not produce sperm properly speaking. First, he argues, sperm is to a man as menstruum is to a woman. A man produces sperm because he does not menstruate; a woman menstruates because she does not produce sperm. This symmetrical picture arises from the asymmetry of heat: sperm is the final form of completely digested food, and women lack the heat to complete the digestion and therefore produce only menstruum. Second, argues Albertus, moving to a higher level of abstraction and citing Aristotle's *Physics*, matter and agent cannot coincide. That which effects a result, that which is the efficient or moving cause, cannot also be the material which is affected, in which the result resides. And since the woman supplies the matter for reproduction and sperm is the agent, the woman cannot produce sperm. Albertus gives only cursory consideration to the contrary position, omitting to deal with what Aristotle himself had treated as among the most serious challenges to his account of reproduction: children's resemblance to their mothers. To the argument that the greatest pleasure occurs as a result of the emission of semen, that women experience the greatest pleasure in intercourse, and that therefore women must emit seed, Albertus replies that this pleasure comes not from sperm produced by the woman but from the touch either of the man's sperm in the womb or of the penis against her sexual part.[33]

So clear-cut a response to the question of female semen is rare, though Giles of Rome propounded in greater detail something very close to it, emphasizing the material nature of the female contribution and the unequivocal passivity of matter.[34] Rarer still is the straightforward defense of the competing position, that there exists a female semen distinguished from menstruum and in some respects analogous to the male semen, which is necessary for conception. Since Galen himself had been sympathetic to Aristotelian philosophy and aware of Aristotle's objections to a two-seed model, since Avicenna had likewise studied and incorporated Aristotle into his medical works, and since medical authors of the scholastic period often had prior training in an arts curriculum full of Aristotle, nothing that might be called a pure medical position existed. Still, Jacopo of Forlì could declare, citing

33 Albertus Magnus, *Quaestiones de animalibus*, bk. XV, q. 19, p. 271. In discussing women's pleasure as a separate subject, Albertus takes a different view, treated later.
34 Hewson, *Giles of Rome*, pp. 67–75.

Avicenna and the pseudo-Galenic *On Sperm*, that Galen's view "seems to me closer to the truth."[35] He summarized that view as follows: "the sperm of both [the man and the woman] contributes to generation materially and effectively alike," the adverb "effectively" referring to the active role of efficient cause which Aristotle had denied to the female sperm.[36]

In the context of attempts to resolve the tensions perceived to exist between the two authorities and in the context of the separate exposition of Aristotelian and medical texts, there evolved not so much a debate as a conversation concerning the nature and role of the female seed. At times the conversation became quite heated, not because two clearly defined sides were doing battle so much as because with many philosophical, medical, theoretical, and empirical issues at stake, the participants were scrambling to arrive at resolutions which were both compelling and consistent with any number of dearly held principles or premises. At stake, for example, was the conviction that nature is economical. If both sexes produce active seed, is nature duplicating its efforts unnecessarily? If only the male produces seed, did nature make the female testes (ovaries) in vain? So although the phrasing of the questions made females the issue, and although many of the specific arguments expressed negative views of women, what was at issue in these works sometimes had more to do with philosophy and physiology than with broader notions of gender and the nature of the feminine. As the next chapter will show, authors taking disparate positions on specific scholastic questions such as the existence of a female seed drew on shared assumptions about the differences between women and men; thus, this set of philosophical and medical concerns highlighted and reinforced gender concepts but did not call them into question. Whatever the implications of the various positions taken on these scholarly discussions, the exchanges and disagreements do not represent a debate between feminists and misogynists.

Several examples of scholastic attempts to mediate between what were taken to be the positions of Aristotle and Galen will illustrate the rich variety and resourcefulness of scholastic arguments. In a late thirteenth-century commentary on one of the works of the *Articella*, the Italian physician and teacher Taddeo Alderotti addressed the question of reproductive contributions narrowly in the *questio* "Whether generative power is in the male's sperm or in the female's sperm."[37] Having asserted that Aristotle and

35 Jacobus Forliviensis, *De generatione embrionis*, fol. 15va: "Ideo breviter primo tractabo positionem Philosophi, secundo Galieni que ut mihi apparet est veritati conformior."

36 Ibid., fol. 2rb: "Secunda autem positio fuit Galieni tenentis utrumque sperma concurrere materialiter simul et effective ad generationem."

37 Thaddeus Florentinus, *In* Isagogas *Joannitianas expositio*, in *Expositiones in arduum* Aphorismorum *Ipocratis, in divinum* Pronosticorum *Ipocratis librum, in preclarum* Regiminis acutorum *Ipocratis opus, in subtilissime* Joannitii Isagogarum *libellum*, ed. Joannis Baptista Nicollinus (Venice: Luca Antonius, 1527), fol. 357vb. On Taddeo's life and work, see Siraisi, *Taddeo*.

Avicenna agree that reproductive power exists only in the male sperm, he proceeded to make and respond to arguments having to do exclusively with the female role. The resemblance of children to their mothers is due only to the passive resistance of the matter supplied by the female to the formative power coming from the male and does not imply any activity on the female side. He simply dismissed the position, which he attributed to Galen, that there is generative power in the female, a position to which he claimed Avicenna had taken strong exception. Taddeo continued in this Aristotelian vein, pointing out that if women had both menstruum, which serves as matter for the fetus, and an active sperm, they would be able to produce offspring by themselves. (Albertus Magnus had recorded what he understood to be Galen's response to this objection: that the female capacity had to be activated by the male sperm.)[38] Thus he rejected the possibility not only of an active female reproductive role, but also of a female sperm. Why, then, do Constantine, Avicenna, and many other authors hold that women do have sperm? How can they and Galen and Aristotle all speak of the pleasure women derive from the emission of their own seed in intercourse? They are, Taddeo answered rather dismissively, not using the word "sperm" in its strict sense.

This notion, borrowed from Avicenna, that the inconsistencies among and within the works of authorities could be resolved by postulating two interpretations of "sperm," took on a more positive tone in the work of one of Taddeo's students, Dino del Garbo, himself a prolific medical writer.[39] In his commentary and questions on the Hippocratic *On the Nature of the Embryo*, Dino addressed the twofold question, Do women have sperm properly speaking, and (if so) is it a necessary principle of generation?[40] Dino's answers did not differ dramatically from Taddeo's, but the way in which he arrived at and phrased them accorded much more significance to the female contribution. Dino started with the premise that three things are necessary for reproduction to occur: two sperms and a womb. In the face of contemporary scholarship, including both a plethora of authoritative sources and a system of analysis which demanded greater precision and consistency, Dino could not, as Constantine had, leave the necessity of female seed unqualified. Thus he too was to conclude that what women produce is not sperm in the strict sense of the term, but he nevertheless gave it a certain prominence. His first arguments, which he would later modify by implication but not refute, were designed to show that women do indeed produce sperm. Although he might, like Taddeo, have mentioned Aristotle's references to female seed, he preferred to appeal to the authority of Hippocrates and

---

38 Albertus Magnus, *De animalibus*, bk. XI, tr. ii, ch. 1, §83. p. 707.
39 On Dino's life and work, see Siraisi, *Taddeo*, pp. 55–64 and passim.
40 Dinus de Florentia, *Recollectiones super libro Hypocratis* De natura fetus, in Bassanius Politus, comp., *De generatione embrionis*, fols. 46rb–48rb.

Avicenna – perhaps because they took its existence more seriously than Aristotle had. Authorities established, Dino proceeded to his treatment "from reason," starting with the argument that women have what is necessary to produce sperm. Since, like men, they produce a superfluity of the ultimate form of nutriment, they can make sperm, which Aristotle characterizes as just that. (And there is no more reason for a man to have this excess than a woman.) Furthermore, women, like men, have the organs necessary to produce sperm, namely, testes. Even Aristotle admits that menses undergo a whitening conversion, like the production of milk, to make the necessary material for generation. Dino offered ancillary evidence as well. Women have nocturnal emissions like men, and the retention of sperm causes serious ill effects in women, just as it does in men. Dino was not prepared to conclude on the basis of such arguments and evidence that women produce a seed equivalent to men's. The difficulties – such as the implication that females, having both the active principle and the matter, could then reproduce without males – were too grave. Furthermore, although the Hippocratic text on which he was commenting assumed the necessity of a female seed, no authority had argued systematically for so significant a female role.

What Dino was prepared to do was to use the notion that there are several senses of "sperm" to give far more substance and prominence to the female reproductive role than Taddeo Alderotti or Giles of Rome or Albertus Magnus's very Aristotelian *Questions on Animals*. Broadly defined and in common parlance, said Dino, sperm is "any humor having whiteness and thickness and emitted with pleasure and pulsation."[41] Strictly and properly speaking, sperm is "a moisture which is necessary in the act of generation, so that it not only has the four properties mentioned, namely that it is white and viscous and emitted with pleasure and with pulsation, but adds beyond these that it is a moisture capable of generation."[42] Sperm in this second sense has the power to generate something in the likeness of the organism from which it comes. Dino agreed with the more adamant Aristotelians that women lack sufficient heat to produce sperm in the stronger sense, but unlike them, he went on to discuss in some detail what women do produce, that is, sperm in the first sense, and what purpose it serves. What may be called the female sperm is a substance which descends from the womb (and which, for that reason, may very loosely be called "menstruum"). It is involved in women's nocturnal emissions, and we may suppose that it possesses the four qualifications for sperm in the broad sense – whiteness, viscosity, pleasure, and pulsations. Dino had already given the reason this substance cannot contain the active

41 Ibid., 47ra: "Large quod dicitur de omni humido habente albedinem cum viscositate emisso cum delectatione et pulsu."
42 Ibid., fol. 47ra: "Et hoc modo dicitur sperma solum prout est humiditas que est necessaria in actu generationis, ita quod non solum habet proprietates quatuor predictas, scilicet quod sit album et viscosum cum delectatione emissum et cum pulsu, sed super hec addit, scilicet quod sit humiditas apta generationi."

principle of generation: the female heat is insufficient to give it that power. Can it be necessary for generation in some other way? The only other necessary component in the reproductive process is matter, but that role is played by the menstruum proper, a point to which Dino returned later.

Having insisted on the existence of this female sperm, Dino then had to face the possibility that it has no purpose. Nature, however, does nothing in vain. Although not *necessary* for generation, this fluid may *aid* the process in four ways. First, it can enhance the pleasure of coitus in the way that saliva, which comes to the mouth when one is hungry, enhances the pleasure of food. Second, in those cases in which the male semen is too hot for generation, the female semen can moderate it, making it suitable. Third, it provides lubrication which allows the male sperm to be more easily drawn into the womb. And finally, by filling up the space in the womb, it helps to keep the male sperm in place there. Other scholastic authors who, like Dino, affirmed the existence of some sort of nonessential female sperm offered variations on these functions. Albertus Magnus, for example, distinguished a separate fluid, which is not in any sense seed, and which he called "sweat," operating in the manner of Dino's "saliva." He agreed that in some cases the female sperm's incorporation with the male sperm makes it possible for the womb to draw in the seed, but whereas Dino saw the function of the female semen in this case as mere lubrication, Albertus saw it as counteracting the overlubrication caused by the sweat.[43] Dino does not take advantage of the additional point made by Constantine the African, that female seed moderates too-powerful male seed.[44]

The female sperm that Dino del Garbo thus described would seem to be white, thick, and associated with pleasure and pulsation, but not, in spite of his first assertion, necessary for generation. He added, without much elaboration, that women do have a "seed" which, although apparently not emitted with pleasure and pulsation, and although in no sense active, is nevertheless essential to reproduction. This is the menstruum properly speaking, which, cooked and recooked, is a "pure and digested superfluity of the ultimate nutriment capable of having a principle (at least a material one) necessarily required for generation."[45] Once again, Dino did not depart from the letter of the Aristotelian insistence that nothing is required of the female in reproduction save the contribution of passive matter. But both

43 Albertus Magnus, *De animalibus*, bk. X, tr. i, ch. 1, §10–11, p. 734. On Albertus's multiplication of fluids, see Luke Demaitre and Anthony A. Travill, "Human Embryology and Development in the Works of Albertus Magnus," in James A. Weisheipl, ed., *Albertus Magnus and the Sciences: Commemorative Essays, 1980*, Studies and Texts 49 (Toronto: Pontifical Institute of Mediaeval Studies, 1980), p. 417. See also Danielle Jacquart and Claude Thomasset, "Albert le Grand et les problèmes de la sexualité," *History and Philosophy of the Life Sciences* 3 (1981): 77–82.
44 Constantinus *Theorica*, III, 34, in idem, *Pantegni*, fol. 14ra.
45 Dino, *De natura fetus*, fol. 47va: ". . . superfluitas ultimi alimenti pura et digesta potest habere principium necessario requisitum ad generationem saltim materiale."

here and with the more elaborate treatment of the fluid associated with female pleasure, he accorded the female contributions the greatest significance possible given their actual roles – in one case merely material and in the other case merely ancillary.

In Dino's view, the merely material role of the female semen precluded its being necessary for generation except insofar as the term applied in its loosest sense to menstruum, for the latter was the necessary and (because of nature's economy) sufficient source of the fetus's matter. But from early in the debate, other authors had extended the role of the nonmenstrual, intercourse-related female semen, even to the point of claiming it was required for reproduction. Taking their cue from Avicenna, who was in turn looking back to Galen, some said the substance of the female seed served as the matter for the membrane which encloses the fetus.[46] It would thus be necessary for the reproductive process without entering into the substance of the fetus's organs and thus without duplicating the role of the menstruum, which is supposed to supply them with matter.

Albertus Magnus, whose set of questions on Aristotle's *On Animals* had stuck close to the Philosopher's doctrines, took the role of the female seed a step further in his more complicated and less narrowly Aristotelian commentary on that same work written later in his career. According to Albertus, Galen had held that what he called "woman's sperm" was drawn out of her testes at the time of intercourse, had to be present for conception to occur, and possessed an "informative" virtue.[47] Albertus objected to much of this picture, but he did hint at the possibility of a certain level of activity on its part when he rehearsed a distinction, which he attributed to Galen, between "formative" power, possessed only by males, and "informative" power.[48] He conceded more positively the likelihood that female semen is necessary for conception, if still only in a material, not a formative, role. He posited not that it constitutes the material for the peripheral membranes but that it supplies the matter for the initial formation of the fetus itself. This position leaves him with a long series of standard objections to meet. He took seriously the Aristotelian objection that in other species the female is not observed to have the analogous emission. Rather than argue that humans are a special case, he suggested it is more probable that female animals do produce such seed, but that it is not observable. To the objection that women who have not experienced the emission of sperm at the time of intercourse nevertheless sometimes get pregnant, he responded that in those cases the male sperm has met up with female sperm which had descended into the womb at some earlier time. (Here Albertus implicitly offered an

46 Avicenna, *Liber canonis*, bk. III, fen xxi, ch. 2, fol. 361vb; Jacobus Forliviensis, *De generatione embrionis*, fols. 3rb–va and 9va–b.
47 Albertus Magnus, *De animalibus*, bk. XV, tr. ii, ch. 11, §142–5, pp. 1055.
48 Ibid., bk. XI, tr. ii, ch. 1, §83, p. 707.

alternative to the position expressed by earlier authors that a raped woman must experience some pleasure to conceive.) And to the objection that his position would involve an uneconomical duplication of the menstruum's function, he argued that the female seed is properly suited to the initial formation, whereas the menstruum is properly suited to the subsequent nourishment of the fetus. The seed, which has undergone a digestion, a whitening refinement, from its original sanguinous state, is already prepared to serve as the matter of a fetus; the menstruum, still in need of conversion, will be assimilated during the gestation process.[49]

Just as the moment of conception afforded room for what were understood to be Galenic or medical revisions of the female's place in the Aristotelian model of generation, so it was the occasion for some adjustment of the male's place. The question, first posed by Aristotle, whether the male semen persists materially in the fetus was, to judge from the frequency of its occurrence in commentaries and *questiones*, much less interesting to scholastic writers than the questions surrounding the female seed. In some respects what was at stake was equivalent to what was at stake in discussions about the female seed: admitting an active role for the female or a passive (material) role for the male erodes the strict Aristotelian distinction between the efficient, agent cause and the material cause, and thus between the sexes. In addition, the question involved the medium by which life was conveyed to the offspring. But the ontological parity of the two questions did not make them equally compelling for medieval authors, for whom the attribution of activity and power to the female was the subject of greater concern and therefore of more extensive discussion. Although keeping women in their place was hardly the main goal of scholastic treatments of the sexual division of labor, the tendency to give more attention to the problem of female activity than to the problem of male materiality may well suggest which case would be more disturbing within late medieval culture and society.

Like those who wrote about the female sperm, authors entertaining the question "Whether the male sperm is a material part of the fetus" sometimes framed it in terms of the disagreement between natural philosophers and medical writers, between Aristotle and Galen. According to Albertus Magnus:

There is a controversy surrounding this question between the Philosopher [Aristotle] and the medical writers. For the Philosopher argues that the sperm is not part of the conceptus, but only the agent [effecting it]. For he says that the sperm is to the conceptus as the craft or the artisan is to what is crafted. But the artisan is not a material part of the artifact. Therefore, the sperm will no more be part of the conceptus than the carpenter is part of the bench. The medical writers, however, argue that the sperm is part of the conceptus. For they hold that the fetus is made

---

49 Ibid., bk. XV, tr. ii, ch. 11, §142–5, pp. 1055–7.

from the mixture of the seed of both – the male and the female – otherwise there would be no part of the father in the child. But in bodily traits a child often resembles its father, which would not be the case were not its matter received from the father.[50]

Like other subjects advertised as points of contention between medical writers and natural philosophers, the topic of the male sperm's material persistence turns out *not* to have divided medieval authors into two camps according to their disciplinary commitments. Taddeo Alderotti, a medical writer commenting on a medical text, was familiar with the medical view that certain parts (especially white ones), such as bones and nerves, take their initial substance from the material part of the male sperm. But he was drawing on his broad and deep familiarity with Aristotelian natural philosophy when he disposed of the claim in short order. After observing that "we say that bone is a member made from sperm, and that what is made from something has that something in it," he countered that "an efficient cause is not a part of that which it effects, but sperm is, as it were, the efficient cause of the conceptus."[51] Taddeo reminded his listeners and readers of Aristotle's point that a carpenter is not part of a house. The male sperm is not, he concludes, a *material* part of the fetus. It is in the fetus only in the incorporeal sense that its virtue, or power, inheres in the embryo, as rennet, the efficient cause of coagulation, may be said to be in the cheese as it forms. Thus, he avoids permitting male semen to duplicate the material, female role, but then he adds almost parenthetically that "sperm" *may* be understood in a corporeal sense, in which case it is indeed part of the fetus.[52]

If Taddeo, a professor of medicine, was dismissive and trivialized the supposedly medical position, Albertus Magnus, lecturing on Aristotelian natural philosophy, took it more seriously. Like Taddeo's, Albertus's position is generally Aristotelian, emphasizing that the essential feature of the male sperm, its power or agency, is not material and is only "in" the fetus in a noncorporeal sense. The arguments he presented to the contrary are almost frivolous, such as the suggestion that, because the sperm is drawn from the male body, the generation which ensues is like the propagation of a plant from a cutting, the cutting persisting materially in the new plant.

50 Albertus Magnus, *Quaestiones de animalibus*, bk. XV, q. 20, p. 272: "Circa istam quaestionem controversia est inter Philosophum et medicos. Philosophus enim ponit sperma non esse partem concepti, sed solum agens. Dicit enim, quod sperma se habet ad conceptum sicut ars vel artifex ad artificiatum; sed artifex non est pars materialis artificii; ergo neque sperma erit pars concepti, sicut necque carpentator est pars scamni. Medici vero ponunt, quod sperma est pars concepti. Ponunt enim, quod fetus fit ex commixtione utriusque seminis, scilicet maris et feminae, alioquin in filio nihil esset de patre. Nunc autem in dispositionibus corporalibus multotiens filius assimilatur patri, quod non esset, nisi materia eius assumpta esset a patre."
51 Thaddeus Florentinus, *In* Isagogas *Joannitianas*, fol. 358ra: "Nos dicimus quod os est membrum factum ex spermate. . . . Causa efficiens non est pars eius quod efficit. Sed sperma est tanquam causa efficiens concepti. . . ."
52 Ibid., fol. 358ra–rb.

Nevertheless, when he came to considering the material component of the sperm, he treated it more seriously than Taddeo. Operating on a different understanding of the relationship between rennet and cheese, Albertus resolved the matter thus:

It seems to me one ought to say that there are two things in sperm, namely, the moisture (or the superfluity of fully digested food) and the power of the father's soul, existing in a certain foamy spirit. Hence, with regard to the moisture, the sperm can be part of the conceptus, just like the menstruum; with regard to the spirit itself, however, it cannot. For that humidity is at first mixed with the menstruum, just as wine [is mixed] with water or rennet with cheese. And it is well established that the rennet is part of the cheese and the water of the wine.[53]

Furthermore, although he denied that this material can be a necessary part of the conceptus – since that role of necessary material is played by the menstruum – Albertus allowed for the possibility that the material part of the male sperm plays a specific role in the composition of the embryo:

Nothing, however, prevents some material part of it from passing into the matter or body of the conceptus, as a result of which it is mixed with the menstruum. And this is how the medical authors understand it. And perhaps the principal and fundamental members are generated from it and the fluid members from the menstruum.[54]

Although he often upheld the Aristotelian view that the heart is the first and central organ, Albertus occasionally employed this medical distinction between the principal organs, which are formed first and which are of primary importance, and the secondary organs, which serve them. The first members of animals, he said at one point, take on substance "from the spermatic superfluity," from which they develop into the dominant parts.[55] In a variation on the medical opinion touched on by Taddeo, he also said that the nerves are generated in this way.[56] Albertus's commitment to this view is equivocal at best. Restrained phrasing ("nothing prevents"), ambiguity

---

53 Albertus Magnus, *Quaestiones de animalibus*, bk. XV, q. 20, p. 272: "Videtur tamen esse mihi dicendum, quod in spermate duo sunt, scilicet humiditas vel superfluitas ultimi cibi et virtus animae patris in quodam spiritu spumoso existens. Unde quantum ad humiditatem potest sperma esse pars concepti sicut menstruum, quantum tamen ad ipsum spiritum non, quia ipsa humiditas primo commiscetur cum menstruo, sicut vinum cum aqua vel coagulum cum lacte. Constat autem coagulum esse partem casei et aquam vini. . . ." On the sense in which water becomes part of wine when mixed with it, see Joan Cadden, "The Medieval Philosophy and Biology of Growth: Albertus Magnus, Thomas Aquinas, Albert of Saxony and Marsilius of Inghen on Book I, Chapter v of Aristotle's *De generatione et corruptione*" (Ph.D. diss., Indiana University, 1971).
54 Albertus Magnus, *Quaestiones de animalibus*, bk. XV, q. 20, p. 273: "Nihil tamen prohibet aliquam partem eius materialem cedere in materiam vel corpus concepti, ex quo commiscetur cum menstruo, et sic intelligunt medici. Et forte ex illo generantur membra principalia et radicalia, ex menstruo fluentia membra."
55 Ibid., bk. XVI, tr. ii, c. 6, §§122–3, p. 1129: ". . . ex superfluitate spermatica. . . ."
56 Ibid., bk. IX, tr. ii, ch. 2, pp. 710–14.

about the relationship between the spermatic superfluity and food, and direct arguments for the sufficiency of menstrual blood accompany his suggestions that there might be a material role for the male sperm. Nevertheless, by making room for these views, which he labels "medical," Albertus Magnus has, albeit grudgingly, undermined the dichotomy he himself had set up between the Aristotelian and Galenic traditions and has in the process slightly muted the Aristotelian dichotomy between female and male.

The question of the material contribution of the male sperm thus complemented those surrounding the necessity and activity of the female sperm in the way in which it posed and then revised the perception of conflicts between the medical and philosophical traditions and in the way in which it reaffirmed yet mitigated the sexual division of labor with respect to reproduction. But the two sets of issues were not of equal concern to medieval authors. Treatments of the former are few, short, and relatively uncomplicated, and treatments of the latter are more numerous, more extensive, and more likely to implicate other dimensions of the reproductive process, such as the means by which a fetus comes to resemble its mother or its father. Furthermore, whereas scholastic discussions of the material persistence of the male seed are contained almost exclusively within the small number of questions specifically devoted to it, discussions of an active female role spilled over into the scholastic treatments of other subjects, most notably into the problem of sex determination: what causes a fetus to be male or female?

FATHERS AND SONS: HOW THE EMBRYO ACQUIRES ITS SEX

Prescholastic authors had expressed a range of views about how a fetus comes to be a male or a female. Constantine the African had, at one point, coordinated two ancient perspectives on the subject, saying that (1) if the united male and female sperms settle on the right side of the womb, the child will be male; if on the left side, female; and (2) if they settle in the middle, the child's sex will depend on the quantity of the two sperms. At another point he added another pair of theories, saying that males result (1) from the dominance of sperm from the father's right testicle and (2) from the heat associated with strong sexual appetite. Hildegard's perspective was simpler and slightly different, being consistent with Aristotle's view while showing no indication of having been directly influenced by it: the child's sex depends on the strength of the father's seed. *On Human Generation* preferred the left–right inclinations of the medical tradition, emphasizing the fetus's position in the uterus. Even as late as the early thirteenth century, Michael Scot, whose translations and writings had an important effect on scholastic natural philosophy but who was writing outside the incipient university environment, did not hesitate to string together varying explanations for sex determination. Without feeling compelled to explain further, he asserted that it is not left and right in general, as some say, but the left and right male testicles which cause females and males respectively. (Witness, he suggested, the situation in which a wounded soldier has only one testicle and only produces children of the corresponding sex.) But then he added that if a lot of seed enters the womb and settles in its seven cells, the embryos on the right will be males, those on the left will be females, and the one in the middle will be a hermaphrodite.[57]

These authors felt free to collect or select causes without extensive comment or justification. In general, before the assimilation of the full range of Greek and Arabic authorities and before the rise of the comparative and systematizing impulses of scholasticism, all the juxtaposing, harmonizing, distinction making, and determinations characteristic of thirteenth- and fourteenth-century university circles were unfamiliar and uncalled for. More specifically, the earlier authors' choices were not seriously limited by their opinions on the role of the female seed, from which they remained more or less separate. Later authors, like Albertus Magnus or Jacopo of Forlì, on the other hand, had not only to meet the general demands of the scholastic method but also to coordinate their opinions on sex determination with their specific conclusions concerning the reproductive contributions of males and females. Although Albertus and Jacopo both mentioned a vast array of factors in connection with sex determination, they turned their serious attention to only a small cluster of them. Thus while their writings pass on some of the diversity of the older traditions, the thrust of their work largely focuses and crystallizes the subject around the male semen. The systematic understanding of female and male reproductive contributions weighed heavily in favor of, if it did not always logically imply, certain conclusions about sex determination, such as the notion that females are the result of insufficiently warmed and concocted male seed.

In spite of their differences on what lines to draw where, scholastic authors generally agreed that the role of the female seed – if such a thing existed at all – was very limited. Thus, although they might occasionally and momentarily seem to subscribe to some version of the Hippocratic opinion that the male and the female seeds compete to determine the offspring's sex,[58] in their serious discussions of the subject they had to take their conclusions about the female semen into account. Taddeo Alderotti argued, for example, that no matter how great a female's physiological power, no matter how strong her animal, natural, or spiritual virtues, *with respect to sperm* she cannot be stronger than a male. Even when commenting

---

57 Michaelis Scotus, *De secretis naturae*, in *Alberti Magni De secretis mulierum. Item De virtutibus herbarum, lapidum et animalium. De mirabilibus mundi. Michaelis Scoti libellus De secretis naturae* (Amsterdam: I. Ianssonius, 1643), pt. I, ch. vii, pp. 243–5.
58 Thaddeus Florentinus, *In Isagogas Joannitianas*, fol. 372rb.

on a medical text, Taddeo took what was probably the simplest course: he supported the Aristotelian position that the father's heart, as the source of greater or lesser warmth, is the ultimate cause of the offspring's sex. The heart determines the heating and refinement of the male semen, which in turn gives the seed its strength, its virtue. "The strength of virtue of the male's sperm over the woman's sperm produces a male; and its weakness over it makes a female."[59] The phrasing here, emphasizing the strength or weakness of the male component, rather than the relative strength of female and male, stresses the Aristotelian passivity of the female contribution, the matter.

Taddeo offers more abstract (and equally Aristotelian) reasons to preclude a determinative role for the womb, the other potential source of female influence. The formation of the sexual organs may take place in the womb, but those members, although they are essential to the *operations* of males and females, are not the source of the determination of male and female. In other words, Taddeo marginalized the concrete anatomical manifestations of sex difference and placed at its center the abstract teleological principles. The sexual members are at the service of the purpose, the final cause of maleness and femaleness. In this more fundamental sense, sex difference is determined in a primary and formal way by the seed, even before the development of the embryo. Thus, even though male and female principles cannot be realized without the appropriate reproductive organs, the final cause, the defining purpose of an embryo's sex, is logically and chronologically prior to the formation of the organs: "The end disposes those things which exist for the end."[60] Likewise supporting the notion that sex is determined from the beginning by the father's seed, Albertus Magnus pointed to the absurdity of the implication that the conditions of the womb could *change* a male fetus into a female and vice versa.[61]

Not all authors allowed abstract considerations of cause and form to limit their ideas about what makes a child female or male. Jacopo of Forlì, a physician, citing Giles of Rome, a philosopher, named a variety of factors that affect the outcome, including some inconsistent with Albertus's and Taddeo's views.[62] One brief treatise, "Chapter on the Cause of Masculinity and Femininity," enumerates the various levels at which the question can be addressed, associating the appropriate authority with each: (1) the ability of males and inability of females to effect full digestion of seed (Aristotle); (2) the warm male complexion and cool female (Aristotle); (3) the heart

59 Ibid., fol. 372ra: "Fortitudo virtutis spermatis maris super sperma mulieris facit masculum, et eius debilitas super ipsum facit feminam."
60 Ibid., fols. 371vb–372ra: "Finis ordinat ea que sunt ad finem" (372ra).
61 Albertus Magnus, *Quaestiones de animalibus*, bk. XVIII, q. 1, p. 296. Cf. bk. IX, q. 18, p. 210.
62 Jacobus Forliviensis, *De generatione embrionis*, fol. 10ra–va.

(Avicenna); (4) the heart and genitals (Aristotle); and (5) various accidental causes (Hippocrates, Galen, and others).[63] But the center of academic treatment (including Jacopo's) was the father's seed.

The premise that sex determination originates with the father's semen (or, ultimately, with the father's capacity to concoct semen, which resides in his heart) is also the basis of the Aristotelian notion that every female child is a failed male child. If taken to mean that girls are essentially birth defects or monstrosities, the employment of the phrase *mas occasionatus* – a ruined or defective male – would seem less an incidental implication of ideas about reproductive roles and more a salvo of medieval misogyny. But the scholastic philosophers who employed the term thus translated from Aristotle's *Generation of Animals* invoked it in an explicitly limited sense and with larger principles of natural philosophy in mind.[64] According to Albertus Magnus, since the father's sperm is determinative, and since whatever reproduces seeks as much as possible to create a likeness of itself, the goal of the male sperm is to produce sons. But the father's heat is not always sufficient to prepare the sperm adequately for the task, and thus females are frequently born.[65] Speaking of the blindness of moles, Albertus insists that such regular deficiencies cannot be treated as "failures" in the strict sense. Although ordinarily eyes are for seeing and thus blindness is a defect, in moles, which hunt for food in the darkness underground, sight would be superfluous.[66] There is thus a reason for the mole's apparent deficiency, the failure of its eyes to be realized and perfected. The medieval natural world encompassed varying degrees of perfection, including defects which occurred with some persistence. Female offspring, although the result of some material necessity, such as a lack of seminal warmth, had, nevertheless, their own purpose, their own final cause. (In this respect they differed from hermaphrodites, whose occurrence could be explained on a material level but not on a teleological level.) For Thomas Aquinas, not simply the natural order but rather divine intention is at stake. If females were simply accidents or monsters, they would not have been among those first things that, according to Genesis, God created. With respect to their specific nature in relation to the active virtue of the male seed, females may be said to be deficient or failed. "But with respect to universal nature, the female is not something failed but

63 Nicolaus Florentinus, "Capitula de causa masculinitatis et femininitatis," in *Excerpta*, British Library, Sloane 336, fols. 156r–159v. The author may be the Nicolas of Florence identified by Thorndike (*History of Magic and Experimental Science*, vol. 3, p. 565) and Wickersheimer (*Dictionnaire des médicins*) or a later writer.
64 Albert Mitterer catalogues and explicates the connotations of *occasionatus* in Aristotle, Albertus Magnus, and Thomas Aquinas in "*Mas occasionatus* oder zwei Methoden der Thomasdeutung," *Zeitschrift für katholische Theologie* 72 (1950): 80–103.
65 Albertus Magnus, *De animalibus*, bk. XVI, tr. i, ch. 14, §72–3, pp. 1099–100.
66 Ibid., bk. I, tr. ii, ch. 3, §140–1, p. 51.

is ordained for the purpose of generation by the intention of nature," which proceeds from God.[67]

These views on the way sex is determined resonate with values – active and passive, strong and deficient. But in the context of academic teaching and scholarship they were not consciously, much less willfully, chosen to denigrate women. Rather, they formed part of a coherent system of reproductive theory, which, in spite of differences between the "medical" and "philosophical" versions, provided a common ground for scholastic authors. Abstract considerations, such as form and matter or activity and passivity, and concrete considerations, such as the regular occurrence of male and female children or the resemblance of offspring to their parents, all fit more or less comfortably into the framework that thirteenth- and fourteenth-century authors constructed in the course of answering questions on the female seed and related subjects. Although not constructed as instruments of a misogynist agenda, the extent and contents of scholarly production on the subject of sex determination had implications for more general attitudes toward masculinity and femininity treated in the next chapter.

THE RISE AND DIVISION OF PLEASURE

The scholastic treatment of female seed and sex determination owed much to the classical traditions that had been preserved in or reintroduced into medieval Europe. The consciousness of differences between a medical and a philosophical school helped to determine the appropriate topics for discussion, even though the differences themselves were not really the basis for significant divisions among medieval thinkers. In addition, views that were reported and dismissed by the dominant ancient authorities added intricacy and importance to the debates. Such was not the case for the subject of sexual pleasure, which, like the question of reproductive contributions, helped to shape late medieval notions of sex difference: the function of sexual pleasure and the distinction between male and female pleasure were not matters of special interest to the classical authors with whom the scholastics were conversant. Ancient authors had spoken of desire, appetite, and attraction, but they seldom linked these phenomena to broader aspects of sexuality. Thus, when late medieval authors began to take an interest in these matters, they sometimes hung their treatments on incidental remarks by the ancient authors, such as Aristotle's assertion in *Physics* (where he is explaining the relationship of form and matter) that matter desires form as

---

67 Thomas Aquinas, *Summa theologiae*, bk. I, q. 92, art. 1, p. 654: "Sed per comparationem ad naturam universalem, femina non est aliquid occasionatum, sed est de intentione naturae ad opus generationis ordinata."

female desires male.[68] Arabic authors had somewhat more to say about specifically sexual appetite.[69] But with the exception of a passage in Avicenna's *Canon* that discusses male and female pleasure in the context of overcoming impediments to conception,[70] such works explored the subject of desire more than the subject of pleasure, insofar as the two were distinguished[71] and were concerned almost exclusively with the experiences of men. Late medieval authors, therefore, had only a few authoritative texts to draw upon, and no ancient controversy around which to frame a set of questions. These considerations help to explain why the subject of sexual pleasure commands far less attention in scholastic works than, say, the subject of the female seed. Yet, if not at the center of a persistent controversy, the nature of sexual pleasure and the possibility of distinguishing female and male pleasure nevertheless figured prominently in a good number of medical and natural philosophical works of the thirteenth and fourteenth centuries. Passing comments by Aristotle that a woman can conceive without having experienced pleasure and that female humans, unlike the females of other species, are always sexually receptive, as well as Galen's concept of an appetitive virtue in the womb, may have helped to direct and legitimate these discussions, but for the most part they were medieval in origin and content.

Writings of the preceding centuries contributed significantly to scholastic interest in pleasure. As we have seen, Constantine the African, Hildegard of Bingen, and *On Human Generation* all raised questions about pleasure. What is it for? What is its relation to conception? Is it manifested differently in men and women? Although not always explicitly acknowledged, the influence of the earlier medical literature and especially of Constantine is frequently detectable in the later discussions.

The purpose of pleasure

The idea of Constantine most often invoked is his opening justification of intercourse and its pleasures as part of the divine plan of Creation in *On*

---

68 Aristotle, *The Physics*, ed. and trans. Philip H. Wicksteed and Francis M. Cornford, 2 vols., Loeb Classical Library (Cambridge: Harvard University Press; London: William Heinemann, 1957–60), I, ix, 192a20–23, vol. 1, p. 94.

69 See Avicenna, *Liber canonis*, bk. III, fen i, tr. 5, chs. 24–5, fol. 190va–b; Mary Frances Wack, "The *Liber de hereos morbo* of Johannes Afflacius," pp. 324–44; 344; and idem, *Lovesickness in the Middle Ages: The* Viaticum *and Its Commentaries*, Middle Ages Series (Philadelphia: University of Pennsylvania Press, 1990).

70 Avicenna, *Liber canonis*, bk. III, fen xx, tr. 2, chs. 43–5, fol. 358ra–b.

71 Pleasure and desire continued to be closely related in the Latin tradition. See, e.g., Johannes de Sancto Amando, *Die Concordanciae des Johannes de Sancto Amando nach einer Berliner und zwei Erfurter Handschriften . . . herausgegeben*, ed. Julius Leopold Pagel (Berlin: Georg Reimer, 1894), p. 391; and Helen Rodnite Lemay, "William of Saliceto on Human Sexuality," *Viator* 12 (1981): 166, n. 3.

Coitus: "As Constantine says, pleasure is attached to intercourse so that it will be more desired, and thus generation will continue."[72] (Late medieval academics chose not to cite Constantine's phrasing elsewhere, which brought out the irrationality of pleasure.)[73] This straightforward teleological explanation, although it never became a disputed proposition, attracted a certain amount of attention among scholastic authors and even became the subject of mild contention in their hands. By the second half of the thirteenth century, the teleology had taken on a more explicitly Aristotelian cast. From the psychological perspective, the imagination, memory, or judgment of pleasure might give rise to sexual appetite.[74] From the metaphysical perspective, every agent takes pleasure in fulfilling its own proper purpose; ensuring the eternity of the species was a very noble end; and the higher the purpose, the greater the pleasure.[75]

In addition to expressing Constantine's dictum in up-to-date philosophical language, scholastic authors suggested two different understandings of what it was that pleasure was designed to overcome. The first and more pragmatic reading highlighted reasons females in particular might be reluctant to have intercourse. Albertus Magnus pointed out that animals would otherwise have good reason to abhor coitus, given the burden of pregnancy, the pain of childbirth, and the trouble of caring for offspring.[76] Likewise, Giles of Rome, writing in a theological context, suggested that women receive greater pleasure in intercourse to encourage them to engage in it in spite of the pain of childbirth.[77] The second reading did not distinguish between males and females but stressed the suspect associations of sexual behavior. Gilbert the Englishman, a physician writing in the midthirteenth century, gave Constantine's preface a slightly moralistic tone, taking it to mean that without desire and pleasure, creatures might find intercourse disgusting, and thus their lines might perish.[78] Writing a few decades later, Bernard of Gordon, professor of medicine at the university in Montpellier, cited Ovid to support the view that pleasure enabled animals to overcome their aversion in order to perpetuate their kind. But he seemed to suggest that human beings *ought* to have ample motivation for intercourse without

72 Albertus Magnus, *De animalibus*, bk. IX, tr. 2, ch. 3, §303, p. 716: ". . . sed delectatio, ut dicit Constantinus, apponitur coitui ut plus appetatur et sic continuetur generatio."
73 Constantinus, *Theorica*, V, 107, in idem, *Pantegni*, fol. 25ra.
74 Bernardus de Gordonio, *Practica dicta Lilium* (Venice: Bonetus Locatellus, 1498), pt. VII, ch. i, fol. 87vb; Albertus Magnus, *Quaestiones de animalibus*, bk. V, q. 6, p. 157. This formulation is linked in turn to the Galenic view that the process starts in the brain. Bernardus de Gordonio, *Lilium*, pt. VII, ch. i, fol. 88ra.
75 Johannes de Sancto Amando, *Concordanciae*, p. 328. John is refuting the argument that the pleasure experienced by the whole body in intercourse constitutes evidence in favor of pangenesis.
76 Albertus Magnus, *De animalibus*, bk. XXII, tr. i, ch. 1, §2, p. 1350.
77 Hewson, *Giles of Rome*, p. 91, referring to his commentary on Peter Lombard's *Sentences*.
78 Gilbertus Anglicus, *Compendium medicine* (Lyon: Jacobus Saccon, 1510), bk. VII, ch. [i], fol. 287va.

the addition of pleasure, when he (falsely) attributed to Constantine the following epigram: "Few have intercourse for the sake of offspring, more for the sake of health, and many more for the sake of pleasure."[79] Bernard's formulation highlighted the social and moral aspects of the issue by distinguishing elements which Constantine's formulation had fused: it suggested that the species would not in fact perish without sexual pleasure – if the example of the righteous few were followed.

The introduction of a moral dimension into the discussion of pleasure's natural function, discussed more fully in Chapter 6, suggested to some authors a distinction between the human situation and that of animals – a distinction explicitly precluded by Constantine, who had introduced his treatise on human intercourse with the Creator's plan for animals' perpetuation.[80] John of St. Amand, another thirteenth-century medical writer, noting that the authorities do not agree, held that animals have intercourse, not for pleasure, but because nature compels them to do so in order to relieve a buildup of seed. Pious men likewise have intercourse to relieve a superfluity, but unlike animals, they are capable of pleasure and therefore of exercising restraint.[81] Distinguishing humans from animals would suggest that the reluctance which, according to Gilbert the Englishman, had to be overcome, might be specific to human beings, perhaps related to their postlapsarian sense of shame. But Gilbert himself held, to the contrary, that, "This force [pleasure] is common to beasts and humans, the foolish and the wise, men and women."[82] An anonymous Aristotelian treatise on animals mentions that horses enjoy coitus more than any other animal except humans, thus offering yet another perspective: animal–human differences are a matter of degree.[83] As a scholastic interested in the concord and dissonance of authorities, John of St. Amand acknowledged disagreement on this point, citing Isaac Israeli and Galen.[84]

Statements about the ultimate purpose of pleasure, even those that incorporated a moral dimension, did not usually distinguish between male pleasure and female pleasure: both were designed for the same end, procreation. But if the final cause of sexual pleasure is essentially the same for men and women, the mechanisms of pleasure and the conceptualization of pleasure as

---

79 Bernardus de Gordonio, *Lilium*, pt. VII, ch. i, fol. 87vb: "Et dicit Constantinus quod pauci coeunt propter prolem sed plures propter sanitatem sed plurimum valde propter delectationem."
80 Constantinus, *De coitu*, p. 299: "Creator volens animalium genus fermiter ac stabiliter permanere. . . ."
81 Johannes de Sancto Amando, *Concordantie artis medicine*, Bayerische Staatsbibliothek, MS CLM 8742, fol. 9rb.
82 Gilbertus Anglicus, *Compendium medicine*, bk. VII, ch. [i], fol. 287va: "Communis enim est hec virtus bestiis et hominibus, stultis et sapientibus, viris et feminis."
83 *Propositiones de animalibus*, Cambridge University Library, MS Dd.3.16, fol. 74va.
84 Johannes de Sancto Amando, *Concordantie artis medicine*, Bayerische Staatsbibliothek, MS CLM 8742, fol. 9rb.

an efficient cause or as a sign of sexual function sometimes presented themselves differently for the two sexes.

The mechanisms of pleasure

For the most part, scholastic authors commented only casually on the anatomy and physiology of pleasure. Differences of opinion on those subjects did not give rise to debates or attempts at resolution, except insofar as they played some part in arguments about pangenesis, expositions of lovesickness, or the question whether women or men experience more pleasure. Notions about the causes and sites of pleasure were closely tied to notions about the origins and pathways of desire or semen. These links arose, among other things, from the idea that pleasure was an incentive and thus acted as an immediate end in the service of the larger final cause, procreation. The idea or memory of pleasure was widely held to be the motive cause of arousal, seed production, and, ultimately, pleasure itself. Gilbert the Englishman gave a well developed account of the process. The appetite for intercourse arises from thought, which produces a motion toward sexual pleasure. This, in turn, effects an excitation of spirit in the heart, which passes to the penis, where, made subtle by a virtue there, it enters the hollow nerves of the penis, filling and extending it. Gilbert goes on to say that the brain is the organ which ultimately sends the semen to the penis, and the liver is the origin of the appetite and pleasures.[85]

Like most such accounts in antiquity and the Middle Ages, Gilbert's turns out to be concerned with men. Although occasional references to women's thoughts and memories in connection with sexual pleasure suggest that the early stages of the process were understood to be similar in women, no scholastic author took on a comparison of the anatomy and physiology of male and female sexuality as Hildegard had at the end of the twelfth century. The subject did arise in the context of comparisons of the amount of pleasure men and women experience in intercourse, discussed later, but otherwise the clues are scattered and undeveloped. Thomas of Cantimpré, a contemporary of Gilbert's, in a work that belonged to the older encyclopedic tradition rather than the newer scholastic modes, described male sexual arousal as an interaction among mind, heart, liver, kidneys, and penis, and mentioned elsewhere that the *umbilicus* is the seat of lust in the female, as the kidneys are in the male.[86] John of St. Amand held otherwise. Calling on Galen's notion of a natural faculty of attraction, he says, "There is a strong

85 Gilbertus Anglicus, *Compendium medicine*, bk. V, ch. [i], fol. 287va.
86 Thomas Cantimpratensis, *De naturis rerum*, bk. I, chs. 61 and 56, edited in Christoph Ferckel, *Die Gynakologie des Thomas von Brabant. Ein Beitrag zur Kenntnis der mittelalterlichen Gynäkologie und ihrer Quellen: Ausgewählte Kapitel aus Buch I* [De anatomia corporis humani] *De naturis rerum beendet um 1240*, Alte Meister der Medizin und Naturkunde 5 (Munich: C. Kuhn, 1912), p. 47. See also Albertus Magnus, *De animalibus*, bk. X, tr. i, ch. 5, §65, p. 756.

appetitive power in the sex organ [*vulva*], for by nature it possesses strength of the faculty in ejecting sperm with great desire and pleasure."[87] In part, the lack of clarity and agreement about the geography of pleasure is the result of the different contexts in which the comments are made – sometimes speaking of immediate causes, for example, and sometimes of less proximate causes. In part, too, the differences can be traced to different sources, which the scholastic authors did not attempt to resolve or harmonize.

From the turn of the thirteenth century, one medical concern did, however, focus some attention on the origins and mechanisms of pleasure. This was the complaint known as *amor heroicus*, or lovesickness, mentioned by Constantine in his *Viaticum* and the subject of considerable elaboration in commentaries on that work. In a study of these commentaries, Mary Wack argues convincingly that in the course of exploring the etiology of lovesickness, Peter of Spain, an expert on both medicine and philosophy, shifted the balance of interpretation from an emphasis on the somatic, implicating the testicles (and, one might add, the liver, site of the lower functions, and the penis), to an emphasis on the psychological. The more somatic, material, and directly sexual aspects of lovesickness retain significance, but they are not the locus of the pathology. The disorder results from a failure of reason or judgment, in particular of the imaginative, estimative, cognitive, or other faculties.[88] This reorientation, as developed a few decades later by Arnald of Villanova, who was to become a professor of medicine at Montpellier, brought pleasure directly into the picture: the patient has imprinted in his imagination and memory the form of an object of desire with which he associates great pleasure and which he hopes to obtain. The pleasure sought and judged a good worthy of pursuit is, however, a harmful one – not because it is a sexual pleasure per se, but because of the pathological effects of the obsession.[89] The psychological emphasis in turn led Peter of Spain, both philosopher and physician, to mediate between the Aristotelian seat of the psyche, the heart, and the Galenic seat of the mental functions, the brain. The former, he concluded, is the origin of passionate love, neither harmful in itself nor conducive to lovesickness, but the latter can give rise to the disorder. Thus Peter of Spain and a number of authors who followed him found reason to sort out some of the anatomy and physiology of pleasure in order to deal with this complaint, which, at least partly because of its social and literary associations, had attracted their attention.

---

87 Johannes de Sancto Amando, *Concordanciae*, p. 391: "In vulva est fortis virtus appetitiva, quia natura fortitudinem habet virtutis in spermate ejiciendo cum nimio desiderio et delectatione."

88 Wack, *Lovesickness*, pp. 90–8. The history of the term itself is revealing: see Wack, pp. 46–7 and 60–1; and Danielle Jacquart and Claude Thomasset, "L'amour 'héroïque' à travers le traité d'Arnaud de Villeneuve," in Jean Céard, ed., *La folie et le corps* (Paris: Presses de l'Ecole Normale Supérieur, 1985), pp. 150–4.

89 Jacquart and Thomasset, "L'amour 'héroïque,'" pp. 147–8.

Lovesickness in particular, like late medieval comments about sexual pleasure in general, had mainly to do with men. In addition to the general presumption that the patient is male, the definition of the condition came to include the specification that it primarily afflicts noble men, and the remedies involve such practices as distracting the patient with women other than the object of the obsession. Yet, perhaps as a result of Peter of Spain's innovative approach to the subject, scholastic authors developed a minor interest in women's susceptibility as well. Albertus Magnus regarded women as more susceptible to apparent or misguided love (as opposed to true love) because of the weakness of their reason. On account of a corruption of their judgment, they desire intercourse more.[90] Peter of Spain himself held that women were prone to lovesickness because they were, according to Aristotle, less hopeful and more easily depressed than men (a characteristic related to their moistness). Men, on the other hand, were prone to this suffering because of their ability to retain the image of the desired woman (a characteristic related to their dryness).[91] Thus the inclusion of women in the scholastic treatment of lovesickness signaled not a conflation of the male and female pathologies associated with this suffering in the pursuit of imagined pleasure but rather a distinction between male and female susceptibilities and experiences. This distinction is more fully manifested when these authors respond to the question, Who experiences greater pleasure?

The special case of lovesickness has implications for discussions of pleasure in other contexts. For example, the psychological dimensions, especially the role of imagination and memory, are present in many scholastic texts not directly related to the illness. In addition, while clarifying and specifying some of the anatomical and physiological aspects of pleasure, authors writing about lovesickness tended to confirm the diversity of the experience of pleasure and of academic reasoning about it. Thus Peter of Spain, ranging from the mechanical to the metaphysical, responded to the question, "Why is there so much pleasure in intercourse?":

There are four causes. The first is the disposition of the members, which are very sensitive, since [they are] of a nervous nature. The second cause concerns its operation, since every power takes pleasure in its own operation. . . . The third cause is the spermatic moisture's coursing through the members, for it brings on a certain tickling and pleasurable motion. The fourth cause is the nerve-filled members rubbing against each other, from which a temperate heat arises. And those are the causes of pleasure in intercourse. Some also assign a fifth cause regarding the purpose, saying that God placed a great pleasure in such an act lest, on account of its uncleanness, animals should loath it, and thus generation would fail.[92]

90 Albertus Magnus, *Quaestiones de animalibus*, bk. V, q. 4, p. 156.
91 Wack, *Lovesickness*, pp. 114–15.
92 Peter of Spain, *Questions on the* Viaticum, Version B (ed. in Wack, *Lovesickness*, pp. 244, 246): ". . . quattuor sunt cause: Prima est dispositio membrorum que sunt valde sensibilia quia nervosa. Secunda causa est a parte sue operationis quia quelibet virtus delectatur

These late medieval views on the anatomy and physiology of pleasure in general and on lovesickness as a specific disorder illustrate two sets of tension or ambiguity. First, whereas some discussions, like the one just cited, apply to both sexes, others distinguish between them or take the male to be the norm. Second, whereas the mechanisms of pleasure are sometimes connected with their ultimate purpose, they nevertheless retain a certain autonomy. Peter of Spain's list of the five causes of pleasure does not accord hierarchical privilege to its ultimate purpose. On the contrary, it includes procreation rather grudgingly. These two sets of tensions – the equivalence and differences between the sexes and the association and dissociation of pleasure and procreation – also play themselves out in the ways in which pleasure was understood to function. In particular, the possibility, and even naturalness, of nonreproductive sexual pleasure undermined the simple teleology of Constantine's formulation; and the isolation of certain instances of female pleasure bestowed dark undertones upon women's sexuality.

The functions of pleasure

For men, even though the emission of seed was separable from sexual pleasure in several ways, late medieval authors generally linked pleasure with ejaculation and with the ability to effect conception. At the very least, the male sensation of pleasure was identified with that which impelled his seed in the direction of the womb. Although, strictly speaking, male pleasure per se was neither necessary nor sufficient for conception, its association with the emission of seed made it an accepted sign of male sexual function. On a theoretical level, Albertus Magnus insisted specifically on a difference between pleasure and the essential "seminitive power" of seed. He took Constantine's dictum to imply that sexual pleasure is something distinct. It is attached to intercourse but is not naturally inherent in it: "Not pleasure according to nature but, as Constantine says, pleasure attached to coitus so that it is more sought after, and thus generation is continued."[93] Not only is pleasure intellectually separable from seed, but there are regular occasions on which men emit seed without pleasure, specifically in nocturnal emissions. Medical writers agreed with ecclesiastics concerned to distinguish between these "pollutions," as they called them, and waking ejaculations, which could

in propria operatione. . . . Tertia causa est discursus humiditatis spermatice per membra; inducit enim quandam titillationem et motum delectabilem. Quarta causa est confricatio membrorum nervosorum ad invicem ex qua provenit calor temperatus, et iste sunt cause delectationis in cohitu. Quintam etiam causam assignant aliqui a parte finis dicentes quod magnam posuit deus delectationem in opere tali ne propter eius immundiciam ab animalibus abhominaretur et sic deficeret generatio."

93 Albertus Magnus, *De animalibus*, bk. IX, tr. ii, ch. 3, §103, p. 716: ". . . nomen spermatis est ex ratione virtutis sementivae: et ad hoc non intenditur delectatio secundum naturam, sed delectatio, ut dicit Constantinus, apponitur coitui ut plus appetatur et sic continuetur generatio."

pose a threat to chastity. (Jean Gerson, preacher, humanist, and Church politician, wrote a tract, *On Pollution*, at the turn of the fifteenth century, which cited Thomas Aquinas and other authors, "both theological and scientific," in favor of his position that a priest who has had a nocturnal emission is not forbidden to celebrate mass.)[94] Just as there may be emission without pleasure, so there may be pleasure without the production of true semen, as was held to be the case with the emissions of adolescent boys. But the situations in which pleasure and emission are dissociated take place outside the context of intercourse. Where intercourse and reproduction are concerned, most late medieval authors assumed or asserted the regular connection with male pleasure. Although John of St. Amand and Bernard of Gordon both held that men could and should engage in intercourse for purposes other than pleasure, they did not deny that pleasure would be (incidentally) involved. Some theologians did entertain the possibility of reproductive intercourse without pleasure.[95] But from the twelfth-century canonist who insisted sex was always somewhat sinful because it was always pleasurable[96] to the fifteenth-century medical writer who listed insufficient pleasure as a cause of reproductive failure,[97] scholars confirmed the commonplace conjunction between the ejaculation of active semen and the experience of pleasure in men. Nevertheless, the notion that male pleasure is in some sense an efficient cause or necessary condition of conception is rare. Perhaps for that reason, as well as because of the uncontroversial nature of the pleasure–seed connection in men, scholastic authors, whether in medicine or in natural philosophy, did not regard male sexual pleasure per se as a matter of any serious interest.

Because pleasure and the emission of seed were so closely associated, the role of pleasure in conception was more controversial with respect to women than with respect to men: it raised, in another way, the problem of the female seed. William of Conches had explained prostitutes' infertility in terms of their lack of pleasure in intercourse and had gone so far as to insist that raped women, all appearances to the contrary, must experience some pleasure, since they sometimes conceive. This position was repeated in later compilations that carry on the earlier traditions.[98] As scholastic authors placed limits and qualifications on the character and function of female "seed," they tended to take the position that women could indeed conceive

---

94 Johannes Gerson, *De pollutione* (Cologne: Ludwig von Renchen, n.d.), fols. [5]vb–[6]ra. See also Brundage, *Law, Sex, and Christian Society*, pp. 400–1.

95 Huguccio suggested that a man could fulfill his marital debt to his wife and still avoid the sin of pleasure by refraining from ejaculation. See Brundage, *Law, Sex and Christian Society*, pp. 281–3; Jacquart and Thomasset, *Sexuality and Medicine*, p. 218, n. 40.

96 See Brundage, *Law, Sex, and Christian Society*, p. 429.

97 Christoph Ferckel, "Zur Gynäkologie und Generationslehre im Fasciculus medicinae des Johannes de Ketham," *Archiv für Geschichte der Medizin* 6 (1913): 208.

98 See, e.g., [*De generatione humana*], Bibliothèque Nationale, MS lat. nouv. acq. 693, fol. 183r.

without experiencing pleasure.[99] At the turn of the thirteenth century, even before Aristotle's *Generation of Animals* had been translated in full, David of Dinant was paraphrasing this aspect of the Philosopher's argument against female semen: not only do women frequently conceive without experiencing pleasure, but the sexual pleasure which (some) women do experience is like that of boys before they become fertile, that is, unassociated with true seed.[100] The concept of female pleasure dissociated from the emission of seed solved several problems at once: it disqualified female pleasure as evidence for female seed; it absolved men of a reproductive interest in women's sexual satisfaction; and at the same time it permitted emphasis upon women's strong sexual impulses. Albertus Magnus suggested that "woman does not always have intercourse with emission, but she also has other pleasures in intercourse and is always prepared for intercourse."[101] Other scholastic authors treated a woman's pleasure as inessential to reproduction, although it might be usual and helpful.[102] For these authors female pleasure was, therefore, a part of the divine plan insofar as it promoted coitus and thereby reproduction. It did not, however, serve in any way as a necessary efficient cause in conception. This understanding represents a mild contrast with views on the efficacy of male pleasure. For although there was not complete agreement on the absolute necessity of male pleasure, most authors implicitly or explicitly associated it with the emission of active seed, which is indeed required for conception.

Does female pleasure serve any purpose, beyond bringing the sexes together? Answers to this question paralleled the opinions of scholastic authors on the function of female sexual emission in general, with which it was closely associated: pleasure is, in one way or another, adjuvant. Aristotle had suggested that female secretion and the accompanying pleasure leave the mouth of the uterus open, thereby facilitating the male seed's entry into the womb.[103] Avicenna had said more generally (in the context of recommendations on enlarging a man's penis) that the lack of pleasure on the woman's part often gave rise to her failure to emit semen and ultimately to produce a child.[104] Late medieval authors did not concern themselves

99 Jacquart and Thomasset cite Giles of Rome and Averroes to this effect (*Sexuality and Medicine*, p. 66). Cf. Laqueur, who sees the "biological possibility of a passionless female" as originating with the dissociation of conception from female orgasm in the eighteenth century (*Making Sex*, p. 161).
100 Kurdziałek, "Anatomische und embryologische Aeusserungen Davids von Dinant," p. 10.
101 Albertus Magnus, *De animalibus*, bk. X, tr. i, ch. 1, §1, p. 730: ". . . tamen mulier, quia non semper coit emittendo, sed etiam alias habet coitus delectationes, semper parata est ad coitum. . . ."
102 [Johannes] Buridanus, *Questiones super* Secreta mulierum, Wissenschaftliche Bibliothek, Erfurt, MS Amplon. Q 299 (II), fol. 171r–v; see also Hewson, *Giles of Rome*, pp. 87–9.
103 Aristotle, *Generation of Animals*, II, iv, 739a32–36.
104 Avicenna, *Liber canonis*, bk. III, fen xx, tr. 2, ch. 44, fol. 358ra–b. The Latin translation here says, "Non fit filius," which could be interpreted to mean she does not produce a

seriously or systematically with the question, but a thirteenth-century medical writer held that "such [female] desire or pleasure is not required in intercourse, except to effect better reproduction in a better way."[105]

The vagueness and ambiguity associated with the functions of female pleasure also pervade medical recommendations, recipes, and signs. The enhancement of male pleasure was a subject in thirteenth- and fourteenth-century chapters and treatises on sterility, as it had been in Constantine's *On Coitus*, where it was regularly treated as a necessary element in male sexual and (therefore) reproductive function. Whether or not that framework was, in some cases, a mere pretext for the conveyance of aphrodisiacs for more hedonistic purposes, it served as an organizing and legitimizing principle. The scrutiny and promotion of female pleasure enjoyed no such recognized niche. Nevertheless, the topic appears occasionally in contexts which hardly help to clarify the function of sexual pleasure in women. Sandwiched between a set of remedies for postpartum ailments and a set of aids to conception, one treatise gives recipes for ointments to increase desire and pleasure in men and women and for a laudanum-based vaginal suppository specifically to ensure the woman's enjoyment of intercourse.[106] Are the recipes intended to aid in the recovery of sexual activity after childbirth or to promote the conception of the next child? Are they aphrodisiacs for their own sake, tucked unobtrusively into the text? Michael Scot included in his physiognomic treatise the signs by which women who gladly have intercourse and women who don't may be recognized. Those who do, in addition to having traits indicative of sexual maturity, are proud, not pious, and bold in their speech. Furthermore, they have scant and irregular menses and are thus less likely to conceive; when they do bear children, they have little milk. Cooler and more sexually reticent women are mild and soft. They believe what they are told and thus are good and pious. They, in turn, have ample menses, become pregnant quickly, and produce a lot of milk.[107] In these cases, women's sexual indulgence seems to be inversely related to their reproductive capacity; adherence to social norms is rewarded by respectable and healthy fertility. In other cases, late medieval authors include the woman's sexual satisfaction in their formulas for healthy and successful reproductive intercourse.[108] The ambiguous function of sexual pleasure is highlighted by the specific associations of female sexual pleasure, with its

son. Usually, however, when speaking of the sex of a child, the translator used the word *masculus*.

105 William of Saliceto, *Summa conservationis et curationis*, cited in Lemay, "William of Saliceto," p. 166, n. 3: "Tale desiderium vel delectatio non requiritur in coitu nisi ut generation melius et meliori modo fiat."

106 Arnaldus de Villanova, *De ornatu mulierum*, in *Opera omnia cum Nicolai Taurelli . . . annotationibus* (Basel: Conrad Waldkirch, 1585), col. 1672.

107 Michaelis Scotus, *De secretis naturae*, bk. I, chs. iv and v, pp. 240–1.

108 Lemay, "William of Saliceto," pp. 169–71.

ambivalent undertones. These emerge again in discussions of nonreproductive sexual activities, such as intercourse during pregnancy.

Nonreproductive pleasure

The complications and exceptions surrounding the association of pleasure with reproduction in scholastic medicine and natural philosophy served to undermine Constantine's crisp and unproblematic teleology. Indeed, unlike their predecessors, who, aside from cases of sterility, usually linked pleasure, intercourse, and reproduction, late medieval writers commented repeatedly on the exceptions to the rule. The ambiguous state of puberty provided several types of example, and the special case of pregnant women occasioned a variety of speculations.

Medieval authors often treated the beginning of sexual maturity, not as a phase, but as a moment, usually at the age of fourteen (or sometimes twelve for girls and fourteen for boys).[109] Understood in this way, the first emission of semen, the onset of menstruation, the beginning of intercourse, and the arrival of fertility all converged.[110] On the other hand, because neither the body in general nor the reproductive parts and capacities in particular were fully perfected, no one recommended that boys or girls have children at that age, and some specifically recommended otherwise on various grounds, including the weakness of the resultant child and the danger to the young mother.[111] Before they were capable of producing offspring, adolescent boys and girls were capable of engaging in sexual activities and experiencing sexual pleasure. These reservations, along with the common observation of the years of maturation, which included changes in voice, hair, and other features as well as the production of semen and menses, left room for authors who wished to comment on puberty as a period of transition with its own peculiar characteristics, not a few of which had to do with sexuality. Writing about problems related to child rearing, one thirteenth-century author warned about the ill effects on boys of too much intercourse. He refers specifically to boys with a hot, dry complexion, who "desire a lot but can do little" and whose emissions consist of insufficiently converted

---

109 See Elizabeth Sears, *The Ages of Man: Medieval Interpretations of the Life Cycle* (Princeton: Princeton University Press, 1986).
110 See, e.g., *Propositiones de animalibus*, Cambridge University Library, MS Dd.3.16, fol. 74rb.
111 *Propositiones de animalibus*, Cambridge University Library, MS Dd.3.16, fols. 74rb, 75rb; *De impedimentis conceptionis*, in Carl Eduard Arlt, *Neuer Beitrag zur Geschichte der medicinischen Schule von Montpellier*, Friedrich-Wilhelms-Universität (Berlin: Gustav Schade [Otto Francke], [1902]), p. 17; Albertus Magnus, *De animalibus*, bk. IX, tr. i, ch. 2, §§16–17, p. 681. Aristotle held that the production of seed preceded the ability to reproduce (*Historia animalium*, ed. and trans. A. L. Peck [Cambridge: Harvard University Press; London: William Heinemann, 1965], V, xiv, 544b12–19).

blood.[112] Although the nature of their emissions indicates that they are not producing fully actualized semen, yet they seek frequent intercourse, because the pleasure involved is vividly fixed in their memories.

Albertus Magnus, who gives the fullest medieval account of puberty and who treats it as a process and a period, rather than just a moment, mentioned a number of specific situations in which sexual pleasure is dissociated from reproduction and even from intercourse.[113] Aside from the statement made in another context that pleasure is not essentially connected with seed, Albertus made no specific argument that pleasure was distinct from its usual function, yet his discussion of prereproductive sexuality in general and masturbation in particular strongly suggests that he regarded sexual pleasure as an independent phenomenon. For him, puberty involved a complex of changes, which are, for the most part, either the same or parallel in girls and boys. These parallels extend to the domain of sexual awakening:

Also at this time, there begin to be frequent titillations in the head of the penis, as if an emission of seed should follow; because, however, it does not pour out . . . there is a certain pain. . . . A girl also begins to desire coitus then, but in [this] desire she does not have an emission.[114]

This is a period of life when both girls and boys practice masturbation, from which pleasure and "pollutions" (some sort of emission) may arise. Whether speaking of masturbation or of intercourse, to which young people – especially girls – are attracted, Albertus seldom mentioned semen and did not entertain the possibility of conception. For example, after speaking of the development of girls' breasts and of the change in their voices, he explained the relationship between sexual activity and growth for many (though not all) adolescents:

For in this period of puberty women as well as men distill a lot of humidity in their genitals and are greatly moved to seek coitus. And in many, if they practice moderate intercourse at that time, their bodies will grow faster than before. . . . For in those in whose bodies there are many, thick humidities, these same [humidities] impede the heat augmenting the body, which is not able to overcome and dissolve [the moisture]. And when it exits in part from the rubbing of intercourse, the body is better able to be nourished by the remaining portion, in males as well as in females.[115]

112 Petrus Gallegus, *In regitiva domus* [*Economica*], in Auguste Pelzer, "Un traducteur inconnu: Pierre Gallego, franciscain et premier évêque de Carthagène (1250–1267)," *Miscellanea Francesco Ehrle: Scritti di storia e paleografia*, vol. 1, *Per la storia della teologia e della filosofia*, Studi e testi 37 (Rome: Biblioteca Apostolica Vaticana, 1924), p. 451: ". . . et pueri colerici, quia multum appetunt et parum possunt . . . spermatizant sanguinem indigestum. . . ."
113 See Jacquart and Thomasset, "Albert le Grand," pp. 85–7.
114 Albertus Magnus, *De animalibus*, bk. IX, tr. i, ch. 1, §§6–7, p. 676: "Incipiunt etiam illo tempore frequenter esse titillationes in capite veretri, quasi debeat sequi emissio seminis, cum tamen non effundatur, . . . est quidam dolor. . . . Incipit etiam tunc puella desiderare coitum, sed in desiderio non emittit. . . ."
115 Ibid., §10, p. 677: "In hoc enim tempore pubertatis multa in inguine distillant humiditate tam feminae quam viri, et moventur multum ad quaerendum coitum: et ut in pluribus si

Albertus was explicit about the shared experience of early sexual activity and, in this particular case, about the nonreproductive effects of intercourse on both sexes. The sexual enthusiasms of both boys and girls are encouraged not only by the physiological changes which they are undergoing but also by their mental state, for their enthusiasm for intercourse is reinforced by their memory of its pleasure.[116]

Albertus did, however, make some distinctions between sexual development in boys and girls, though these are differences in degree and not in kind. He made special mention of the psychological dimension of sexuality in girls, saying that fourteen-year-old girls are more likely to get satisfaction by masturbating while imagining men than by having intercourse.[117] Furthermore, he found males and females differentially susceptible to specific dysfunctions:

There are some men to whom semen does not come, because of a coldness and dryness of complexion during puberty, and to these the ability to have intercourse never returns at any age, but rather, because of coldness, they are forever impotent. And it is the same in certain women, but it is very rare.

. . . .

When girls are chaste and shun [intercourse or other causes of emissions], for the rest of their lives they never have pollutions or experience the pleasure of intercourse. And this also happens to males, but very rarely. Some women have this from a defect in their complexion, as we said before, and they cannot reproduce.[118]

Albertus was suggesting that conditions and behaviors during puberty have implications for individuals' sexual and reproductive futures. His distinctions between predominantly male and predominantly female disorders highlight sexual impotence in men and generative impotence in women. Both these points have implications for the question of infertility, discussed in Chapter 5. Here they serve to underscore the extent to which medieval authors regarded adolescence as a moment of sexual activity and import, without attributing reproductive capacity to boys and girls at this transi-

---

utantur coitu moderato in illo tempore, velocius corpora eorum accipiunt incrementum quam prius, . . . quia illi in quorum corporibus multae sunt et grossae humiditates, ex ipsis eisdem impeditur calor augens corpus non potens eam vincere et dissolvere: et cum exit in parte per confricationem coitus, ex remanente melius augetur et nutritur corpus tam in maribus quam in feminis."

116 Ibid., §11, p. 678.

117 Ibid., §7, p. 676.

118 Ibid., §10, 11, p. 678: "Et quidam sunt quibus ex frigiditate et siccitate complexionis in annis pubertatis non accidit semen, sed illis numquam redibit potentia coeundi in aliqua aetate, sed potius ex frigiditate impotentes erunt in aeternum; et in feminis quibusdam est similiter, sed est valde rarum.

. . . .

. . . et ideo quando puellae castae sunt et avertunt animum, stant usque ad antiquitatem ultimam, quod numquam polluuntur neque experiuntur coitus delectationem: et hoc fit etiam in maribus, sed perraro. Quaedam autem habent hoc ex vitio complexionis sicut ante diximus, et illae non generant."

tional moment. Puberty is thus one framework within which sexual pleasure is without any immediate necessary connection to reproduction.

The possibility of this separation bore an ambiguous relation to the Constantinian teleology that naturalized and justified the experience of pleasure.
On the one hand, it was consistent with the interpretation that pleasure was
something added on to intercourse; on the other hand, it dissociated pleasure from its final cause – the perpetuation of the species. If adolescents
provided an example of nonreproductive sexuality that was, at worst,
slightly unruly, other instances had a darker tone. One reason for the condemnation of contraceptives and of certain coital positions was that they
served pleasure without serving generation – that they made pleasure an
end in itself. If masturbation and prereproductive intercourse could be enjoyed by both males and females, some aspects of adult nonreproductive
sexual pleasure called attention to women's sexuality in particular. In the
course of an argument about whether men or women derive greater pleasure from intercourse, Gerard of Brolio, a fourteenth-century commentator
on Aristotle, offered the view that "woman derives pleasure from emitting a
vacuum or a superfluity and from retaining what is appropriate; but man
only from expelling what is harmful."[119] The very marginality of women's
emissions, in other words, suggests her pleasure has a certain scope and
independence. According to Bernard of Gordon, animals' sexual appetite
"is for the species and not for pleasure. In women it is the contrary. They
desire [intercourse] not only on account of the species but also on account of
pleasure."[120] Scholastic authors revised Aristotle's observation that humans
and horses, both male and female, have the greatest sexual appetites of all
animals, asserting that women are unlike other female animals in their
perpetual receptivity to intercourse.[121] Furthermore, in contrast to animals,
only women (or only women and mares) are willing to have intercourse
after they had conceived.[122] Bernard of Gordon gave an Aristotelian physiological reason: most animals use up their useful residues in the production of
fur, horns, or claws, rather than for extra seed, but women have abundant
menses, which stimulate them.[123] Albertus Magnus's psychosocial explana-

---

119 Gerardus de Brolio, *Super librum* De animalibus, Bibliothèque Nationale, MS lat. 16166,
bk. V, fol. 44rb: "Item mulier delectatur emittendo vacuum vel superfluum et retinendo
conveniens. Vir autem solum expellendo nocivum."
120 Bernardus de Gordonio, *Lilium*, pt. VII, ch. ii, fol. 88rb: "Quarto notandum quod cetera
animalia abhoret coytum post conceptum. . . . et quia appetitus est ad speciem et non ad
delectationem. In mulieribus est contrarium. Appetunt enim non solum propter speciem
sed propter delectationem."
121 The subject is discussed, for example, in many of the commentaries on and compilations
of the *De secretis mulierum*; e.g., Bibliothèque Nationale, MS lat. 7106, fols. 21r–22v;
Aristotle, *Historia animalium*, VI, xxii, 575b30–1.
122 Bernardus de Gordonio, *Lilium*, pt. VII, ch. ii, fol. 88rb; *Propositiones de animalibus*, Cambridge University Library, MS Dd.3.16, fol. 74va; [ps.-]Th[omas], *De coitu*, Bibliothèque
Nationale, MS lat. 16195, fol. 25ra; Aristotle, *Historia animalium*, VII, iv, 585a2–3.
123 Bernardus de Gordonio, *Lilium*, pt. VII, ch. i, fol. 88rb.

tion is more unusual. After citing an opinion (certainly not widespread) that women abhor intercourse when they are pregnant, he went on to report, "However, women themselves say they experience greater pleasure in intercourse when they are pregnant than when they are not."[124]

Although it by no means denies men's sexuality, the focus on women's capacity for sexual pleasure creates the impression that it is women's sexuality which deviates from the ideal course of nature. No one calls attention to men's willingness to have intercourse with pregnant women. Women's experiences and inclinations did not so much undermine the widely accepted teleological explanation for sexual pleasure as they demonstrated the contingent character of the natural order. Many conditions and accidents could interrupt the fulfillment of any natural purpose. In the case of the sexual pleasures of girls and boys in puberty, the realization of the adult through the process of maturation itself deflected pleasure's reproductive goal. In the case of pregnant women's pleasure, no countervailing purpose or contingent necessity provided an explanation or excuse. Women experience pleasure when the reproductive purpose is already being actualized – when they are pregnant. The overtones and consequences of intercourse during pregnancy were generally negative. Although not prohibited by Scripture and never considered a serious sin, it was proscribed by canon law.[125] Some held it would have dire consequences, such as the death of the fetus.[126] Others who commented on the subject suggested rather milder complications, such as premature parturition or multiple births.[127] One compilation, following and adding to Aristotle, enumerated a variety of potential outcomes:

No female among animals is receptive to coitus after impregnation except the woman and the mare. A certain woman miscarried twelve children in successive pregnancies. A certain woman committed adultery after having become pregnant [by her husband]. She gave birth to two sons, of whom one resembled the husband and the other the adulterer. Certain women miscarry and become pregnant at the same time, so that one [fetus] leaves the womb and the other is conceived.[128]

Bernard of Gordon also tells the story of the adulterous woman. Lest the lesson be lost, he takes care to specify that the adulterer and, more to the

---

124 Albertus Magnus, *De animalibus*, bk. X, tr. ii, ch. 3, §56, p. 753: ". . . tamen mulieres ipsae dicunt se magis delectari in coitu quando sunt impregnatae, quam quando non sunt impregnatae."
125 Brundage, *Law, Sex, and Christian Society*, pp. 91–2, 155–6, 451–2.
126 Jacobus de Vitriaco, cited in D. L. d'Avray and M. Tausche, "Marriage Sermons in *ad status* Collections of the Central Middle Ages," *Archives d'historie doctrinale et littéraire du Moyen Age* 47 (1980): 99, 107; cf. Hildegard of Bingen, *Scivias*, pt. I, vis. ii, ch. 22, pp. 28–9.
127 Bernardus de Gordonio, *Lilium*, pt. VII, ch. ii, fol. 88rb.
128 *Propositiones de animalibus*, Cambridge University Library, MS Dd.3.16, fol. 75rb: "Nulla femina animalium recepit coitum post impregnationem nisi mulier et equa. Quedam mulier aborsit xii filios quorum impregnatio erat successiva. Quedam mulier post impregantionem fornicata fuit et peperit duos filios quorum unus assimilabatur coniugi et alter fornicatori. Quedam mulieres abortiunt et impregnantur simul ita quod unus quod [sic] exit a matrice et alius concipitur." Aristotle, *Historia animalium*, VII, iv, 585a8–23.

point, the illegitimate child were wicked.[129] These accounts show that intercourse during pregnancy might not always be nonreproductive in the sense of having no potential for conception. Indeed Bernard suggests that the conjunction of pleasure, conception, and abortion occurs because all involve the opening of the womb. Such a conjunction does, nevertheless, betray the larger purpose and natural course of reproduction.

Sexual behaviors distanced from their proper ends presented a variety of challenges to late medieval authors. From the use of contraceptives to sodomy, pleasures detached from reproductive intent met with varying degrees of disapproval. The cases treated here, such as masturbation, intercourse before full sexual maturity, and intercourse during pregnancy, were, to natural philosophers and physicians, natural manifestations of human sexuality in specifically defined situations. For that reason they often escaped direct condemnation in scientific and medical texts. Yet even the relatively neutral tones of an author like Albertus Magnus do not mask an uneasy preoccupation. To demonstrate that the motion of the womb is a source of female pleasure, Albertus argued, "It is on account of this that some women take the neck of a vessel in their vagina and draw it [in and out], so that they may thus derive pleasure by the womb's having been moved."[130] The special attention given to women's experience of nonreproductive pleasure and the general tension such pleasure creates with the teleological view of sexual satisfaction reveal the subject's potentially disruptive dimensions.

Scholastic authors did not always treat male and female pleasure separately, but when they did, the distinction was multivalent. Women's pursuit and enjoyment of pleasure were associated explicitly with a willfulness that distinguished them from animals, with a weakness of judgment that distinguished them from men, and with negative reproductive consequences that separated them from the optimal fulfillment of their procreative functions. The emphasis here on the special appetites of female humans accords with an older tradition that women have greater sexual desire and pleasure than men. But when scholastic authors addressed directly the question of female and male pleasure, they incorporated the older formula into one that at once reinstated the sexual force of men and created a kind of incommensurability between men's and women's pleasure.

THE MEASURE OF PLEASURE

Before the awakening of the scholastic interest in determining which sex derives more pleasure from sexual intercourse, several authors had men-

---

129 Bernardus de Gordonio, *Lilium*, pt. VII, ch. ii, fol. 88rb.
130 Albertus Magnus, *De animalibus*, bk. IX, tr. ii, ch. 6, §132, p. 728: ". . . propter quod quaedam feminae apprehendunt collum vesicae in vulva et trahunt, ut sic mota matrice delectentur."

tioned the subject in passing. William of Conches's *Dragmaticon* and the tract *On Human Generation* derived from it had paused to explain woman's greater sexual heat in the light of her generally cooler constitution and had followed Constantine in asserting that women had greater pleasure from intercourse because they both emitted and received seed. One twelfth-century author had alluded to the story told by Ovid about Tiresias, who had been turned into a woman because he had insulted some serpents, and, after seven years in that state, had gotten himself turned back again. Jupiter and Juno called upon him to settle an argument: Jupiter held that women enjoyed greater pleasure; Juno, that men did. Tiresias, the only one in a position to compare the experiences, agreed with Jupiter.[131] Although Hildegard had offered a more equivocal account, presenting the male experience as more focused and the female experience as more diffused, the issue had not been the subject of much debate or comment, and the consensus was in accord with Tiresias. There were surely moral overtones associated with female weakness and passion, implications that may have contributed to Hildegard's revisions, but they were no more the subject of discussion in medicine or natural philosophy than was the topic of differential pleasure itself.

A number of scholastic authors, however, beginning in the mid-thirteenth century, found the comparison of men's and women's pleasure of sufficient interest to treat it as a problem. In doing so, they connected it with standard physiological themes, such as the operations of heat, and with reproductive issues, such as the nature of the female seed. They also brought into relief the ambiguous position of pleasure. On the one hand, it was a link between sexuality and reproduction, which provided an avenue for the appreciation of male potency and primacy; on the other hand, it was an expression of irrationality and lack of control, which suggested a dimension of female weakness. Thus, even though the scholastic treatments of Jupiter and Juno's question were seldom bluntly moralized, they reverberated with these overtones, which occasionally came explicitly to the fore.

With this question as with others, the authors of thirteenth- and fourteenth-century commentaries and *questiones* did not leave behind the older formulations, but rather appropriated and reformulated them. Peter of Abano, in the learned compilation of current medical and philosophical questions that he wrote in the early part of the fourteenth century, named Ovid among his authorities.[132] Furthermore, once the issue took shape, additional authorities were mustered. The most significant of these was

---

131 Ovid, *Metamorphoses*, III, 316–33, alluded to in an anonymous twelfth-century interpolation in a manuscript of William of Conches's glosses on Macrobius, cited in Lemay, "William of Saliceto," p. 172, n. 46.

132 Petrus de Abano Pativinus, *Conciliator differentiarum philosophorum et precipue medicorum* (Venice: Gabriele de Tarvisio for Thomas de Tarvisio, 1476), diff. 34, fol. 57ra–b.

Avicenna, whose formulation was frequently cited, although, like the other authors often invoked, he himself did not have much to say on the subject. In a widely read and commented chapter of the *Canon*, "On the Generation of the Embryo," Avicenna mentioned that women "derive pleasure from the motion of the sperm which is in them; and they derive pleasure from the motion of the man's sperm in the mouth of their uterus descending to the cavity of the uterus; or rather, they experience pleasure on account of that motion which happens to the uterus."[133] The passage is not comparing women's pleasure with men's: it is an aside within a discussion of conception. Yet scholastic authors used it to weigh in favor of the proposition that women get more pleasure from intercourse than men. (Most took Avicenna to be enumerating two, not three, separate sources of female pleasure.) In Peter of Abano's presentation, Avicenna joins Ovid, Constantine, Aristotle, and Galen on that side of the argument. Thus authorities ancient and modern joined the consensus of the eleventh and twelfth centuries as the basis for a new interest in and a new perspective on sexual pleasure in women and men.

Questions concerning which sex has greater pleasure in intercourse and whether women have greater pleasure than men occurred in both medical and natural philosophical settings. Peter of Spain entertained the problem in his commentaries on Constantine's *Viaticum*, on Aristotle's *On Animals*, and on Johannitius's *Isagoge*.[134] Albertus Magnus and a fourteenth-century commentator, Gerard of Brolio, also addressed it in their treatments of Aristotle's *On Animals*.[135] A number of Italian academic medical writers included it in their commentaries and *questiones* on various texts: Taddeo Alderotti on Johannitius, and Mondino de' Luzzi and Jacopo of Forlì on the chapter in Avicenna just quoted.[136] It was by no means unusual for scholastic authors to import questions raised by one text into their commentaries on other texts, but unlike the existence of a female seed (which was also entertained in a number of settings), this question was one that was not firmly grounded in any particular set of authoritative texts. It was an essentially medieval question, which an author might (but certainly need not) raise on a variety of occasions.

The question was who experienced greater pleasure (*delectatio*), though it was sometimes accompanied by discussions of love (*dilectio, amor*) or desire

---

133 Avicenna, *Liber canonis*, bk. III, fen i, tr. 1, ch. 2, fol. 362ra–b: "Ipse enim delectantur ex motu spermatis quod est in eis; et delectantur ex motu spermatis viri in ore matricis earum descendendo ad ventrum matricis; immo delectantur propter ipsum motum qui accidit matrici."

134 Wack, *Lovesickness*, pp. 244, 246, 309, n. 42.

135 Albertus Magnus, *Quaestiones de animalibus*, bk. V, q. 4, pp. 155–6; see also q. vi, pp. 156–7; Gerardus de Brolio, *Super librum de animalibus*, Bibliothèque Nationale, MS lat. 16166, bk. V, fols. 44rb–45ra.

136 Thaddeus Florentinus, *In Isagogas Joannitianas*, ch. X; Jacobus Forliviensis, *De generatione embrionis*, fol. 11rb; Siraisi, *Taddeo*, p. 340.

(*appetitus*). The scholastic project was to unpack the word "greater" (*maior*). The result was twofold: on the one hand, the refinement and elaboration of the concepts of "pleasure" and "more" and, on the other hand, the attribution of new meanings to women's and men's roles and experiences.

The lack of meaty authoritative texts and the scholastic habits of comparison and synthesis led authors to link the question of differential pleasures with the larger frameworks of sex difference in general and reproductive roles in particular. For example, Albertus Magnus cited Aristotle's view (expressed in *Physics*) that matter seeks form as female seeks male and as bad seeks good to argue that because of her greater lack or need, "pleasure is greatest and desire is greatest in woman."[137] However, he also argued that men, who contribute form to the offspring, must have more pleasure, since everything takes pleasure in its proper operation, and the more "formal" the operation, the greater the pleasure.[138] In a similar way, some authors introduced into their treatment of pleasure a vocabulary of quantification developed in other medical and philosophical contexts. The engagement of abstractions of this sort and the general process of analysis and distinction making, in addition to creating a legitimate niche for discussing differential pleasures, served to distance the subject somewhat from lurking moral entanglements of sexual matters. Like other scholastic questions, this one was as much an opportunity to display technical expertise as it was to express deeply held views. At the same time, as the value hierarchy implicit in the Aristotelian framework illustrates, the exercise of scholastic virtuosity and the communication of assumptions about sex difference were not mutually exclusive, especially in a situation in which there existed no strong independently established orthodoxy.

Scholastic authors developed and enhanced the differences between male and female pleasure in part simply by reiterating and highlighting earlier formulations: "Women experience more pleasure than men, since women take pleasure in emitting and receiving, but men only take pleasure in emitting."[139] The succinctness of this statement (especially the author's elliptical omission of "coitus" and "seed") is indicative of the familiarity of the question. Although Avicenna had stressed the motion of the womb either as the basis of or in addition to the reception of the male seed, even some authors invoking the authority of Avicenna tended to read the passage cited as equivalent to the earlier Latin phrasing, "emitting and receiving." Taddeo Alderotti, who took up the issue in connection with the argument about the existence

---

137 Albertus Magnus, *Quaestiones de animalibus*, bk. V, q. 4, p. 155: ". . . maxima est delectatio et maximus appetitus in ipsa muliere." Peter of Spain cites the same passage to the same end in his commentary on *De animalibus* (Wack, *Lovesickness*, p. 117).

138 Albertus Magnus, *Quaestiones de animalibus*, bk. V, q. 4, p. 155.

139 Ps.-Isidorus, *De spermate*, Oxford, Bodleian Library, MS Bodley 484, fol. 46r: "Sciendum est quod mulieres plus delectantur quam viri, quia delectantur in emittendo et in recipiendo, sed vires solum delectantur in emittendo."

and nature of the female sperm, cited Avicenna (along with Constantine, Aristotle, and Galen) as an authority for the view "that the woman experiences more pleasure in coitus than the man. And this is because women derive pleasure from their own emission of sperm and in the reception of the man's sperm."[140] (Pursuing his purpose, Taddeo explained that this observation does not contradict the Aristotelian position that women have no seed, for as Avicenna says, "sperm" has a narrow, proper meaning and a broad meaning, and only the latter is intended in this case.) Jacopo of Forlì, in a commentary on Avicenna, attempted to resolve the ambiguity of Avicenna's text and to bring it into accord with the simpler emission–reception model. Was Avicenna suggesting the motion of the womb as a substitute for the reception of male seed or as a third source of pleasure for women? Jacopo suggested woman's pleasure comes from (1) the motion of her own sperm and (2) the motion of the man's sperm, which she experiences (a) in the mouth of the womb and (b) at the cavity of the womb.[141] Unsatisfactory though it may be, this attempt to consolidate the argument for greater female pleasure is a product of the repeated consideration of the problem.

If the repetition and elaboration of the standard view of the several forms of female pleasure underscore the extent to which the question of comparative pleasures had caught on, the introduction of a set of counterarguments gives the question full scholastic status and reorients the medieval academic perspective on pleasure. The new view – that there was an important sense in which men had more pleasure – was a vehicle for the exercise of a fashionable mode of analysis which may loosely be called "quantitative" and at the same time an expression of a new emphasis on male sexual pleasure. The two dimensions of the development reinforced one another.

The investigation of "more"

In explicit response to Constantine's assertion that women had more pleasure because theirs came from two sources, Peter of Spain, writing in mid-thirteenth-century Siena, where he was teaching medicine, responded:

To this it must be said that, as we believe, pleasure is greater in males than in females. And it is apparent because they emit more and are consumed more in intercourse. On the woman's part there is twofold pleasure – in emitting and receiving – however, it is not qualitatively as much.[142]

---

140 Thaddeus Florentinus, *In* Isagogas *Joannitianas*, fol. 357vb: ". . . quod mulier magis delectatur quam vir in coitu. Et hoc est quia mulieres delectantur in emissione propria spermatis et in receptione spermatis viri."
141 Jacobus Forliviensis, *De generatione embrionis*, fol. 11rb.
142 Petrus Hispanus, *Questiones super* Viaticum, Version B (Wack, *Lovesickness*, p. 146): "Ad hoc dicendum quod sicut credimus maior est delectatio in maribus quam in feminis. Et patet quia plus emittunt et plus consumuntur in cohitu. Sed a parte femine est duplex delectatio in emissione et in receptione; et tamen non est tanta qualitate."

Peter was clearly struggling to sort out the possible meanings of "more" pleasure in an attempt to shift the weight to male enjoyment without directly and completely discarding the commonplace about the double nature of female enjoyment. His attempt took him in two not entirely consistent directions. On the one hand, "emit more" (and perhaps also "consumed more") places a continuous, extensive quantity against the woman's discontinuous, numerical quantity: she has a greater *number* of pleasures but he has a greater *amount* of pleasure. On the other hand, the claim that female pleasure "is not qualitatively as much" contrasts not the amount of male pleasure but its quality or character with female pleasure. The latter notion of qualitative muchness was to be the basis for the emergent idea and measure of yet another sense of "more," namely, intensity.

In Peter of Spain's distinctions concerning amounts of pleasure, Mary Wack detects the application of terminology borrowed from philosophical and theological discussions of the quantification of qualities.[143] Against the position that "in women the desire for coitus is greater and love is greater and more intense than in men," Peter held "that love is more intense on the part of man than on the part of woman; however, as Constantine would have it, pleasure is greater on the part of woman."[144] Peter made use of the word "intense," connected with the developing vocabulary of quantification, in his attempt to reconcile the Constantinian sense in which women had more pleasure with the new inclination to believe that men did. He did not, however, pair the terms "intension" and "remission," used by later philosophers and theologians to indicate the waxing and waning of a property, such as heat, in an object, or even the terms "intension" and "extension," used to distinguish the strength of a property inhering in an object from the measure of the object in which it inheres. His concerns did, however, bear on the establishment of the latter distinction between, say, increasing the hotness (temperature) of the water already in a pot and increasing the amount of warm water there, which in turn laid a foundation for the quantification of a variety of properties – from heat to charity – by later physicians, philosophers, and theologians.[145]

---

143 Wack, *Lovesickness*, pp. 115–20.
144 Petrus Hispanus, *Questiones super* Viaticum, Version B (Wack, *Lovesickness*, p. 244): "Ergo maior est appetitus coitus et maior est amor et intensior in feminis quam in viris. . . . quod intensior est amor a parte maris quam a parte femine, tamen maior est delectatio, sicut vult Constantinus, a parte femine." See Wack, *Lovesickness*, p. 116.
145 There were important differences among various systems of quantification, including the philosophical analysis of intensity, the philosophical quantification of qualities, and the pharmacological system of degrees. See Edith Sylla, "Medieval Quantifications of Qualities: The 'Merton School,' " *Archive for History of the Exact Sciences* 8 (1971): 9–39; and Michael McVaugh, "The Development of Medieval Pharmaceutical Theory," in Introduction to Arnaldus de Villanova, *Opera medica omnia*, vol. II, *Aphorismi de gradibus* (Granada: Seminarium Historiae Medicae Granatensis, 1975), pp. 3–136 (on Peter of Spain, see esp. p. 100).

From the midthirteenth century on, some ways of expressing the difference between the two senses of "more pleasure" do reflect a few elements of the developing language of quantification. For example, in his question "Whether Pleasure in Intercourse Is Greater in Men than in Women," written shortly after Peter's, Albertus Magnus directly applied the intension–extension distinction, arguing:

> The cause of desiring to have intercourse is heat and a multitude of seed. Since heat moves from center to circumference, heat is thus the mover in the emission of seed. But heat is more abundant in man than in woman, and so is seed. For although in women there is a great quantity of superfluous and undigested fluid, yet that is evacuated through the flow of the menses, which does not occur in men. Hence pleasure is intensively greater in men than in women, though in a woman it is perhaps extensively greater than in a man, since she experiences pleasure in several ways, namely, both by receiving and by emitting.[146]

Based on the involvement of the sense of touch in the generation of pleasure, Peter of Abano, writing in the early fourteenth century, used similar language. He said man's enjoyment is more intense, whereas woman's pleasure is extensive but "rarer" (i.e., less concentrated).[147] The role of the sense of touch provided the opportunity to introduce other terms associated with the quantification of natural philosophical language. Peter of Spain had entertained the simple syllogism that "the male's member has greater sensation. Where there is greater sensation of a pleasurable thing, there is greater pleasure. Therefore pleasure is greater in males."[148] The Aristotelian understanding of touch involved the notion of balance, which came to be expressed as ratio or proportionality. Thus Peter of Abano could argue that since sexual pleasure derives from touch, man's pleasure is stronger. For man is more temperate than woman, and his sense of touch is therefore more perfect and more intense. Put slightly differently, "Pleasure or delight is caused by a proportionate conjunction of like with like, but this

146 Albertus Magnus, *Quaestiones de animalibus*, bk. V, q. iv, p. 155: "Praeterea, causa appetendi coire est calor et multitudo seminis, quia calidum movet a centro ad circumferentiam, et ideo calidum est movens in emissione seminis. Sed calidum est abundantius in viro quam in muliere et similiter semen. Licet enim in mulieribus multum sit de humido superfluo et indigesto, illud tamen evacuatur per fluxum menstruorum, qui non accidit in viris, et ideo intensive maior est delectatio in viris quam in mulieribus, extensive tamen forte est maior in muliere quam in viro, quia pluribus modis delectatur, scilicet et recipiendo et emittendo."
147 Petrus de Abano, *Conciliator*, diff. 34 (fol. 57rb), contains such phrases as "intensior igitur voluptas in viro" and "intensive voluptatur peramplius," in contrast to "extensive plus delectatur mulier" and "rarius." He also took up the question in his *Expositio* Problematum *Aristotelis*, ed. Stephanus Illarius (Mantua: Paulus Johannis de Puzpach, 1475), pt. IV, probl. 15, fols. [68]vb–[69]rb.
148 Petrus Hispanus, *Questiones super* Viaticum, Version B (Wack, *Lovesickness*, p. 246): "Membrum masculini est maioris sensus. Sed ubi maior est sensus rei delectabilis est maior delectatio. Ergo in maribus maior est delectatio."

will be more powerful in the man, since he is of a more temperate complexion than the female."[149]

Other examples of the use of such words as "extensive," "intensive," "double," "several," and "rarer" confirm the absorption of a certain level of quantitative vocabulary as a means of explicating the concept of "more pleasure." But alternative formulations, such as the idea that woman's pleasure was quantitatively greater and man's pleasure was qualitatively greater, also appeared.[150] Furthermore, neither the philosophical nor the medical authors who entertained the question of male and female pleasure made much of the technical capabilities of such language. Their applications never seriously approached either the kind of quantitative language which developed in the context of pharmacology or that which developed in the context of theology and other problems of natural philosophy, such as the study of motion.[151] Though the flavor is there, the authors are using the terms loosely and do not regard this particular question as an occasion to display their expertise in the analysis of quantities and qualities. Even when the concepts are fairly complicated, the quantities involved are relative, vague, and often casually expressed. So, for example, when Albertus Magnus offered his version of Avicenna's view, he added to the number (or extension) of female pleasure the notion that each separate element may vary in strength (or intensity). He used words that convey proportionality, but his phrasing included neither the terms "intension" and "extension" nor any formal representation of proportionality or measure of intensity:

Woman has these three pleasures in intercourse, namely, (1) by ejaculating a fluid similar to sperm, and then however much she ejaculates, so much does she experience pleasure, just like a man; (2) by the adhesion of the man's sperm, and then however much adheres, so much does she experience pleasure; and (3) when the womb moves, and then however much motion the womb makes, so much does she experience pleasure.[152]

---

149 Petrus de Abano, *Conciliator*, diff. 34, fol. 57rb: ". . . delectatio seu delicia causatur ex coniunctione proportionata convenientis cum convenienti, sed hec vehementior erit in viro cum sit temperatioris complexionis femella. . . ."

150 [Ps.-]Th[omas], *De coitu*, Bibliothèque Nationale, MS lat. 16195, fol. 24vb.

151 See McVaugh, "Pharmaceutical Theory" in Arnaldus de Villanova, *Aphorismi de gradibus*; and John E. Murdoch, "From Social into Intellectual Factors: An Aspect of the Unitary Character of Late Medieval Learning," in John Emory Murdoch and Edith Dudley Sylla, eds., *The Cultural Context of Medieval Learning: Proceedings of the First International Colloquium on Philosophy, Science, and Theology in the Middle Ages – September, 1973*, Synthèse Library 76; Boston Studies in the Philosophy of Science 26 (Dordrecht and Boston: D. Reidel, 1975), esp. pp. 280–9.

152 Albertus Magnus, *De animalibus*, bk. IX, tr. ii, ch. 6, §132, p. 728: ". . . mulier in coitu tres istas habet delectationes, scilicet proiciendo spermati similem humorem, et tunc delectatur totiens, quotiens proicit, sicut vir, et glutiendo sperma virile, et tunc totiens delectatur quotiens glutit, et quando matrix movetur, et tunc totiens delectatur quotiens motum dat matrix. . . ."

Even by the end of the fourteenth century, when the technical vocabulary was more fully developed and widely applied, it does not seem to have entered more than casually into the treatment of pleasure.[153]

Male strength

Far more significant within the scholastic comparisons of women's and men's pleasure than the faint aura of quantification is the promotion of male strength and the means by which that promotion was effected. The authors who entertained the question in the thirteenth and fourteenth centuries were in even more agreement that the greater pleasure belonged to the man than the earlier, less involved authors had been that it belonged to the woman. As was often the case, scholarly explorations of the subject consisted less in debating the answer to the question posed than in devising a variety of supporting evidence and arguments for the agreed-upon answer: as Gerard of Brolio very simply put it, "The single mode of delectation which exists in the man is greater than the double which exists in the woman."[154] In taking up this dimension of sex difference, the discussions therefore provided a survey of male strengths – constitutional, reproductive, and sexual. They explicated the notion of "more pleasure" by elaborating on the generally held understanding that for women, "more" has to do with "many" (forms, occasions, ways, causes) and that for men, "more" has to do with "stronger" and "more intense."[155]

Support for the weightiness of male pleasure included several arguments already touched on. Man's physiological balance is more temperate than woman's, which makes his sense of touch and therefore his sense of pleasure more acute. Desire and, therefore, pleasure arise from heat, and men are hotter than women. Other points build upon other generally accepted differences between the sexes. Pleasure from the emission of more perfect seed is greater than pleasure from the emission of less perfect seed, and man's semen is unquestionably more perfect. Similarly, pleasure comes from certain acts, and the more formal the operation, the greater the pleasure: in the act of generation, the male role is more associated with form.[156]

Still other sources of support are specific to the mechanisms of pleasure. Several authors commented on the duration and timing of pleasure. Whereas Albertus Magnus saw men and women as equivalent in this regard, observing that both experience the emission of seed in a series of successive impulses,

---

153 See Jacobus Forliviensis, *De generatione embrionis*, fol. 11va.
154 Gerardus de Brolio, *Super librum* De animalibus, Bibliothèque Nationale, MS lat. 16166, bk. V, fol. 45ra: ". . . ille unicus modus delectationis qui est in viro est maior quam duplex qui est in muliere."
155 Bernardus de Gordonio, *Lilium*, pt. VII, ch. ii, fol. 88rb.
156 Albertus Magnus, *Quaestiones de animalibus*, bk. V, q. 4, p. 155; see also Wack, *Lovesickness*, p. 117.

others denied the parallel in a manner which supported the intensive–extensive distinction.[157] According to Peter of Abano, one sense in which women have more pleasure extensively is that with the motions of the two sperms and the various motions of the womb, her pleasure is a succession of events and thus lasts longer. Men's emission is faster and more sudden; his pleasure is undivided and takes place in a shorter period of time, and it is therefore more intense.[158] The temporal interpretation of extensive pleasure may possibly refer to authors' impressions of the length or multiplicity of women's orgasms, but the evidence is slight. Jacopo of Forlì says simply: "Man experiences pleasure more intensely; however, woman [experiences pleasure] in several ways and over a greater period of time in the emission of her own sperm in intercourse, as is felt."[159]

Beneath the variations and idiosyncrasies of specific accounts lies a fundamental theme: the differences between the sexes with respect to their experiences of pleasure. As with male and female reproductive roles, distinctions in pleasure which may arise from a difference of degree along a continuum, such as the greater heat of the male or the greater refinement of his reproductive fluid, take on a qualitative significance. Sometimes, as when the active and formal roles are contrasted with the passive and material, the differences become oppositional. At other times, the differences are rather a sort of incommensurability: female and male pleasures are measured on separate scales, so that "more" means something different in each case. At the same time, and somewhat paradoxically, the structure and tone of the academic literature of comparative pleasures clearly declared the male the winner: his "more" is greater, better, higher; the scale on which it is measured is more significant.

The values of pleasure

The arguments that man has greater pleasure were mainly based on male strength and reproductive primacy. Even a straightforward assertion like "the male's member has greater sensitivity"[160] turns out to be based on male physiological superiority. These correlations alone express and reinforce a cluster of values which, although neither the motivation nor the subject of the discussions of pleasure, nevertheless color the changes in ideas about the experience of sexual pleasure. Whereas earlier statements about the plurality

---

157 Albertus Magnus, *De animalibus*, bk. IX, tr. ii, ch. 3, §103, p. 716; see also bk. IX, tr. i, ch. 7, §66, p. 700.
158 Petrus de Abano, *Conciliator*, diff. 34, fol. 57rb.
159 Jacobus Forliviensis, *De generatione embrionis*, fol. 11va: ". . . vir intensius mulier aut pluribus modis et pluri tempore delectatur in emissione proprii spermatis in coitu ut tactum est."
160 Petrus Hispanus, *Questiones super* Viaticum, Version B (Wack, *Lovesickness*, p. 246): "Membrum masculini est maioris sensus."

of female pleasure had neither accorded women any implicit status nor reflected negatively on men's sexuality, the new formulation, which set up a kind of competition, revolved around properties of the male that clearly enhanced his image. The shift was a complex one, for it did not reorient the standing of sexual pleasure per se: the message had not become, "Pleasure is good, and men have more of it," but rather, "The intensity of male pleasure is a manifestation of male strengths." Furthermore, the new focus on men's pleasure did not simply redefine women's pleasure accordingly.

To be sure, in connection with such matters as heat or refinement of seed, female incapacity was the obverse of male strength. Discussing the greater intensity of male pleasure, Albertus Magnus commented that greater female love and lust are more apparent than real in the sense that they arise from women's misjudgments, from the weakness of their reason.[161] In addition, women's sexual pleasure could be characterized in terms of remedying a lack:

Matter is said to seek form and woman man not because woman should desire intercourse with man. Rather, this is the meaning: that everything imperfect naturally desires to be perfected. And woman is an imperfect human in comparison to man; thus every woman desires to exist under [the form of] manliness. For there is no woman who would not naturally want to shed the definition of femininity and put on masculinity.[162]

But the new discussions of pleasure did not simply emphasize female weakness and incapacity. They also perpetuated the older formulation more or less intact: as Constantine and Avicenna had said, women had multiple pleasures. And, in the course of exploring the comparison, they elaborated on the specific mechanisms of the plurality. For example, after having reviewed the standard sources of female pleasure according to the authorities – emitting seed, receiving seed, drawing seed into the womb, various motions of the womb – Peter of Abano added that on the contrary, in his opinion, women derive no small amount of pleasure from the rubbing of the part situated at the mouth of the womb. "For this [part] corresponds to the head of the penis, where extreme pleasure flourishes."[163] Another text that addresses the comparison of men's and women's pleasures speaks of "the great pleasure that she has, since, through the presence of the penis in the woman's sexual part

161 Albertus Magnus, *Quaestiones de animalibus*, bk. V, q. 4, p. 156; cf. Petrus Hispanus, *Questiones super* Viaticum, Version B (Wack, *Lovesickness*, p. 244).
162 Albertus Magnus, *Quaestiones de animalibus*, bk. X, q. 4, pp. 155–6: ". . . materia dictur appetere formam et femina virum, non quia femina appetat coire cum viro, sed iste est intellectus, quod omne imperfectum naturaliter appetit perfici; et mulier est homo imperfectus respectu viri, ideo omnis mulier appetit esse sub verilitate. Non enim est mulier, quin ipsa vellet exuere rationem femininitatis et induere masculinitatem naturaliter."
163 Petrus de Abano, *Conciliator*, diff. 34, fol. 57ra: "Ipsa enim balano correspondet virge, ubi viget delectatio grandis. . . ."

[*vulva*], the nerves and veins in that part are rubbed and moved."[164] In keeping with the ways in which Constantine and Avicenna had spoken of female pleasure, these later authors also perpetuated the formula according to which man's pleasure came from the emission of his semen, whereas woman's pleasure derived only partially from her own emission and depended for the rest upon the man.

The tendency to treat female pleasure as something different from a pale version of male pleasure contains the residue of earlier treatments of sex difference not only in the sense that some of the substance of the beliefs has been transferred but also in the sense that a certain eclecticism persists. Although scholastic writing was by its very nature logical and systematic, although it had as one of its goals to expose and resolve inconsistencies, it nevertheless retained (and, given the challenge of juggling an impressive array of authorities, even developed) the ability to draw from a variety of sources and represent topics from a number of different perspectives. Thus medical and philosophical views concerning women's pleasure were not simply mirror images of those concerning men's pleasure. In particular, the associations of women with pleasure were occasions for reflection on the negative and dangerous sides of sexuality in a way that the associations of men with pleasure were not – even though men's greater pleasure had been established.

For academic writers on medicine and natural philosophy in the thirteenth and fourteenth centuries, the structures, functions, and mechanisms of sexual pleasure were, in many respects, fundamentally similar in men and women. The procreative purpose of pleasure and the existence of pleasure outside the procreative process; the physiological and psychological cycle of imagination (or memory), desire, act, and pleasure; and the relationship of this pleasure to others and of humans' pleasure to animals' were all subjects that encompassed the operations and experience of both women and men and that commanded the interest of scholastic authors. What accounts for this remarkable expansion of pleasure as a domain of inquiry in this period? It may be explained in part by the general extension of scholarly interests and the enormous increases in scholarly production which took place with the rise of the universities and the development of commentaries and *questiones* as academic genres. It also may be explained in part by its connections with other issues, such as the existence and function of a female seed, the relations between form and matter, or the distinction between intensity and

---

164 H. Vorwahl, "Die Sexualität im Hoch-Mittelalter," *Janus* 37 (1933): 294: ". . . propter magnam delectationem, quam habet, quia per virgam virilem existentem in vulva nervi et venae in vulva confricantur et moventur. . . ." Vorwahl's attribution is simply to Albertus Magnus, *De animalibus*, X, 2. The passage does not correspond to anything in book X of Albertus's work (nor to book X, question 2, in Albertus's *Quaestiones de animalibus*) and appears to have been transcribed from some other commentary on Aristotle's text attributed to Albertus.

extension. And it may be explained in part by the desire of scholars who were not only Christian but who were also witnessing (and in many cases participating in) a broad-based effort in theology, canon law, and other fields to identify, explore, and resolve questions about the relationship between nature (including human nature) on the one hand and Christian doctrine and discipline on the other. But at least some of the content and direction of these investigations seems to have been inspired by specific concerns regarding the relations of men and women to each other and by the ambiguous and problematic characteristics of sexual pleasure itself. A fuller view of the content of those anxieties will emerge in connection with the issue of sexual abstinence. Here the most visible aspects are the coexistence of reproductive and nonreproductive possibilities for pleasure, the parallels and disjunctions between the male and female experiences, and the association of "more" pleasure with both superiority and weakness. The incommensurability of male and female existence that characterizes certain aspects of the scholastic understanding of pleasure poses special challenges. In particular, it represents the feminine as at least partially autonomous and thus not fully under control either on the conceptual level or on the level of experience and social life.

The lack of solid guidance from ancient authorities, as well as the force of broader social and cultural implications made scholastic treatments of pleasure less stable and systematic and more ambiguous and unsettled than scholastic treatments of female and male reproductive contributions or the determination of sex in the embryo. But all these subjects were highlighted, organized, and investigated within the university curriculum and according to the structured practices of academic scholarship. The commentaries, *questiones*, and treatises in which they figured afforded teachers and students of medicine and natural philosophy the opportunity and methods for clarifying and emphasizing matters of sexual practice and reproduction. In the process of these investigations, scholars had to deal – sometimes directly and sometimes tangentially – with the similarities and differences between females and males, women and men.

In spite of the great care a number of authors devoted to these subjects, the conclusions on any given topic were not always clear and consistent. The identification of a function for the female emission, for example, or the coordination of the multiple factors involved in causing a fetus to be one sex or another left unanswered questions, and in so doing provided a certain open-endedness that prevents us from seeing late medieval views on sex difference as monolithic or inflexible. Similarly and more strikingly, the concepts of male and female projected by the answers to different questions differed from one another. In discussions of reproductive role and sex differentiation the female is never a fully active partner nor a completely passive vessel but exists and operates somewhere on the continuum between the two. Furthermore, no significant factors distinguish humans from animals. In discussions of pleasure the woman's experience is measured on a different scale from that of the man's, and several elements of inclination and behavior distinguish humans from animals. Scholastic science produced a vast quantity of information and reflection on subjects relating to sex difference, often presented in a thorough and ordered fashion. It drew together ancient as well as older medieval sources, it integrated or juxtaposed the metaphysics and mechanics of specific topics, and it developed and fortified certain orthodoxies. At the same time, it left open a number of choices and possibilities. Thus although there was no significant disagreement with the belief that women were cooler, weaker, less intellectually competent, and generally less perfect than men, there were, first of all, various ways in which those differences could be played out and understood and, second, numerous dimensions of the procreative process and sexual behavior which had little if anything to do with that central continuum of power, activity, and value. Thus, although the medical and philosophical works which dealt with reproductive roles, sex determination, and pleasure articulated a doctrine of the sexes and their interactions, that doctrine was neither monolithic nor all-encompassing.

The significance of this network of scholastic ideas is twofold. On the one hand, it represents the culmination of a process, begun in the late eleventh century, by which Western learning brought to the fore scientific and medical questions involving the differences between the sexes. Technical and sophisticated, it refined the factors that distinguished male and female and at the same time laid bare tensions and inconsistencies contained in them. These developments have been the subject of Part I. On the other hand, it represents a mine of material which, though seldom intended to do so, reveals its connections with broader ideas about masculinity and femininity. Reflecting and influencing opinions beyond the university, it expresses far more than the solutions to certain academic problems. This dimension of scholastic views will come into play in Part II.

The interaction of the highly structured and elaborate university ideas with the larger culture of Western Europe in the later Middle Ages followed several pathways. The participants were not insulated from other aspects of society: some grew up in families of the aristocracy or urban patriciate, others were raised in monasteries; some practiced medicine, others heard confession, and many spent time on the busy streets of growing towns. Thus Albertus Magnus used as evidence for a relationship between heat and female sperm the conviction that black women have more sperm than white women, "since black women are hotter and most swarthy, who are sweetest for mounting, as the pimps say."[165] Furthermore, the work of university scholars reached wide audiences among the literate elite, in no small part through the same educational institutions and literary genres that also carried on the older traditions of Isidore of Seville and Constantine the African. For example, a structured compilation of authoritative opinions on a wide array of medical subjects, the *Compendium of Medicine* written by Gilbert the Englishman in the midthirteenth century, summarized views about the origin of semen attributed to Avicenna, Ali ibn Abbas (Constantine's *Pantegni*), Hippocrates, and Aristotle.[166] Another general work on medicine written by his compatriot John of Gaddesden in the early fourteenth century paused in its matter-of-fact account of the causes of sterility (be sure there is not a pin used by a dead person in your bed) to equivocate about the necessity of female seed to the reproductive process, citing the authority of university philosopher and theologian Giles of Rome.[167] Both Gilbert and John were, in turn, widely known beyond university circles – to Chaucer and his audience, among others.[168] Finally, only a few of the men who spent time as university students went on to academic careers; most made their way as schoolteachers, healers, bureaucrats, or preachers, and as such they were vectors for the new learning.

Thus, although the evolution of academic ideas about specific problems like the female seed has been represented chronologically in terms of groups of texts and in terms of the processes, such as translations and institutional changes, that affected them, an examination of the relationship between learned opinions and the notions about males and females entertained in the culture at large demands a more fluid and less linear approach. The following chapters present a thematic portrait of scientific and medical views which reflects the accretion and coexistence of layers of understanding compounded over centuries and assembled from the rubble of antiquity, the intrusions of Arabic learning, and the strata of medieval thought. It includes old views which continued to be learned, as well as new views which were being rapidly disseminated; it includes opinions expressed by and for a wider intellectual elite, as well as those expressed by experts. Seen in this way and given the diversity of positions taken even within the university

165 Albertus Magnus, *Quaestiones de animalibus*, bk. XV, q. 19, p. 271: "Et tale sperma magis invenitur in feminis nigris . . . quam albis; quia nigrae sunt calidiores et maxime fuscae, quae sunt dulcissimae ad supponendum, ut dicunt leccatores. . . ." The language of skin colors in the Middle Ages has not been seriously studied, so it is difficult to evaluate the sense of this passage in relation to modern concepts of "race." Certainly more is involved here than relative lightness and darkness.

166 Gilbertus Anglicus, *Compendium medicine*, bk. VII, ch. [i], fol. 287ra–b.

167 Johannes Anglicus, *Rosa Anglica practica medicine* (Venice: Bonetus Locatellus, 1516), fols. 74vb, 75ra. See also Thomas Cantimpratensis, *Liber de natura rerum*, pt. 1, *Texte*, ed. H. Boese (Berlin and New York: Walter de Gruyter, 1973), bk. I, ch. 71, p. 72.

168 Geoffrey Chaucer, "General Prologue" of *The Canterbury Tales*, vol. 1 of *The Complete Works*, Group A, ll. 429–34.

tradition, late medieval views of sex difference are much richer and more complex than the stereotypical dichotomies of active/passive, soul/body, superior/inferior sometimes imputed to them. At the same time, for all its elasticity, the picture of female and male created by this agglomeration of medical and philosophical sources had sufficient integrity to maintain its distinctness from other forces, particularly social and religious, which asserted themselves in the later Middle Ages.

PART II

Sex difference and the construction of gender

Learned Latin discussion reflecting ideas about sex difference became more detailed, more explicit, more complex, and more complete during the period from the late eleventh through the fourteenth century. The elaboration of male and female reproductive roles provided a firm, if not solid, base for defining male and female natures. Most authors occupied the ample middle ground between the position, encouraged by Hippocratic ideas of pangenesis and the interaction of two seeds, that males and females played essentially comparable roles in generation and the position, encouraged by Aristotle's strongest formulations, that all significant work was done by the male. Furthermore, the new emphasis that both medical writers and natural philosophers placed upon the subject of pleasure expanded the scientific conceptualization of sex difference beyond reproduction itself into the domain of sexual impulses, behaviors, and experiences. This network of ideas offers specific clues to medieval notions about women and men, and about femininity and masculinity. The attribution of special appetites and pleasures to women, for example, developed far beyond the requirements of the particular questions about the role of female semen within which it originated, suggesting at least one dimension of medieval images of women. Furthermore, some aspects of the intellectual and institutional settings within which these ideas developed had a bearing on their formation. Thus, for example, the opening of some versions of pseudo–Albertus Magnus's *Secrets of Women*, addressed by a cleric (probably a Dominican friar) to his colleagues, cites women's dangerous nature as the reason for presenting a work that deals with sexual, gynecological, and embryological topics.[1]

Systematic thinking about these subjects was not simply a straightforward reflection of a broader social and cultural understanding of what women and men were supposed to be and do, or of what traits, inclinations, and habits

---

1 For several relevant openings, see Lynn Thorndike, "Further Considerations," pp. 413–43.

were quintessential features of femaleness and maleness. Authors writing about gynecology or generation or coitus were subject to many forces that, though not unrelated to gender, had strong connections with other dimensions of the medieval world. That university students and teachers were all men, and that the universities themselves participated in a number of masculine power structures certainly shaped and limited the perspective of academic writing about sex difference in a general way. The content of the curriculum was affected by considerations as different as the course of medieval ecclesiastical careers and the opinions of ancient authorities; the forms of pedagogy and therefore of literary production were affected by considerations as diverse as the politics of medical licensing and the love of dialectic. Each of these dimensions was gendered, involved in a system of power, authority, success, and the reproduction of knowledge in ways that divided women and men, but each also incorporated other interests and forces operating in medieval culture. Thus there are links between scholastic science and medicine on the one hand and medieval gender concepts on the other, but the relationships are not neat: the choices and ambiguities generated by the many and various sources carry over into the network of gender meanings; the taxonomy of masculine and feminine is undermined by the very explanatory system which supports it, when, for example, intermediate forms disrupt the clear distinctions between hot and cold or left and right; and the cases of sterility and abstinence reveal tensions within and among the religious, social, medical, and natural philosophical axes.

4

Feminine and masculine types

GENDERED MEANINGS

The interests and traditions of scholastic authors led them to explore and debate specific questions related to sex difference and reproduction. They contributed to but by no means exhausted the ways in which Latin writings on nature and medicine represented females and males. An array of traits differentiated the sexes in the late Middle Ages, not all of which fit neatly into the repertoire of theoretical systems upon which scholastic arguments drew to sort out such specific puzzles as the existence of a female seed or the kinds and degrees of pleasure. One treatise, borrowing selectively from Aristotle, lists many differences. Among non-egg-laying animals, the male is larger; among such egg-laying animals as snakes and frogs, the female is larger. All females have higher and subtler voices – except cows. Female deer lack horns. Males are stronger – except among bears and leopards.[1] The lists of sex-linked characteristics become longer and the construction of "female" and "male" becomes more complicated (and sometimes elusive) when we look at a wider range of sources. The more open style and less carefully delineated content of the prescholastic works, along with a large number of sometimes haphazard and omnivorous compendia and epitomes deriving from the scholastic literature itself, added choice, flexibility, and ambiguity to the by no means simple or settled results of scholastic discussions.

A number of the distinguishing features of females and males, such as strength and voice, bear with them medieval concepts of behaviors, temperaments, and social roles understood to be typical of women and men. Straight eyebrows, for example, are a sign of femininity, implying, in this case, both wickedness and adaptability.[2] Natural philosophy and medicine thus provide bridges among reproductive roles of females and males, social roles of women and men, and typologies of feminine and masculine. Few

---

1 *Propositiones de animalibus*, Cambridge University Library, MS Dd.3.16, fols. 73ra–74vb.
2 Ibid., fol. 73ra.

texts take as their explicit task the project of constructing gender ideas, but when a medical author calls intercourse with the woman on top "usurpation" in a discussion of unhealthy sexual practices, the bridges between nature and society are visible.[3] Even when the subject at hand is not remotely related either to reproduction or to social roles, gender implications may be lurking. Male fish are better to eat than females, because they have firmer flesh, and the meat of males, females, and castrati differ with respect to fat, facts that reflect on the vigor and robustness of the groups in question. In general, the meat of the male is better and more digestible (except for goat meat), a fact that recalls the more perfect balance of the male.[4] This kind of piecemeal information about nature, as well as more systematic ideas about male and female build, constitution, and disposition, produced a framework and vocabulary for medieval gender attributions – an array of ideas and images grounded in understandings of nature. These in turn shaped the way in which medieval authors spoke of the genesis of sex difference, whether framed in embryological or biblical terms. Elements of the various levels of analysis converged to create polarized sets of characteristics which were remarkably powerful in spite of the variety and malleability of their particulars. Challenges arising from the presence of hermaphrodite features, transvestite acts, and homophile inclinations in the experienced or imagined world were not only socially suspect but also conceptually unstable: an instance or its parts would usually be labeled "male" or "female," qualified as "feminine" or "masculine." Underlying these assertive constructs were certain basic principles of male and female existence. "First," said Jacopo of Forlì, "it must be noted that male differs from female in three [ways], namely, complexion, disposition, and shape. And among these complexion is the most fundamental."[5]

BEING FEMININE AND BEING MASCULINE: COMPLEXION, SHAPE, AND DISPOSITION

Complexion

Although some authors, especially those interested in obstetrics and gynecology, represented the uterus as the defining feature of the female, many agreed

3 Enrique Montero Cartelle, ed., *Liber minor de coitu: Tratado menor de andrología anomino salernitano,* Lingüística y filología 2 (Valladolid: Universidad de Valladolid, 1987), pt. II, ch. 2, p. 98; see Natalie Zemon Davis, "Women on Top," in *Society and Culture in Early Modern France: Eight Essays* (Stanford: Stanford University Press, 1975), pp. 124–51.

4 *Propositiones de animalibus,* Cambridge University Library, MS Dd.3.16, fol. 74ra; [Constantinus Africanus, *De dietis universalibus*], Bibliothèque Nationale, MS lat. 7036, fols. 28v and 23r.

5 Jacobus Forliviensis, *De generatione embrionis,* fol. 9vb: "Notandum primo quod masculus differt a femella in 3, scilicet complexione, moribus et figura. Quamvis complexio inter hec principalior existat."

with Jacopo that sex differences were founded on – and thus could best be explained by – the distinction between male and female complexions. Complexion was the balance or ratio of qualities, especially hot, cold, moist, and dry, which characterized an individual or group. Fish have a cooler complexion than cattle, and that difference explains why the former lay eggs and the latter bear live young. Insects have a drier complexion than birds. Females are moister than males, which can explain why the meat of male animals is firmer and the meat of females (and emasculated males) more lax. Heat, however, was the most fundamental physical difference between the sexes, and a cause of many other differences.[6] It is their greater heat that allows men to make their nutritive superfluities into hair and beards, and it is their greater heat that (whatever the differences in *pace* of maturation) permits them to grow to a higher stage of completion and perfection than women. The general belief was that the coldest man was still warmer than the warmest woman.[7] Indeed, from the very beginning, males are warmer than females, which is one of the reasons male embryos grow more quickly in the womb.[8] Or did girls mature faster than boys? William of Conches thought so. Disagreement on such points was less important than the consensus that heat was a profoundly powerful explanatory principle. For some of the most subtle and thoughtful authors, the exact nature of this heat was a matter of some interest. William of Conches, a learned and encyclopedic natural philosopher of the twelfth century, agreed that females were colder but held that when something cold burns, it is hotter and harder to extinguish, which may be why females mature faster.[9] And a fourteenth-century scholastic commentary on a basic medical text explained that we are not to understand "heat" in the material sense but rather in the formal sense, since some women are *physically* hotter than some men.[10] Most texts, less sophisticated and less anxious to preserve explanatory consistency or explore philosophical subtleties, simply held that males were warmer than females.

That general constitutional difference gives rise to more important results than maturation speed or beards. It is the basis of the Aristotelian perspective on the sexes that the male is characterized by the ability to cook nutri-

6 Authors formulated and interpreted the heat differential differently but agreed on its importance. Cf. Maclean, *Renaissance Notion of Woman*, pp. 32–33.
7 *Secreta mulierum maior*, Cambridge University, Trinity MS O.2.5, fol. 76va, cites Hippocrates to this effect. See also (without mention of an authority) ibid., fol. 130 vb; Trinity MS
R.14.45, a version of the same text, that says there can be exceptions to the rule (fol. 25r);
and Peter of Abano, *Conciliator,* who summarizes opinions (Bibliothèque Nationale, MS lat.
6961, fol. 40ra).
8 Jacobus Forliviensis, *De generatione embrionis*, fol. 5ra.
9 Guilelmus de Conchis, *De substantiis physicis,* bk. VI, p. 238; Lemay, "William of Saliceto,"
p. 172; see also Jacobus Forliviensis, *De generatione embrionis*, fol. 5ra–rb. This observation
probably refers to different ages of puberty, not to embryonic maturation.
10 *Versus Egidii* [a commentary on a commentary], Oxford, Exeter College, MS 35, fol. 85va;
see similarly Jacobus Forliviensis, *De generatione embrionis*, fol. 5ra.

tional residues in order to produce seed and the female by the inability to do so. Even those who believed that females too produce seed still held both that heat is the instrument by which the body refined nutriment into semen and that females have less or weaker heat for this purpose. There were more abstract principles of which heat was merely the vehicle or instrument – the soul or the vital principle. Dante, in his concise summary of Aristotelian reproductive theory as conveyed by the Arabic commentator Averroes, alluded only briefly to heat, speaking instead of the "formative virtue" which derives from the father's heart.[11] Still, it is heat to which medieval authors, especially the less systematic among them, appealed with the greatest regularity when attributing causes to female and male functions.

The importance of heat as an instrument and as a manifestation of sexual differentiation illustrates both the extent and the complexity of the tangle created by notions of sex difference and the gender constructs with which they interact. Heat is explicitly or implicitly linked to several principles of differentiation that participate in the definition and explanation of sex and contribute to the characterization of gender. The relative firmness of the male's breast, for example,[12] and the relative weakness of women[13] participated both in the scientific analysis of sex as related to heat and in the cultural meaning of gender. The notion that women are soft and smooth and weak had to do with the inability of their bodies' heat to produce semen and at the same time with a more general aura of incapacity, with the sense that women do lead and should lead a more sedentary life, and with the idea that women lack the vehemence which men possess. Hildegard of Bingen, for example, introduced a long discussion of the various types of female temperament with these observations on the effects of exercise:

A male who is of sound body is not much harmed if he walks or stays standing for a long time. . . . A man who is weak should sit, since if he were to go or stand, he would be harmed. Woman, however, since she is more fragile than man, and since she has a divided skull, should walk and stand in moderation, but should sit more than she runs around, lest she be harmed.[14]

According to this view, women's constitution requires rest; according to another, women's practice of resting affects her constitution. The medical writer Bernard of Gordon suggested that women are more harmed by

11 Dante Alighieri, *Purgatorio*, in *The Divine Comedy*, ed., trans., and comm. Charles S. Singleton, 6 vols., Bollingen Series 80 (Princeton: Princeton University Press, 1970–75), XXV, ll. 37–99: "virtute informativa" (l. 41); "virtù" (l. 89).

12 *Propositiones de animalibus*, Cambridge University Library, MS Dd.3.16, fol. 73rb.

13 Ibid., fol. 74vb; Hildegard, *Causae et curae*, bk. II, p. 77.

14 Hildegard, *Causae et curae*, bk. II, pp. 86–7: "Masculus autem, qui in corpore sanus est, si diu ambulat aut si diu erectus stat, inde non multum laeditur. . . . Qui vero debilis est, sedeat, quia, si iste multum iret aut staret, inde laederetur. Mulier autem, quia fragilior viro est, et quia diversa calvariam habet, moderate ambulet et stet, sed magis sedeat, quam discurrat, ne inde laedatur." On women's divided skull, which allows menstruation to occur, see bk. II, pp. 107–8.

sexual abstinence than are men because women get less exercise.[15] Are habits the source of the medical condition or is the constitution the source of behavior? That this question did not occur to medieval authors is an indication of the extent to which medical and scientific ideas about sex were integrated with gender constructs and also of the cultural assumption that the integration was appropriate, requiring no explanation or justification.

At the convergence of the constitutional differences in heat and the constitutional differences in the processing of physiological superfluities stood the production and expulsion of seed and menses. Within the terms of the academic debates, there were two general ways of representing this constellation of processes and products. Either men, because of their superior heat, were able to refine their superfluous blood completely into semen, and women, unable to do so, were left with menses; or men, because of their superior heat, produced more, more refined, warmer, less watery semen than women, while women produced inferior semen – and also menses. With respect to their gender implications, however, the two positions did not differ much in practice. Even those who held that menses in women were homologous to semen in men nevertheless set menstruation apart as a female idiosyncracy; and even those who held that women did produce some kind of seed nevertheless gave it much less attention than either male seed or menstruation. Menstruation was the specific feature of the female constitution which attracted the most attention among natural philosophers and medical writers. Although it was sometimes depicted as the equivalent of some male function, whether the production of semen or of sweat, menstruation was, like the womb, singularly and remarkably female. Like the womb in anatomy, the physiological fact of menstruation characterized the female and the feminine in two ways: first as an aspect of the reproductive function and second as a more general principle of the female constitution or temperament.

Obstetrical texts illustrate and underscore the place of menstruation in medical thinking about reproduction. The female ailment most discussed both in general medical works and in those devoted to the diseases of women is menstrual retention, which was regarded as a common impediment to conception: "no menses, no conception" was a tenet widely held without reference to the specific reproductive role attributed to menstrual fluid. Thus, remedies for menstrual retention abound. A twelfth-century formulary recommends a powder of burnt deer's horn to be taken with old wine;[16] a thirteenth-century source suggests a number of remedies, including pills, baths, herb drinks, phlebotomy, charms, and pessaries.[17] (Since remedies often include only recipes without reference to causes or to the

15 Bernardus de Gordonio, *Lilium*, pt. VII, ch. i, fols. 87vb–88ra.
16 Vienna, Nationalbibliothek, MS CVP 2532, fol. 71v.
17 [Ps.-]Trotula, *De passionibus mulierum*, Cambridge University Library, MS Dd.11.45, fols. 62v–63r, 68r; British Library, MS Sloane 1124, fols. 172ra, 177rb–va.

relationship among symptoms, it is difficult to distinguish remedies aimed at curing menstrual retention per se from those promoting conception.) Excess menstrual flow was also a significant, though less prominent, concern. The emphasis on menstruation, like the emphasis on the womb, thus reinforced the centrality of women's function as childbearers. "Be fruitful and multiply" and, to an even greater extent, "in sorrow thou shalt bring forth children"[18] gave depth and breadth to the medical concern with reproduction and its connection with menstruation. Thus, although "female" is nowhere defined as "the sex which menstruates" (or even as "the sex which bears young"), menstruation is a prominent factor in defining both her sex and her social and cultural functions.

The significance of menstruation is larger than its connection with reproduction. Although compared and even homologized with certain male functions as a refinement of blood or a purgation of excess, menstruation distinguishes women from men, as well as from other female animals. It is a specifically womanly mark of the Fall.[19] From this perspective, menstruation is a blemish, a sign of imperfection, just as in Aristotelian natural philosophy it is the result and token of the female's inability, due to the inadequacy of her heat, to refine blood into semen. In Paradise there was no menstruation, and in the higher realms of nature, which are not subject to change, there is no need for sexual differentiation (i.e., for the imperfect female). But in the world in which we live, these things must be as they are. Menstruation is no sin, and the existence of the female serves the higher purposes of nature, but both are marks of a natural falling away from perfection.

Theologians often regarded menstruation as a stain (though not a sin).[20] Systematic theologians struggled with the problem of the Virgin Mary's physiological status. Dominican writers preferred to preserve her humanity, holding that she bore the full burden of womanhood. And even those who promoted the notion (later doctrine) of the Virgin's Immaculate Conception believed that she condescended to be Eve's heir in this respect.[21] That Mary's menstruation posed such a problem demonstrates the extent to which the Fall and the stain of womanhood haunted that physiological process. That late medieval theology was able to reconcile monthly bleeding with the status of the Virgin was a tribute both to the convergence of Christian and Aristotelian teleology (according to which God had created nothing in vain) and to new emphasis on Incarnation, which asserted Christ's humanity and countered heretical rejection of the physical world.

18 Genesis 1:28 and 3:16.
19 Charles T. Wood, "The Doctors' Dilemma: Sin, Salvation, and the Menstrual Cycle in Medieval Thought," *Speculum* 56 (1981): 710–27.
20 Carolly Erickson, *The Medieval Vision: Essays in History and Perception* (New York: Oxford University Press, 1976), pp. 195–6.
21 Wood, "Doctors' Dilemma," pp. 718–23.

Medical writers and natural philosophers were more likely than others to put menstruation in a positive light, because of its purgative as well as its reproductive functions, but even naturalists sometimes represented menstruation darkly. Isidore of Seville, the influential encyclopedist of the sixth century, was probably reflecting popular belief, as well as Pliny, when he wrote that in the presence of a menstruating woman, crops do not germinate, wine sours, grass dies, trees lose their fruit, and iron rusts.[22] These notions recur in later texts, such as a commentary on the *Secrets of Women* that justified addressing a scientific work on women to a monastic audience by observing not only that priests may need to know about such things when they take confession from women, but also that they may need the information to protect themselves, since menstruating women are dangerous.[23] In other words, the misogynistic possibilities of menstruation did not go unexploited.

Menstruation thus casts a shadow over woman but does not leave her in total darkness. The beneficial effects of menstruation were widely recognized. These were related to its purgative function, which was effective beyond any of the analogues attributed to men. Few medical or scientific texts pressed the notion of an important female advantage based on menstruation, since the general view was that female weakness included ill health,[24] but Hildegard of Bingen, one of the few women we can identify who wrote in Latin on medical matters, observed that women were less susceptible to hernias and attributed the low incidence of gout among women directly to the purgative effects of menstruation.[25] And Heloise, in one of her famous letters to Abelard, called on the authority of an early medieval encyclopedist to support her view that women get drunk less easily than men because of their frequent purgations and moist constitutions.[26] Recognizing the social resonances of beliefs about women's nature, Heloise used them in her arguments for the institution of a moderate and humane set of rules for the nuns she supervised.

One example from the work of Albertus Magnus serves to illustrate the restorative power attributed to menstruation and to assure us that we are dealing with medieval – not with warmed-over classical – opinion. Albertus faces what he regards as a fact: that, contrary to the assertions of Aristotle, women live longer than men. The problem was not that Aristotle seemed to have been mistaken about a detail of nature but that the observa-

22 Isidorus, *Etymologiae*, bk. XI, ch. i, §141; cf. Pliny, *Natural History,* bk. VII, ch. 15, §64–5 (vol. II, p. 548).
23 Thorndike, "Further Considerations," p. 430. See also Cambridge University Library, MSS O.2.5, fol. 130va–vb; R.14.45, fol. 24v.
24 *Propositiones de animalibus*, Cambridge University Library, MS Dd.3.13, fol. 75ra.
25 Hildegard, *Causae et curae*, bk. II, pp. 99–100, 102.
26 Abelard and Heloise, *Lettres*, ed. Victor Cousin and trans. Octave Gérard, 2d ed. (Paris: Garnier Frères, 1875), pp. 150, 152, citing Macrobius, *Saturnalia*, bk. VII, ch. 6, §16–17.

tion contravened a principle of natural philosophy. Males are warmer than females, and life is associated with heat, death with the failure of heat.[27] The male body contains the essential causes of long life. But females actually live longer on account of accidental causes: they menstruate, they are less taxed by intercourse, and they work less.[28]

Albertus's strategy, distinguishing the essential from the accidental, permits him to get around Aristotle without contradicting him. It also illustrates the integration of sex and gender in medieval scientific writing. What we would identify as physiological, sexual, and socioeconomic reasons combine to provide an explanation for female longevity. First of all, menstruation cleanses women's bodies, leaving them less polluted by harmful residues or less burdened by excess of useful residues than men. Second, intercourse is harder on men than on women. The differences in reproductive roles partially account for this effect: even those who asserted the existence and importance of a female seed nevertheless regarded the male role as preeminent, and therefore as more taxing. For example, the male contribution is consistently regarded as warmer, and men therefore emit more of their vital heat in intercourse than women. (The relatively slighter female sexual expenditure has other explanations, rooted more clearly in the medieval understanding of women's roles. Whereas men are aged by frequent intercourse, women are aged by frequent childbirth:[29] men's efforts, in other words, are sexual; women's are reproductive.) Perhaps the passive and sedentary aspect of femininity also comes into play here, since overexertion was deemed inappropriate for women, and a passive role in intercourse was prescribed by canonists as well as by medical authorities – women were not, for example, to assume the superior position.[30] Albertus's third reason for female longevity – that women do not work as hard as men – is likewise a reflection of gender definitions. The notion that men do the work may have lurking behind it the distinction between Adam's curse (the labor of food production) and Eve's (the labor of reproduction), but since it is stated without scriptural fanfare, it is more likely a reflection of social perceptions. It reveals what was taken to constitute labor (a significant issue in any culture), for there were few idle women in the Middle Ages.

27 Peter H. Niebyl, "Old Age, Fever, and the Lamp Metaphor," *Journal of the History of Medicine* 26 (1971): 351–68; Joan Cadden, "A Matter of Life and Death: Water in the Natural Philosophy of Albertus Magnus," *History and Philosophy of the Life Sciences* 2 (1980): 241–52.
28 Wood, "Doctors' Dilemma," p. 724, cites Albert's *Quaestiones de animalibus*. On perceptions and realities of female longevity, see Vern L. Bullough and Cameron Campbell, "Female Longevity and Diet in the Middle Ages," *Speculum* 55 (1980): 317–25; and David Herlihy, "Life Expectancies for Women in Medieval Society," in Rosemarie Thee Morewedge, ed., *The Role of Women in the Middle Ages: Papers of the Sixth Annual Conference of the Center for Medieval and Renaissance Studies, State University of New York at Binghamton, 6–7 May, 1972* (Albany: State University of New York Press, 1976), pp. 1–22.
29 Cambridge University Library, Trinity MSS O.2.5, fol. 131ra; R.14.45, fol. 25r.
30 Cartelle, ed., *Liber minor de coitu*, pt. II, ch. 6, p. 98; James A. Brundage, "Let Me Count the Ways: Canonists and Theologians Contemplate Coital Positions" (unpublished paper).

The constitutional differences between male and female could be simply stated in terms of hot and cool complexions, but on that foundation was built a complex set of meanings. Not only did the basic principles explain the differences of appearance – from genitals to hair – but they also had ramifications for the expectations and images of women and men. With respect to work or drunkenness, with respect to health and the effects of the Fall, the complexions of the two sexes suggested and explained a network of gender constructs. Some of these were built around the opposition of male ability and female inability, but others, such as menstruation, which was both a healthful purgation and a threat to others, were more complex and unsettled.

Shape

Males and females are, medieval authors agreed, built differently. Many texts about animals in general (mostly about mammals) mention anatomical differences without dwelling upon them. The more systematic works, especially those derived from Aristotle's *Generation of Animals* and *Parts of Animals,* distinguish *essential* anatomical differences, which were directly tied to reproductive functions, from *secondary* or accidental differences. Many authors accepted the Aristotelian way of conceptualizing one difference: males have external genitals; females, internal genitals. They agreed, too, that this difference had meaning, though not on what the meaning was. The difference might be understood to demonstrate that male and female were opposites (inside as opposed to outside, imperfect as opposed to perfect) or that they were essentially equivalent and just a little differently arranged: both models were widely recognized and applied.[31]

The organs mentioned as characteristic of the sexes are the penis and the uterus: the *matrix* is to the female as the *virga* is to the male. Although some authors believed that females had testes which produced seed, the strong association of woman with uterus, of *mater* with *matrix,* inclined writers to deviate from a strict insistence on parallels between anatomy and physiology such as female seed is to male seed as female testes are to male testes. In her visionary work *Scivias,* Hildegard of Bingen alluded to the contrast between external penis and internal uterus when she explained why men but not women had to be circumcised under the Old Law: "Woman does not need to be circumcised, since she hides the maternal temple in her body . . . and," she went on to add, "since she is under the power of man." [32] (Hildegard, no social egalitarian, nevertheless promoted

---

31 Nemesius, *De natura hominis,* ch. XXIV, p. 109; cf. Laqueur, *Making Sex.*
32 Hildegard, *Scivias,* pt. II, vis. iii, ch. 21, p. 147: ". . . mulier non est circumcidenda, quia maternum tabernaculum latet in corpore eius, . . . et quoniam ipsa est sub potestate viri. . . ."

the interests of women in many contexts. Under the New Law, she held, the Son of God gives women and men alike the circumcision of all bodily members: baptism is efficacious at any time for persons of any age and of either sex.)[33]

The comparison of uterus and penis fit and enhanced two different views of female sexual identity and, in turn, of the feminine gender. On the one hand, the emphasis upon the womb as the central female organ was in harmony with the view of women as essentially passive vessels. The word *vas* in the sense of "jar" or "vessel" occurs in medieval texts as a synonym for woman,[34] and the image of the womb as an upside-down jar (dissociated from any person) is repeated in frequently copied illustrations of fetal positions.[35] (See Figure 5.) On the other hand, the association of the womb with the penis suggests it is an active, sexual organ (as distinguished from a passive, reproductive organ) and is in tune with the view that the womb and therefore (by metonymy) the woman are dominated by an insatiable sexual appetite. The womb has an appetitive faculty in the Galenic sense that it draws to itself the male seed or the combined seed of the male and female; the woman is all appetite in the more colloquial sense that she craves all the pleasures of the flesh.[36]

These two perspectives, the more passive and the more active, coexisted in late medieval culture. Though they appear inconsistent, they share the underlying suggestion that women are empty, void, lacking – that by not having the male principle they both lack masculine activity and need (and therefore desire) men's active principle, semen. Each, by defining the female, placed limits on the feminine, and each was capable of misogynistic expression. The notion of the female as imperfect male entered into philosophical discussions. Thomas Aquinas, for example, entertained it when he discussed "whether woman ought to have been made in the first production of things," considering that she is a "defective" male.[37] But the appetitive woman was the one most frequently played upon in the antifeminist literature of the period. For example, all women, even nuns, are sworn enemies

33 Ibid., ch. 29, 31, pp. 152–3.
34 Charles du Fresne du Cange, *Glossarium mediae et infimae Latinitatis*, suppl. D. P. Carpenter and G. A. L. Henschel, new ed. Léopold Favre (Niort and London: L. Favre and David Nutt, 1882–7), s.v. *vas*, in one instance misinterpreting Paul. See also Hildegard, *Causae et curae*, bk. II, p. 77.
35 The illustrations commonly accompanied Muscio's version of Soranus and eventually made their way into early printed editions of that work. Karl Sudhoff reproduces thirteenth-, fourteenth-, and fifteenth-century examples in "Drei noch unveröffentlichte Kindslagenserien des Soranos-Muscio aus Oxford und London," *Archiv für Geschichte der Medizin* 4 (1911): plate III.
36 See, e.g., the invective of Andreas Capellanus, *De amore libri tres*, ed. E. Trojel (Copenhagen: G. E. C. Gad, 1892; repr., Munich: Eidos, 1964), bk. III, esp. pp. 353–4.
37 Thomas Aquinas, *Summa theologiae*, pt. I, q. 92, art. 1: "Dicit philosophus . . . quod *femina est mas occasionatus.* Sed nihil occasionatum et deficiens debuit esse in prima rerum institutione."

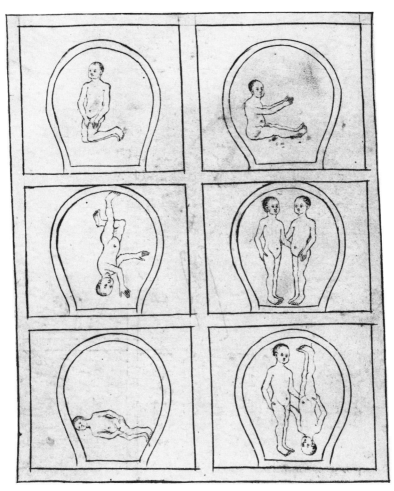

Figure 5. Fetuses in utero. To illustrate fetal positions, manuscripts of obstetrical works, especially Muscio's Latin version of Soranus, showed series of disembodied wombs and their occupants. This is an English example from about 1400. (Oxford, Bodleian, MS Laud. misc. 724, fol. 97v. Reproduced by permission of the Bodleian Library, Oxford.)

of Chastity, and all women are whores, if not in deed at least in desire, according to the Jealous Husband in *The Romance of the Rose*.[38]

Beyond these primary attributes, medical and scientific authors mentioned other features of the female and male which they regarded as charac-

---

38 Guillaume de Lorris and Jean de Meun, *Le roman de la rose*, ed. Ernest Langlois, 5 vols., Société des anciens textes français, (Paris: Firmin-Didot, 1914), ll. 9013–24 and 9155–8, vol. 3, pp. 104–5 and 110.

teristic. In contrast to modern expectations, mammae are not often mentioned in the context of sexual differentiation, although breasts are the subject of various instructions and remedies in obstetrical treatises.[39] Nor do testes serve as an important point of contrast. (Although Galen had accorded them a role in the final refinement of seed, that function applied in both sexes, though to different degrees.) Likewise, in contrast to modern expectations, the kidneys attracted some attention. Because of the belief that the origin of male sexual pleasure was the kidneys, whereas the origin of female sexual pleasure was sometimes said to be the navel (*umbilicus*),[40] some held that the penis had its root in the kidneys, and the uterus had its root in the umbilicus.[41] Hildegard of Bingen was probably resisting this distinction when she took the trouble to insist that the kidneys had the same basic structure in women and men and asserted that man's loins (*lumbi*) are situated *in* the kidneys and that woman's womb is *joined to* them.[42] She held that female desire was different from male desire in degree and disposition but not in kind, and her position on the kidneys is consistent with that view. She appears to have been confronting not a specific argument about the role of female kidneys but rather the failure of medieval authors to trace the path of female sexual arousal. The *Prose Salernitan Questions* are typical in that regard: what starts out looking like a description of the geography of human desire turns out to be the geography of male desire – the relevant humor, produced by the liver and transmitted as nutrient to the whole body, descends along the classical route from the brain through the veins behind the ears, to the kidneys, and then to the testicles, where it is refined into sperm and whence it is emitted through the penis.[43]

If the pattern of the male norm is common, its significance is not always obvious. Several authors mention differences in the head and brain. Hildegard of Bingen says women's skulls are divided, like children's, whereas men's are whole. And when she is describing different types of men and women, she comments on men's, but not women's, brains.[44] The most frequently noted difference is that males have larger heads and brains.[45] Although it is tempting to assume that frequent allusions to this particular anatomical difference are linked to the Aristotelian view that women's rationality is imperfect (Aquinas explains the subjection of women to men by

---

39 Isidore of Seville held that some human features were for appearance, including men's breasts, and others for differentiation: *Etymologiae*, bk. XI, ch. i, §97–104.

40 Ibid., §98.

41 [Thomas Cantimpratensis], *De proprietatibus et natura rerum*, Munich, Bayerische Staatsbibliothek, MS CLM 3206, fol. 145ra.

42 Hildegard, *Causae et curae*, bk. II, p. 100.

43 Lawn, *Prose Salernitan Questions*, B, 16, pp. 10–11.

44 Hildegard, *Causae et curae*, bk. II, pp. 59, 71–5, and 87–9.

45 Thomas [Cantimpratensis?], *De partibus et membris corporis*, British Library, MS Egerton 1984, fol. 144r; *Physiognomia*, Oxford, Bodleian, MS Ashmol. 399, fol. 1r; *Propositiones de animalibus*, Cambridge University Library, MS Dd.3.16, fol. 76ra.

saying the wiser should rule),[46] these sources offer no explicit evidence for a connection. Perhaps more important, the head and brain, although accorded a place in medieval psychology, were not always regarded as the seat of rationality.[47] Comments on heads and brains, like comments on edibility, nevertheless had an indirect connection with gender constructs: the female was in all of these cases exhibiting less mature features. Women are closer to children – incomplete humans. Indeed the internal disposition of female genitals is also a result of the less than full development characteristic of the female. In a world in which women's economic rights and legal standing were limited, the implicit comparison of women to children reinforced notions of their incapacity and dependency.

Many of the differences perceived between males and females, especially human males and females, had to do with hair, and these too had a place in the characterization of the feminine and the masculine. Prominent body hair not only marked the male among humans but also signified masculinity. In remarks about beards and body hair, the contrast is not simply between males and females but rather between the masculine and the nonmasculine, including children of both sexes and castrati as well as women.[48] The production of beard and body hair followed from the physiological characteristics of the male, and the links between male maturity, the growth of the beard, and the ability to produce semen created a bridge between sexual maleness and gender-linked virility.[49] Once again the completeness of the real man is contrasted with the insufficiency of women, children, and eunuchs.

In spite of the suggestion that hairiness was linked not with the ability to produce semen but with the existence of certain pores in men which obviate the necessity to menstruate by providing alternative purgation through sweat and hair growth,[50] male hairiness was specifically associated with sexual virility. Hair was directly proportional to libido in men,[51] and the quantity and location of hair was therefore one of the features which distinguished men of different temperaments from each other.[52] The image of the wild man, represented with increasing frequency in the late Middle Ages,

---

46 Thomas Aquinas, *Summa theologiae*, pt. I, q. 92, art. 1.
47 Albertus Magnus, who incorporated both Galenic and Aristotelian views of the brain, did not mention rationality in his rather lengthy discussion (*De animalibus*, bk. I, tr. iii, ch. 1, pp. 183–92); he did touch on other psychological functions, such as memory and cogitation, which humans share with animals. The large size of the human brain relative to the head as a whole is a sign of the many and perfect animal virtues which humans possess.
48 Constantinus, *De coitu*, ch. 6, pp. 102–4; Thomas Cantimpratensis, *De natura rerum*, bk. I, ch. i, p. 23.
49 *Secreta mulierum minor*, Cambridge University, Trinity MSS O.2.5, fols. 130v–131r, and R.14.45, fol. 25r; see also Hildegard, *Causae et curae*, bk. I, p. 18.
50 *Secreta mulierum minor*, Cambridge University, Trinity MSS O.2.5, fol. 132rb, and R.14.45, fol. 27.
51 British Library, MS Sloane 282, fol. 53v. See also Hildegard, *Causae et curae*, bk. II, p. 75.
52 Constantinus, *De coitu*, ch. 5, pp. 96–100; Bernardus de Gordonio, *Lilium*, pt. VII, ch. i, fol. 87vb.

embodies the association of body hair with sensuality and lust by contrasting the naked, hirsute men and women with the refinement and restraint of civilization. These creatures, somewhat tamed by a new attitude toward the natural and by new criticisms of society as the medieval period drew to a close, came to haunt scenes with respectable couples as symbols of fertility. The image is not unambiguously sexual. There are stories and images, multiplying at the end of our period, of hairy anchorite saints, grown wild in their isolation from society. Several of these pious figures, however, including St. John Chrysostom and Mary Magdalen, were believed to have been guilty of sexual misconduct. [53] The hairy women in these representations project an ambiguous significance, appearing not only as unrepressed nature but also as unicorn tamers – a role usually reserved for virgins. [54] And while the hair of wild women is associated with sexuality, in another context facial hair on women is associated with masculinity as well as with fecundity. [55]

Isidore of Seville listed woman's soft face and man's beard among the anatomical features whose function is to distinguish the sexes. [56] (Beards, like body hair, were relevant among humans, not other animals. The lion's mane apparently did not provide an analogue. A twelfth-century bestiary remarked that "the short ones with curly manes are peaceful: the tall ones with plain hair are fierce.")[57] The beard is not, of course, a random marker. What in nature's regular manifestations lacked function or meaning in the Middle Ages? Like body hair it corresponded to libido: Hildegard of Bingen characterized phlegmatic men as lacking beards and sexual appetite, among other traits. [58] More important, beards are the result of a set of conditions that define the male in an essential way. This definition has anatomical dimensions, but its fundamental elements are physiological, so the distribution of hair illustrates the principle that, as Jacopo of Forlì said, complexion is the most basic of sex differences. In particular, the links between hair and sex difference (including sexual responses) are manifestations of differences in the ability to process residues, which in turn is dependent on heat. Hair is the product of useful residues of the nutritive and generative processes. These residues, though not in themselves harmful, cause harm if retained within the body. Men and women differ in the degree to which they refine their superfluities, and also in the way they dispose of them. Thus, women lack the special pores through which men

53 Timothy Husband, *The Wild Man: Medieval Myth and Symbolism*, with Gloria Gilmore-House (New York: Metropolitan Museum of Art, 1980), esp. pp. 95–109.
54 Ibid., pp. 83, 114.
55 Hildegard, *Causae et curae*, bk. II, p. 88. See also Thomas Cantimpratensis, *De natura rerum*, bk. I, ch. x, p. 23.
56 Isidorus, *Etymologiae*, bk. XI, ch. i, §148.
57 White, *Book of Beasts*, p. 7.
58 Hildegard, *Causae et curae*, bk. II, p. 75.

produce sweat and beards, because they give off their residues through menstruation.[59] Yet if proper purgation by menstruation does not occur, women may grow little beards.[60] In this context menstruation is an analogue to the production of sweat and hair, though in other contexts, it is an analogue to the production of semen. In both cases the differences are based on heat, the central principle of constitutional differences between the sexes. Since females are cooler than males, they accomplish their bodily functions – including the disposal of superfluities – either differently or less completely. In a chapter on the beard, for example, the thirteenth-century encyclopedist Thomas of Cantimpré incorporated notions about heat and about residues: "The beard in humans distinguishes the virile sex from women. A great beard is born from superfluities in hot men, a smaller one in cool [men]. . . . There are women who have an upper beard, and this is a sign of heat in them."[61] Differences in the distribution of hair, like other apparently superficial features, are thus effects and signs of a more essential difference. More important, they are markers chosen from an indefinite number of possible effects to represent the two sexes.

Facial hair is just one example of the several features correlated with the complexions of women and men. The specific combinations of qualities in the male and female bodies also contribute to the natural characters and behaviors of the sexes. But as with build, sex differences in dispositions are not reducible to degrees of heat or other qualities. As the prominence of menstruation and the singularity of the uterus set women apart, so do their natural temperaments and mores.

Disposition

After quoting Isidore of Seville on the etymology and sense of *masculus* (male) and before reiterating the Aristotelian associations of male–form– activity and female–matter–passivity, Bartholomew the Englishman had this to say about the sexes: "The male passeth the female in perfect complection, in working, in wit, in discretion, in might and in lordship. In perfect complection, for in comparison the male is hotter and dryer, and the female the contrary."[62] Bartholomew, a midthirteenth-century friar whose

---

59 *Secreta mulierum minor*, Cambridge University, MSS Trinity O.2.5, fol. 132rb, and R.14.45, fol. 27r.
60 *Propositiones de animalibus*, Cambridge University Library, MS Dd.3.16, fol. 73vb.
61 Thomas Cantimpratensis, *De natura rerum*, bk. I, ch. x, p. 23: "Barba in hominibus distinguit virilem sexum a feminis. Ex superfluitatibus nascitur. Barba magna in viris calidis, minor in frigidis. . . . Sunt femine que barbam habent superius, et hoc signum caloris in eis est"
62 Bartholomeus Anglicus, *De proprietatibus rerum*, [trans. John of Trevisa], rev. and comm. Stephen Batman (London: Thomas East, 1582), bk. VI, ch. 13, fol. 74va. John's English may slightly misconstrue "sensus discretionem," perhaps better rendered "sensory discrimi-

Latin encyclopedia had been translated into French and English by the end of the fourteenth century, clearly saw a connection between male and female complexions and the economic, intellectual, social, and political roles of men and women. One's disposition, or temperament, was, according to medieval theory, closely related to one's general constitution, or complexion. The four qualities – hot, cold, moist, and dry – lay at the foundation of a system of four elements, four humors, and four temperaments. The element fire, which was primarily hot and secondarily dry, was dominant in the yellow bile, which, if it exercised a controlling influence in the body, gave rise to a choleric disposition. (We are here considering a person's normal, healthy state. Under pathological conditions, such as fever, a normally cooler or moister individual might become temporarily choleric.) Earth, especially dry and secondarily cold, was dominant in the black bile, which produced a melancholy disposition; water, especially cold and secondarily moist, was dominant in the phlegm, which produced a phlegmatic temperament; and air, especially moist and secondarily warm, was dominant in the blood, which produced a sanguine temperament. ("Blood" is an ambiguous word in medieval terminology, referring to a pure, specific, warm, moist humor – as in the present context – and also to the more-or-less balanced mixture of all four humors that flows through the veins.)

The existence of a physical basis for what we might think of as personality types reveals the belief in a strong link between constitution and character. This link provides in turn a fundamental element of the medieval outlook upon which the integration of explicit ideas about sex and implicit gender assumptions is based. Indeed, the word "temperament" itself is ambiguous in this system of understanding, referring both to an individual's particular mixture of humors and to a set of attendant behaviors and attitudes.[63] If women have, as they do, a characteristic complexion or constitution – colder than men – then it is natural for them to differ from men in their patterns of conduct and natural for them to be assigned specific roles. The picture of women as sedentary – harmed by excessive exercise and not normally engaged in hard labor – is implicitly supported by the standard characterization of phlegmatics and melancholics (both cool temperaments) as relatively inactive. Women were especially associated with the cold and moist humor, phlegm, and one medical text even refers explicitly to women and phlegmatic men as associated types.[64]

nation." Bartholomaeus Anglicus, *De genuinis rerum coelestium, terrestrium inferarum* [sic] *proprietatibus libri XVIII*, ed. Georgius Bartholdus Posanus (Frankfurt: Wolfgang Richter, 1601; repr. Frankfurt am Main: Minerva, 1964), bk. VI, ch. xii, p. 244: "Maior enim est masculus foemina quoad complexionem, quoad operationem, & quoad sensus discretionem, & quoad potestatem & dominationem. Quo ad complexionem patet, quod vir sive masculus respectu foeminae calidus est & siccus, ipsa vero è converso."

63 Renaissance psychology and iconography give this system full play. See Raymond Klibansky, Erwin Panofsky, and Fritz Saxl, *Saturn and Melancholy: Studies in the History of Natural Philosophy and Art* (London: Thomas Nelson and Sons, 1964).

64 Cartelle, ed., *Liber minor de coitu*, pt. I, ch. 1, p. 56.

The temperaments and their behavioral implications explained both collective and individual dispositions. In his lectures on Aristotle's zoological works, Albertus Magnus used the four qualities to explain the relative softness of male and female flesh and to answer the question whether male or female animals are better to eat. Before going on to address the classical question "Whether the Seed Comes out of the Whole Body," he asked "Whether the Male Is More Apt at Learning Good Behavior than the Female."[65] He cited two arguments in favor of the female. First, children are more educable than old people, and since women are more like children (an argument from female incompleteness), they are more apt. His refutation of this position is based on the female complexion: since women are colder, their sense of touch and therefore their minds are less acute. Second, Albertus continued, Aristotle says women have more prudence, which is a sine qua non for attaining moral virtue. The refutation: what Aristotle meant was not really "prudence" but "cunning." In an extraordinary burst of misogyny, Albertus provided an example of the conviction expressed by Jacopo of Forlì and Bartholomew the Englishman that complexion is the key to understanding what female and male are:

Woman's complexion is more humid than man's. [The nature] of the humid receives an impression easily but retains it poorly. The humid is readily mobile, and thus women are unconstant and always seeking something new. Hence when she is engaged in the act under one man, if it were possible, she would like at the same time to be under another. . . . In short, I should say, every woman is to be avoided as much as a poisonous snake and a horned devil.[66]

For Albertus and his audience, women's moral, intellectual, and sexual characteristics are inextricably linked as correlative effects of their collective constitution.

Complexional qualities account for individual differences too. From a hot woman, therefore, we may expect attitudes and behaviors unlike those of a more typical, cool woman. Thus women with much choleric humor differ from women in general, who love for a long time.[67] Most accounts, like Constantine's, not only use words of the masculine gender (which might in some cases be construed as inclusive) but also give masculine examples, so there is little direct evidence about the application of the theory of temperaments to women. Only Hildegard of Bingen took the trouble to enumerate and describe the four basic female dispositions, juxtaposing them to four types of men. Although she did not label them as such, the groups may correspond to the choleric, sanguine, melancholic, and phlegmatic tempera-

65 Albertus Magnus, *Quaestiones de animalibus*, bk. XV, q. 11, pp. 265–6.
66 Ibid., p. 265: "Complexio enim feminae magis est humida quam maris, sed humidi est de facili recipere et male retinere. Humidum est enim de facili mobile, et ideo mulieres sunt inconstantes et nova semper petentes. Unde cum est in actu sub uno viro, si esset possibile, in eodem tempore vellet esse sub alio. . . . breviter dicam, ab omni muliere est cavendum tamquam a serpente venenosa et diabolo cornuto. . . ."
67 Petrus Gallegus, *Economica,* in Pelzer, "Un traducteur inconnu," p. 448.

ments. Women of one build and constitution, characterized by large bones, thick blood, and ample menstrual flow, are chaste and faithful wives who suffer ill health from sexual abstinence. Women who are plump and have moderate menstrual flow are skillful and lovable and have good memories. A third type of woman has bluish blood, a dark complexion, and ample menstrual flow. Her character is inconstant and tedious, and she is happier and healthier without a husband. Finally, thin women, with pale blood, dark faces (sometimes with a little beard), and modest menstrual flow are active and useful. They have slightly virile minds and tolerate sexual abstinence well, although when they are with men, they are incontinent like men.[68] Hildegard's typology relates personality and behavior not only to indicators of complexion and physiological temperament, such as the quality of a person's blood, but also to build and facial features. In that respect her treatment anticipates the flowering of physiognomy which occurred in the thirteenth and fourteenth centuries.

Physiognomy, like the theory of temperaments, yields evidence about the relation of physical characteristics to expected roles and behavior patterns. The science of discerning disposition and mores from the build, especially the head and face, of an individual, physiognomy is a branch of medieval knowledge much neglected by historians.[69] It does not fit neatly into the dominant framework of systematic natural philosophy or theoretical medicine with their representation of causes and their shared principles such as qualities and opposites. Nor does it correspond to or represent the origin of any recognized branch of modern science. To make matters worse, it has all the markings of a pseudoscience and does not even have the virtue, as does astrology, of having important empirical content, sophisticated mathematical procedures, or coherent theoretical underpinnings. Nevertheless, from the thirteenth century physiognomy was numbered among the natural sciences. It had a respectable basis in authority, deriving from the existence of a treatise on the subject attributed to Aristotle as well as several other works from late antiquity, which were translated into Latin along with Arabic works on the subject.[70] Treatises on physiognomy were copied and bound together with works on medicine and astrology, as well as with works on divination, chiromancy, and dreams and with works on religion and moral philosophy. Many of the most prolific and prominent scholastic philosophers commented on the *Physionomia* attributed to Aristotle, some of whom sought to systematize and rationalize the science by relating it to astrology.[71]

68 Hildegard, *Causae et curae*, bk. II, pp. 87–9. See Cadden, "It Takes All Kinds," pp. 159–66.
69 Lynn Thorndike, the exception, treats physiognomy in *History of Magic and Experimental Science*.
70 Richard Foerster, ed., *Scriptores physiognomonici Graeci et Latini*, 2 vols., Bibliotheca scriptorum Graecorum et Romanorum Teubneriana (Leipsig: B. G. Teubner, 1893).
71 Lynn Thorndike, "Buridan's Questions on the Physiognomy Ascribed to Aristotle," *Speculum* 18 (1943): 99–103.

The premise of physiognomy was that external features, including not only facial traits and build but also such supposedly innate characteristics as voice and gait, were the outward marks of character, attitudes, and behavior. A person with thin, straight black hair, for example, would be foolish and proud.[72] The science thus forms a part of the constellation of medieval scientific ideas which encourages the belief in a correspondence between physique and mores and therefore supports the assumption that gender roles and sex are bound together by nature. But, as in discussions of the four temperaments, so in works on physiognomy, determining the character of various types of *men* is the central concern. There is no indication of whether a woman with a naturally red nose is, like a man, faithful in friendship. And whereas with the temperaments some plausible inference can be made from the theory of humors and qualities which underlies it, in physiognomy there is no analogous systematic foundation from which to make a reasonable guess.

Fortunately, some treatises on the subject devote a brief section to the comparison of men and women. The most extended medieval treatment occurs in the compilation and elaboration of Greek and Arabic sources prepared by Peter of Abano at the end of the thirteenth century.[73] Peter's main source for this section is the physiognomic text most persistently attributed to Aristotle.[74] He reorganized and changed the material in a number of ways. First, unlike his source, Peter segregated the physical and behavioral traits, so that a behavioral profile of each sex emerges more clearly. Then, although he followed the pseudo-Aristotelian text in describing male and female physical characteristics in *animals*, he departed from it in his now distinct chapter on behavior, in which he is unambiguously talking about *people*. And finally, whereas his source had led with the female and had presented the male as her opposite, Peter led with the male – adding a number of behavioral traits – and presented the female in comparison to the male and less fully. In short, he highlights and strengthens physiognomy's lessons on gender difference and reasserts the medieval practice of presenting the male as the standard against which the female is measured.

In his chapter on the properties of the soul that manifest the differences between males and females, Peter of Abano reports: "The males' spirit is lively, given to violent impulse; [it is] slow getting angry and slower being

---

72 Roger A. Pack, ed. "Auctoris incerti *De physiognomonia libellus*," *Archives d'histoire doctrinale et littéraire du Moyen Age* 41 (1974): §15, p. 132.
73 Thorndike, "Buridan's Questions on the Physiognomy"; idem, *History of Magic and Experimental Science*, vol. 2, Appendix II, pp. 917–18. See also Charles H. Lohr, "Medieval Latin Aristotle Commentaries, Authors Narcissus-Richardus," *Traditio* 28 (1972): 331–2. At least three manuscripts give the date 1295: the late thirteenth- or early fourteenth-century Bibliothèque Nationale, MS lat. 16089, fol. 112vb, and the later MSS Munich, Bayerische Staatsbibliothek, CLM 637, fol. 66, and British Library, add. 37,079, fol. 81v.
74 Richard Foerster, ed., *De translatione Latina* Physiognomicorum *quae ferentur Aristotelis*, inaug. diss. (Kiel: Libraria Academica, 1884), pp. 10–11.

calmed. He is long-suffering at the tasks of labor; in deeds eager, able, noble, magnanimous, fair, confident; less flighty and less assiduous and maleficent [than the female]."[75] Peter holds, neither surprisingly nor entirely consistently, that these differences between the sexes result from the female's being less perfect than and the contrary of the male.

The conclusions of complexion theory and physiognomy are compatible with one another, but they are not congruent. Neither the specific assertions about physical constitution, which for the former are physiological and for the latter are anatomical, nor the specific assertions about behavior correspond completely. The most prominent trait shared by the two systems is one that unites the physical and the behavioral: the male tolerance and female lack of tolerance for physical exertions, a characteristic at least implicitly related to female weakness and coolness. On a more general plane, both systems attribute more clearly negative traits to females than to males, who are not only stronger but more liberal. Nevertheless, the female character is accorded a share of real, if not heroic, virtues, such as constancy and assiduousness, which are not specifically opposed to male traits. Still, the representation of the female type is less positive. The asymmetry is heightened by the shared practice of posing the male as the standard to which the female is compared. Thus, although the perspectives of complexion and physiognomy yield different descriptions of sex and gender differences, providing a range of traits from which writers could choose, they agreed not only in some particulars but also in the general outlines of their characterizations. Perhaps the point of firmest agreement resides in the shared assumption that group differences in personality and behavior are grounded in innate constitutional differences between the sexes, seen sometimes as the product of divine Creation and sometimes as the product of human procreation.

BECOMING FEMININE AND BECOMING MASCULINE: CREATION AND PROCREATION

The creation of the world: "Male and female created He them"

Differences between males and females in general and between men and women in particular were, according to medieval opinion, natural. They were natural both in the sense that they were understood to constitute defining principles and to inhere essentially in individuals, and also in the sense that they formed part of the larger order, the plan or logic of the world. The

75 Petrus de Padua [= Abano], *Liber compliationis physionomie,* Bibliothèque Nationale, MS lat. 16089, fol. 99ra: ". . . marium animus vivax est vehemens ad impetum tarde isracens [sic] tardiusque placatur. Laboris perpessivus, in operibus studiosus, aptus, liberalis, magnanimus, iustus, securus, minus prevoluntarius, minusque sedulus et mali operativas. . . ." See also Albertus Magnus, *De animalibus,* bk. VIII, tr. i, ch. 1, §§5–6, p. 573.

central features distinguishing females and males were, in short, part of their natures and part of Nature. In some realms of discourse, particularly scholastic natural philosophy, what is natural is a given. Insofar as it calls for explanation, it requires above all an account of its final cause – its raison d'être, its role in the scheme of things. Thus Aristotelians emphasized the benefits of sexual division of functions and the purpose of those functions, namely, the perpetuation of natural kinds. The final cause of sexual differentiation is reproduction, and the final cause of reproduction is the achievement by the species of what cannot be accomplished by its individuals – immortality. Even before the translations of Aristotle's works on animals made the details of these arguments available, medieval naturalists shared the general teleological outlook on which they were based.

This version of sexual differentiation, with its emphasis on final cause, did not deter medieval authors from making assumptions about or even inquiring into the origins of the arrangement. Nor did Aristotle's belief in the eternity of the world – and with it the eternity of organic types – prevent them from investigating the beginnings of female and male. The desire to determine beginnings found ample authority in the Latin version of Plato's *Timaeus*, which told of the emergence of nature from formless substance.[76] Attention to this Platonic account of coming-to-be swelled in the twelfth century, when many authors interested in the philosophy of nature commented on it or borrowed from it.[77] The medieval version of the *Timaeus* encouraged medieval thinkers to ask where things came from, but it did not contain the passage at the end of Plato's work which treats the differentiation of the sexes and the basis of reproduction.[78] Perhaps because of this omission, and no doubt because of concerns about the orthodoxy of pagan accounts of creation, medieval authors who wished to address the question of the origin of (as distinguished from the reasons for) sex difference turned to the most obvious authority, Moses.

The first chapters of Genesis provided the texts and thereby the occasion for building a theory of the origins of sexual differentiation. Because the Bible describes the acts of Creation, it differs radically from the Aristotelian assumption of beginninglessness and is concerned with more than final

---

76 Plato, *Timaeus a Calcidio translatus commentarioque instructus*, ed. J. H. Waszink, vol. 4 of *Plato Latinus*, rev. ed., Corpus Platonicum Medii Aevi (London: Warburg Institute; Leiden: E. J. Brill, 1975).

77 Among the most prominent of these were William of Conches (*Glosae super Platonem*) and Bernardus Silvestris (*Cosmographia*). Other authors also participated in the diffusion of Platonic creation. See, e.g., Dales, *Marius*; and Joan Cadden, "*De elementis*: Earth, Water, Air and Fire in the 12th and 13th Centuries" (Master's thesis, Columbia University, 1967). See also Raymond Klibansky, *The Continuity of the Platonic Tradition during the Middle Ages: Outlines of a Corpus Platonicum Medii Aevi* (London: Warburg Institute, 1939).

78 *Timaeus* 90E–91D. Calcidius repeats but does not comment on Plato's assertion that souls which fail to control the passions will be born again in a woman's form, and he links the soul's failure with libido in particular (Waszink, *Timaeus*, CXCV–CXCVI, pp. 217–18).

causes. Yet because the biblical narrative incorporates the notions of divine purpose and plan, it is compatible with the teleological elements of the medieval outlook in general and Aristotelianism in particular.[79] Thus the use of Scripture offered the opportunity to extend, without redefining, the boundaries of natural science. There was, it goes without saying, no impediment to using Scripture as authority, and there was ample precedent for basing scientific investigation upon it, starting with Patristic commentaries on the six days of Creation.[80] In the early Middle Ages, works of several sorts alluded to Scripture when exploring questions about nature and alluded to nature when expounding upon moral and religious subjects. Isidore, Bishop of Seville, writing in the seventh century, had relied mainly on pagan sources for his assertions about the natural differences between the sexes, but after having said that women are softer than, weaker than, and subject to men, he called on the authority of the Bible to defend the word (and, by implication, the category) "woman" against the implication of sexual impurity, pointing out that Eve was called "woman" when she was still a virgin.[81] A bestiary of the twelfth century, building on a tradition that drew upon lore about the animal world to illustrate theological and ethical lessons, cites the female vulture's ability to produce young without copulation as an argument against those who question the Virgin Birth.[82]

Particularly for authors of the twelfth century, enjoying a renaissance of natural philosophy and theoretical medicine largely innocent of systematic Aristotelianism and close to the traditions of Isidore of Seville and the bestiaries, the integration of scientific inquiry with biblical exegesis or religious precepts was appealing and fruitful. Hildegard of Bingen's works – both medical and visionary – illustrate this integration. In a complex passage in her *Book of Divine Works*, Hildegard incorporated the two accounts of human Creation at the beginning of Genesis into an explanation of the purpose of sexual differentiation, the immediate origins of sexual differentiation, the general similarities and differences of the sexes, and their reproductive roles.[83] First, she referred to Genesis 1:26–27: God created male and female in his own image and likeness. She proceeded immediately to distinguish – on the basis

79 The problem of devising a plausible harmony between Aristotelian cosmology and Genesis had challenged Jewish and Christian intellectuals since late antiquity. See, e.g., Harry Austryn Wolfson, *Studies in the History of Philosophy and Religion*, ed. Isadore Twersky and George H. Williams, (Cambridge: Harvard University Press, 1973), vol. 1.

80 Frank Robbins, *The Hexaemeral Literature: A Study of the Greek and Latin Commentaries on Genesis* (Chicago: University of Chicago Press, 1912); Thorndike, *History of Magic and Experimental Science*, vol. 1, pp. 337–501; Pierre Duhem, *Le système du monde* (Paris: Librairie Scientifique A. Hermann, 1913–59), vol. 2, pp. 393–501. The tradition is continued in the late Middle Ages. See, e.g., Nicholas H. Steneck, *Science and Creation in the Middle Ages: Henry of Langenstein (d. 1397) on Genesis* (Notre Dame and London: University of Notre Dame Press, 1976).

81 Isidorus, *Etymologiae*, bk. XI, ch. ii, §20; see also White, *Book of Beasts*, p. 222.

82 White, *Book of Beasts*, p. 109.

83 See Scholz, "Hildegard von Bingen"; Cadden, "It Takes All Kinds."

of Genesis 2:21–3:19 – between the male with his greater strength and the female with her gentler power. For "the man was raised up first, and the woman afterward from the man, and she bears children even as the man generates them through the strength of his forces."[84] Hildegard took a moderate position, balancing the sense of unity and similarity suggested by the "image and likeness" passage with the sense of difference and ranking suggested by the story of successive creations and the Fall. Man and woman have one source and are of one flesh, yet they are distinguished by their essential characters as well as by their reproductive roles:

Through the root of a tree, which has vigor within it, the flower and the fruit are nourished, and they are from one [source]. Thus many [offspring] are procreated through male and female, which, however, proceed from one creator. For if there were only male or only female, no person would be born. Hence man and woman are one, since man is in a sense the soul, [and] woman, truly, like the body.[85]

From the stories of the Creation, Hildegard repeatedly derived the conclusion that man and woman are both necessary for procreation and are mutually dependent, not only in the sense of relying upon one another but in a more transcendent sense – as complementary aspects of being. Thus, reaching beyond the Old Testament, she rehearsed the common formulations that man is to woman as soul is to body and that "man signifies the divinity, woman the humanity of the Son of God."[86] The perspective is reinforced by the belief that Jesus derived his humanity from his mother and his divinity from his Father and introduces a hierarchy of gender into the distinction between the sexes. Hildegard thus at once emphasized and mediated the tension between the equivalence of the sexes as represented by their mutual dependence and oneness, and their radical incommensurability as represented by the dichotomies of body and soul, humanity and divinity. The unity and community of man and woman are reinterpreted in terms of the distinction (though not, for Hildegard, polarity) between the divine and the spiritual, on the one hand, and the mundane and material, on the other.

Hildegard's medical work, *Book of Compound Medicine*, likewise integrates the biblical story of the origins of sex difference with an account of female and male characteristics in the natural world. This integration has, in turn, implications for the notions of masculine and feminine roles. From Hilde-

---

84 Hildegard, *Liber divinorum operum*, pt. II, vis. v, ch. 43, col. 945: ". . . sed masculum . . . prius, feminam vero postea de viro tollens, illaque parit, sicut et masculus per fortitudinem virum suarum generat. . . ."
85 Ibid.: "Per radicem quoque arboris, quae viriditatem in se continet, flores et poma enutriuntur et ab uno sunt, ita per masculum et feminam multi procreantur, qui tamen ab uno creatore procedunt. Nam si masculus solus vel si femina sola esset, nullus homo generaretur. Unde etiam vir et femina unum sunt, quoniam vir esset quasi anima, femina vero velut corpus."
86 Ibid., vis. iv, ch. 100, col. 885: "Et vir divinitatem, femina vero humanitatem Filii Dei significat."

gard's medical perspective, the Fall is an essentially sexual event and serves as an introduction to her discussion of sex difference, sexual types, reproduction, and the sexual differentiation of the fetus.[87] Several of the sex-linked and gender-defining characteristics already discussed acquire genetic explanations in the context of Creation, for example, strength, heat, hairiness, and level of physical activity. She observes that humans are not hirsute, because their rationality provides them with adequate protection. The male has a beard because he was made from earth. He has greater strength and heat, and he moves around more. Woman lacks a beard because she was made from man, and she is subject to him. She remains still for the most part – like reptiles, which, not incidentally, were created to serve man.[88] Once again, this time in the context of a medical work, Hildegard presented the Creation as an explanation for both sex and gender, fusing the physical differences and the social roles.

In the thirteenth century Thomas Aquinas, who also wrote extensively on natural philosophy, effected a similar integration, similarly based on Genesis. In the *Summa theologiae* Aquinas, defending God's decision to include woman among his original creations, stated and then placed strict limits upon the position that woman is biologically inferior to man. Certainly the active reproductive force, which is male, aims to create as perfect a likeness of itself as possible. (Thomas has shifted from Eden to Aristotle's Nature for this phase of the argument.) Only weakness of that force, intractability of the material upon which it works, or the operation of some external influence can deflect its realization of that goal and produce a female. But humanity as a whole benefits from the regular occurrence of these individuals who are in some sense imperfect, since sexual differentiation is good for more perfect kinds of creature, and so (to get back to Eden), the creation of woman was part of God's plan for appropriate human reproduction.

What may appear to have been equivocation on Thomas's part is due to some extent to medieval expectations about nature, which differed significantly from our own. In particular, the ideals of perfection defined by God's intention and nature's purposefulness by no means exhaust or limit what the natural world was understood to encompass. If modern standards of lawfulness, regularity, and predictability applied, each female would be a problematic aberration, but medieval nature comprehended many potentialities, as well as necessities. The sexual division of labor inherent in this version of created nature necessarily implied inequality for Aquinas. On the level of reproduction itself, its purpose was the segregation of the higher principle of

---

87 Hildegard, *Causae et curae*, bk. II, esp. pp. 33–70. The structure of this work is problematic, but it clearly starts in the form of an exegesis of the Creation and reaches the sixth day at the opening of book II.

88 Ibid., pp. 33–4. The Latin *reptiles* is a less precise word than "reptiles" and may be construed to include all land animals. The association with hairlessness, however, suggests the narrower translation.

generation from the lower. Indeed, he made the general argument that inequality and the free subjection of one person to another were present before the Fall, that is, are an aspect of nature in its most perfect state. His first examples of inevitable, appropriate, and beneficial subjection (as distinguished from slavery) are those of the family – wife to husband, children to parents.[89] Thus the fact that God chose to create this not-in-every-respect-perfect human has implications which link reproduction and familial roles. The manner in which God chose to create her both confirms his *reproductive* intentions – "one flesh" signifies carnal union[90] – and at the same time offers insights into his *social* intentions, "that there should be a social union between man and woman."[91] Humans are the only kind of creature for which God made the female from the male, and this was to create the love necessary to secure the natural and sacramental character of human marriage: "the male and female remain together their whole life; which does not happen with other animals."[92] Indeed, the conjunction of the biological and social functions is one of the things that makes humans special: "male and female are joined together in humans, not only on account of the necessity of generation, as with other animals, but also for domestic life, in which there are different jobs for the man and the woman, and in which the man is the head of the woman."[93] The specific character of the relationship, though not the specific domestic duties, was spelled out when Thomas explained why God chose to use Adam's *rib* – using Adam's head would have implied her dominion over him, using his foot would have implied her subjection was that of a slave. Like Hildegard, Thomas took a moderate position on the character and extent of inequality. God created both male and female in his image with respect to the defining principle of humankind, its intellectual nature. In a secondary sense, however, woman's relationship to God is mediated, since every creature is of and for God, but she is also of and for man.[94] Here he parted company with Hildegard, who, modifying Paul's words, held that woman is made for man and man is made for woman.[95]

Aquinas's synthesis of the natural and social meaning of Genesis is, in some ways, less revealing than Hildegard's. It is more abstract and so proj-

---

89 Thomas Aquinas, *Summa theologiae*, pt. I, q. 92, art. 1, and q. 96, art. 3.
90 Ibid., q. 92, art. 1.
91 Ibid., art. 3: ". . . quod inter virum et mulierem debet esse socialis coniunctio. . . ."
92 Ibid., art. 2: ". . . mas et femina commanent per totam vitam: quod non contingit in aliis animalibus."
93 Ibid., art. 2: ". . . mas et femina coniunguntur in hominibus non solum propter necessitatem generationis, ut in aliis animalibus; sed etiam propter domesticam vitam, in qua sunt alia opera viri et feminae, et in qua vir est caput mulieris."
94 Ibid., q. 93, art. 4.
95 Hildegard, *Scivias*, pt. I, vis. ii, chs. 11–12, p. 21: see Marie-Thérèse d'Alverny, "Comment les théologiens et les philosophes voient la femme," in [*La femme dans la civilisation des Xe–XIIIe siècles: Actes du colloque tenu à Poitiers les 23– 25 septembre 1976*], *Cahiers de civilisation médiévale* 20 (1977): 122–3.

ects a vaguer notion of role differentiation. And it draws both implicitly and explicitly on sources from other ages, especially Paul and Augustine, to interpret Scripture, thus making it a less specific reflection of medieval attitudes. But it does illustrate how comfortable medieval authors were both with the blending of these natural and social differences and with the use of Scripture to explain the origins of sexual differentiation.

The amalgamation of religion and natural philosophy might seem inevitable in an age whose world view was so deeply informed by Christian theology, which in turn contained important strains of ancient philosophy. Certainly many late medieval intellectuals had no difficulty operating on the assumption that the divine plan and the natural order coincided and that one could be read from the other. Yet this outlook was subject to severe criticism on a number of grounds. When William of Conches, Hildegard's older contemporary, interpreted the creation of Eve in naturalistic terms (which included an account of her slightly imperfect balance of qualities), he was accused of making light of Holy Scripture. Indeed, in a later work, he felt it necessary to retract his errors on this and other matters.[96] Natural philosophers of Aquinas's time, especially those in Paris, were repeatedly warned by theologians not to presume to limit God's power by supposing the Creator was constrained by Aristotle's natural laws, and not to fall into the trap of entertaining two distinct truths, one theological and the other philosophical or scientific. Few if any medieval intellectuals subscribed to this doctrine of double truth. The fuss about it suggests a recognition that natural explanations and religious doctrines were different kinds of knowledge and a consensus that the two kinds of knowledge necessarily converge – even if the terms of the convergence were hotly debated. Thus, with respect to the gender implications of sex difference, science and religion were neither two faces of the same ideology (for Aristotle and Moses belonged to substantially distinct traditions) nor separate and independent spheres (for they were significantly, though not completely, congruent). Furthermore, there was no clear boundary between science or religion, on the one hand, and social constructs, on the other, for both natural philosophy and theology were understood to encompass judgments about values, dispositions, and behaviors.

Those who had recourse to the Bible as a source of scientific information were often authors whose work incorporated but was not centered on natural philosophy or medicine. Hildegard of Bingen's main body of writings consists of lengthy visionary works, and Thomas Aquinas's theological writings dominate his opus. Although in their significant works on natural subjects they often spoke without reference to religious or spiritual meaning, the connections between the natural and the transcendent are more

96 Guilelmus de Conchis, *De substantiis physicis,* Preface, pp. 5–7. See d'Alverny, "Comment les théologiens voient la femme," pp. 124–5, and Thorndike, *History of Magic and Experimental Science,* vol. 2, pp. 58–60.

obvious than they are in the works of authors who focused more completely on natural philosophy and medicine. The prologues both to Constantine the African's tract on coitus and to the obstetrical treatise *On the Diseases of Women* open with references to divine purpose in the creation of sexual function and sexual pleasure,[97] but most medical and scientific works concerned with sexual matters and reproduction make no mention of Genesis.

More common than building a causal account of sex differentiation upon religious foundations or than objecting to such a procedure was the practice of explaining the origins of female and male in embryological terms – that is to say, in terms of the causes of male and female individuals, rather than male and female types or prototypes. Examined earlier in terms of the scholastic argument about maternal and paternal influence, the question of sex determination, especially as it involves additional layers of causation, conveys a good deal about the values and implications associated with "female" and "male."

Procreation: The seeds and conditions of difference

How does it happen that the same couple may produce now a boy child, now a girl child? The question is at once a classical problem in the science of reproduction and embryology and, as the chapter on sterility will argue, an immediate concern to families, whose sense of social and economic interest was shaped by their culture. Accordingly, sources on the production of female and male offspring range from lengthy and subtle academic treatises, like the *questiones* analyzing Avicenna's chapter "On the Generation of the Embryo," to short recipes with no explicit explanation. The extended formal discussions of sex determination undertaken by scholastic authors articulated and elaborated certain general principles of male–female differentiation which, when entertained in less formal contexts, projected a derogatory notion of the feminine. For example, although Thomas Aquinas had argued that a female child was defective only in a limited sense, the subtle qualifications and circumscriptions were far less widely rehearsed than was the fundamental idea that a girl was a failed boy. And in explaining the inability of the father's seed to form the mother's material contribution into a son, even Albertus Magnus, who was conversant with the niceties of the scholastic argument, employed language evocative of social and political domination when he called the matter "disobedient."[98] Unlike the views of Creation, however, which emphasized the divine plan, views of sex determination both within and beyond the university setting posited an array of

97 Constantinus, *De coitu*, "Prologue," p. 76; [Ps.-]Trotula, *De passionibus mulierum*, Cambridge University Library, MS Dd.11.45, fol. 67.
98 Albertus Magnus, *De animalibus*, bk. XVI, tr. i, ch. 14, §73, p. 1100: ". . . impediatur ex inobedientia materie. . . ."

causes, which, among other things, opened up questions of parental behavior. The sex of an embryo was neither biologically preformed nor metaphysically predetermined: the myriad recipes for producing sons (discussed later in relation to sterility) found theoretical support in the natural philosophical recognition that many of the contributing causes of sex determination were susceptible to modification by the art of medicine.[99] Academic interest focused on the father's seed, but even authors thus preoccupied contributed to a broader view. They not only conveyed the dominant positions but also the minority opinions, the exceptional or peripheral cases, and the secondary conditions or accidents, all of which contributed to the pool from which medieval understandings of male and female were drawn. At the same time, they provided rationales for various more practical approaches to insuring the production of sons. Many late medieval sources were concerned less with the final cause – the plan or purpose – behind sex difference and more with the efficient and material causes – the immediate and instrumental origins – of sexual differentiation. This more local perspective in turn projected a different sort of image of the feminine and the masculine, less related to the *general* shape of social and sexual relations (subject/master or passive/active) than to the *specific* and concrete characteristics that distinguished the sexes.

A variety of conditions and influences come into play, before conception, at conception, and during pregnancy, in the determination of sex. The parents' individual constitutions and their relation to one another, the immediate circumstances of intercourse, the astrological situation, and the conditions and accidents during pregnancy are among the elements invoked in medieval explanations of an infant's sex. Few sources take *all* these elements into consideration, but medieval views about conception and birth in general were consistent with the notion that some such range of causes was at work. One Aristotelian compilation, for example, gives a long list of causes – the parents' complexions, the atmospheric conditions, the phase of the moon, and others, citing not only Aristotle's works on animals but also opinions of, attributed to, or associated with Aristotle on metaphysics, meteorology, physics, elements, and nutrition.[100] Similarly, medieval medical writers, drawing from the works of Galen, Avicenna, and others, elaborated on and gave new weight to a number of ancillary determinants of sex.

Jacopo of Forlì, a physician and philosopher teaching and writing at Padua around the turn of the fifteenth century, presented a widely accepted version of the Aristotelian view as interpreted by Avicenna, upon whose work Jacopo was, in turn, commenting. He was thus a participant in the traditions and practices of scholasticism discussed earlier. His work provides many

---

99 Albertus Magnus, *Quaestiones de animalibus*, bk. IX, q. 18, p. 210.
100 *Extractiones quedam de libris fratris Alberti Teutonici naturalibus*, Bibliothèque Nationale, MS lat. 6524, fol. 47r.

examples of late medieval attempts to produce a clear, consistent theory to account for the phenomena of sex difference, and like that of his academic predecessors, it concentrates on the workings of the father's seed. But seen in the context of medieval gender constructs, his work and the scholastic discussions it exemplifies help to illustrate how broad notions about the essences of the male and the female form a substratum within which specific technical disagreements inhere. In other words, concepts of masculine and feminine did not depend on the outcomes of specific academic debates; rather, those debates took place within the boundaries of acceptable views of gender. Thus the advertised scholastic disagreements between medical and philosophical camps on the existence and role of the female seed turned out, as seen earlier, to have been played out on the basis of broad agreement on the limitations of the female role. Works like Jacopo's *On the Generation of the Embryo* also contained the seeds of a more varied approach to what is feminine and what is masculine.

Jacopo's basic account of sex determination is orthodox: the main cause of masculinity (he is only indirectly concerned with the cause of femininity) is "the complexion of the [fetus's] heart received from the principle of generation" (i.e., from the male parent's contribution).[101] The father's semen is responsible for the constitution, especially the strength and warmth, of the fetal heart. And it is the heart, the first organ to develop, which produces both the masculine complexion (the defining characteristic of maleness) and the masculine parts in the rest of the body. But having affirmed this standard picture, Jacopo went on to glean from his sources as many other explanatory factors as he could find. For example, he listed ten causes borrowed from Giles of Rome, a late thirteenth-century Paris master and promoter of Aristotelian natural philosophy:

1. Quality of (male) sperm: warm produces male child.
2. Quantity of (male) sperm: more produces male child.
3. Age (of father): a man just past youth produces male child.
4. Place and disposition of testicles: warm right testicle produces male child.
5. Fetus's place in womb: right side produces male child.
6. Complexion of menstruum: warm produces male child.
7. Food and drink (of father or of both parents) before intercourse: warm produces male child.
8. Air: cold season or region produces male child.
9. Winds: north wind produces male child.
10. Celestial influence: more influence produces male child.[102]

Although several of these points, emphasizing as they do the male sperm, are clearly grounded in the Aristotelian view of the male active principle

---

101 Jacobus Forliviensis, *De generatione embrionis*, fol. 9vb.
102 Ibid., fol. 10ra; see Hewson, *Giles of Rome*, esp. pp. 182–7, 228–30. Point 10 seems to be a misreading of Giles.

working upon the female passive material, and others, insofar as they relate to heat, are at least consistent with Aristotelian physiology, the list is eclectic and expands substantially the range of factors making significant contributions to the process of sex determination. These factors are not surprising – many of them are influential in the process of conception and gestation in general – but they are not specifically unified in any one theoretical system. Cold seasons, regions, and winds favor the masculine, for example. Furthermore, they leave much more room for maternal influence than do the extended scholarly investigations of the female seed.

The womb, for example, has an influence on fetal sex as it does on other aspects of development. The right side of the womb, being warmer because of the proximity of the liver, tends to form male children, whereas the left side, being cooler because of the spleen's proximity, tends to cradle female children. (Why was the left side, where the heart resides, not warmer? Because its heat blows toward the right side and warms it.)[103] The strings of association, right–warm–male and left–cool–female, return us also to the gender implications of medieval views of sex difference. Certainly we are dealing with a consistent scientific theory that takes heat to be a defining principle and an instrument in the creation of maleness, but we are also in the presence of a general hierarchy of value, in which the better alternatives are ranged against the worse. Thus, although the fact of the womb's influence elevates the female role and status, the terms of that influence undermine them.

The association of the right side with warmth and with males, which finds specific expression in this view of uterine influence, is common in classical and late ancient philosophy and medicine. Medieval authors showed more than a passive acceptance of the doctrine when they repeated it again and again in their own works, and they frequently adopted a more elaborate form of it in the doctrine of the seven-celled uterus.[104] The uterus, so the theory goes, is divided into seven cubicles, three on the left side, three on the right side, and one in the center. A conceptus housed in one of the cubicles on the left, the cooler side, would, of course, be a girl; on the right, a boy. A fetus that developed in the middle cell would be a hermaphrodite. The anatomists of twelfth-century Salerno secured a place in medieval medicine for the theory by presenting it in their general anatomical tracts, and the fact that slightly later some authors argued that the number of cells was five (because a woman could not possibly bear more than quintuplets) suggests both that the doctrine of seven cells was widely known and that at least some version of this elaboration on left and right – some odd-numbered division of the womb – was widely accepted in medical circles.

103 Lawn, *Prose Salernitan Questions*, P, 143, p. 259.
104 Kudilen, "The Seven Cells of the Uterus"; Jacquart and Thomasset, *Sexuality and Medicine*, pp. 34–5.

The currency of the theory went beyond medicine, perhaps because in the early thirteenth century the natural philosopher Michael Scot mentioned it several times in his well-circulated work *On the Secrets of Nature*.[105] The anatomical question, What does the human uterus actually look like? was apparently not as important as the conceptualization of multiple births and the explanation of hermaphroditism which the seven cells provided. The general association of left with female and right with male also gave rise to a number of diagnostic methods for determining the sex of a fetus before birth. A pregnant woman will be more swollen on the right side if she is about to bear a male child, and, when asked to walk, will start with her right foot.[106]

Like the attribution of an active role to the womb in the determination of sex, the influence of the external factors in Jacopo of Forlì's list, such as climate, diet, and celestial motions, was widely accepted. If sheep face north when mating, the lamb will be male; if south, female.[107] As we shall see, cures for sterility may be aimed at the production of a child of one sex or the other: use the right (of course) testicle of a cock if you wish to have a boy; the left if you wish to have a girl.[108] There are many recipes that tell how to have a boy or a girl, and more that simply tell how to have a boy. (None that I have found just tell how to have a girl.) In general, medieval opinion held that human seed would be altered according to the hours, planets, and zodiacal signs.[109] There were specific celestial signs that predicted the birth of a male child.[110]

Even Jacopo's more conventional academic concerns, when looked at from the point of view of the elaboration of cultural concepts of sex, reflect a rather decentralized outlook, a rather indecisive theoretical perspective. Though he preferred to view the origins of sex in the fetus in terms of the operations of the active male principle, he added that there is a second way of looking at the matter, Galen's way. Jacopo's presentation of the Galenic alternative, as it was understood, is slightly more complete and more sympathetic than that of some other late medieval writers,[111] but its inclusion is typical of the scholastic impulse to leave no stone unturned. One can, he says, look at the matter from the point of view of general causes, especially

---

105 Michaelis Scotus, *De secretis naturae*, pt. I, ch. vii, p. 245; see Thorndike, *History of Magic and Experimental Science*, vol. 2, p. 329.
106 Thorndike, "Further Considerations," p. 441.
107 *Propositiones de animalibus*, Cambridge University Library, MS Dd.3.6, fol. 74va.
108 Julius Pagel, "Raymundus de Molieriis und seine Schrift *De impedimentis conceptionis*," *Janus* 8 (1903): 533; however, one collection of recipes claims that if a woman eats cocks' testicles, she will bear a son (*Experimenta*, Vienna, Nationalbibliothek, MS CVP 2532, fol. 28v).
109 See Thorndike, *History of Magic and Experimental Science*, vol. 2, p. 586. This belief was reinforced by the widely known ps.-Galen, *De spermate* (ed. Tavone Passalacqua).
110 See, e.g., the nativities in British Library, MS Harley 5402, fol. 31r.
111 Siraisi, *Taddeo*, pp. 195–202.

the disposition of the semen and the menstruum, or one can ask, as Galen does, about the disposition of the sperm both actively and materially. From that perspective, a male child results from the dominance of the father's sperm, a female child from the dominance of the mother's, and a hermaphrodite in case of a draw. Jacopo was without doubt familiar with the scholastic arguments that laid bare the inconsistency between the two perspectives, yet he contented himself with raising and answering just one objection. How can the female sperm dominate the male sperm, when the male sperm is warmer (and therefore, by implication, stronger)? Maybe the female sperm does not have to dominate in the absolute sense, and perhaps too the menstruum may be more disposed to receive the impression of the female than of the male.[112]

The eclecticism of Jacopo of Forlì's approach to the causes of sex determination in the individual has two implications which illustrate common, indeed perhaps prevalent patterns of understanding. First, although some authors, especially those involved in university education toward the end of the Middle Ages, sought either to decide between systematic alternatives or to create a consistent synthesis, many were more content to collect than to reject opinions and were more likely to gloss over than to address problems of system and consistency. This eclecticism is typical of most of the compendia, handbooks, and collections of excerpts so common throughout the Middle Ages, especially as the number of authorities available in Latin multiplied and as ownership of manuscripts broadened. It is also common enough in the scholastic literature like Jacopo's work on the embryo and like the debates on seeds and pleasures. Although it was the job of university teachers to identify and resolve conflicts within and among the great texts of medicine and natural philosophy, only the best regularly succeeded. It was not a simple matter to sort out the opinions, satisfy the requirements of commentary and disputation, acknowledge elements of common experience, and come up with an acceptable and consistent position. If Jacopo did not quite manage, he was in good company. When Taddeo Alderotti, an eminent medical teacher at Bologna in the late thirteenth century, addressed the role of the female sperm, "he concluded," according to a modern scholar, "with a flourish of argument in which his contradictory sources are not so much reconciled as thoroughly muddled."[113] If the scholastic methods and the intensification of higher learning had made the older naive eclecticism obsolete within the more refined genres of commentary and *questiones*, the residue of unresolved problems, along with the habit of listing as many opinions as possible, helped to perpetuate (and in some cases expand) an array of concepts and a diverse pool of vocabulary. This richness permitted the rationalization of multifaceted approaches to such problems as infertility.

112 Jacobus Forliviensis, *De generatione embrionis*, fol. 10va.
113 Siraisi, *Taddeo*, p. 198.

At the same time, writings like Jacopo of Forlì's multicausal explanation of sex determination did not offer the basis for a radical reorientation of gender constructs. On the contrary, the spirit in which he admits the Galenic presumption of two seeds reveals and reinforces medieval notions of gender: if the female seed wins the contest, it is not because it is truly stronger but rather because of the scoring system or the conditions of the match. Whereas, in the seventeenth century William Harvey characterized the "medical," or Galenic, view of female and male contributions much more symmetrically,[114] Jacopo, along with many other scholastic medical authors, diluted the active force attributed to the female semen with various qualifications and disclaimers, such as the suggestion that if the mother's influence wins out and the child is female, it may be because the mother had a "masculine" heart.[115] In part, of course, Jacopo's interpretation serves the medieval academic impulse to harmonize divergent authorities, but it also reflects a set of notions about the masculine and the feminine that reaches beyond the realm of biological form and function. It suggests that some roles are so essentially unfeminine that if a female performs them, she must be masculine.

FEMININE AND MASCULINE TYPES: THE POSSIBILITIES AND LIMITATIONS OF A BINARY CONSTRUCT

The notion of a masculine female or a feminine male is not uncommon in the late Middle Ages. Such an individual was supposed to have been constituted by the natural processes we have been considering. An English didactic work in question-and-answer format from around 1200 asks, for example, why some couples have more boys than girls, others more girls than boys. The answer combines the view that the parent contributing more seed will prevail with the view that position in the womb determines sex and concludes:

If more of the womanly sperm is set in the right part [of the womb], a manly woman [*femina virago*] will be generated. If more in the left than the right, and there is more of the manly seed than the womanly, an effeminate man [*vir effeminatus*] will be born. If [the sperm is] in the middle chamber, so that it is subject to the impression of both parts, there will be a hermaphrodite, since it will have and produce the equipment of the body of both one [sex] and the other.[116]

---

114 Harvey, *Generation of Animals*, exercises 31–4, pp. 293–300.
115 Jacobus Forliviensis, *De generatione embrionis*, fol. 10va.
116 Lawn, *Prose Salernitan Questions*, B, 193, p. 103: "Si vero plus de muliebri spermate in dextra parte collocetur, femina virago generatur. Si plus in sinistram quam in dextram, et si plus sit de virili semine quam muliebri, vir effeminatus nascitur. Si in media cellula ita ut utriusque partis suscipiat impressionem, hermafroditus erit, quoniam et unius et alterius corporis habebit et geret supplementa."

Likewise alluding to multiple causes (placement in the womb, left and right testicles, menstruum, strength of male and female seeds), a commentary on a physiognomic text includes one chapter on the generation of "womanly males and hermaphrodites" and another chapter on "manlike women and hermaphrodites."[117] Thus, within the process of generation, which depended on the existence and operation of two distinct sexes, was the basis for more than two possibilities, not so easily distinguishable. Since being feminine or masculine entailed, not as incidental effects but as defining characteristics, dimensions of disposition, character, and habit, the variations had to do not only with complexion and appearance but also with behavior, including sexual conduct. Medieval authors writing both within and beyond the domains of medicine and natural philosophy developed and extended those aspects of feminine and masculine typology that had to do with personality and deportment as well as those that had to do with anatomy and physiology. Furthermore, they extended the meaning of the terms well beyond their already broad primary applications to plants and planets, cruel mothers and kind confessors, and, consequently, they heightened the duality by elevating and applying the two types, feminine and masculine. Hence the extension and abstraction of gender constructs, in part by incorporating such paradoxes as masculine women and mother abbots, worked to contain experience and expression within the two-term system, in spite of the possibility of middle terms admitted by medical theory. One of the effects of this binary typology, however, was to underscore the problematic character of individuals and acts that did not fit neatly into it. Medieval authors used ecclesiastical, scientific, and other language and concepts to understand and evaluate hermaphrodites, eunuchs, women dressing as men, and men engaging in sexual activities with other men – sometimes grouped together and widely seen as not comfortably encompassed by the duality of sex.

Extension and abstraction

Unlike the biblical Creation, which resulted in two clearly distinguished sexes (whatever the common human elements might be), the act of procreation admitted of degrees. Although Aristotle had insisted that a fetus failing to become a male would become its *opposite*,[118] medieval natural philosophers and medical authors who treated the subject in detail often saw sex determination as involving more variables. Once again, a clear, simple representation yields to a more complex and ambiguous one, reflect-

---

117 Guilhelmus de Mirica, *Physionomia*, Bodleian Library, MS canon. misc. 350, fols. 94v–96v. (The second of the two chapters includes a long discussion of the causes of sex determination in general.)

118 Aristotle, *Generation of Animals*, IV, i, 766a19–24.

ing the confluence of several perspectives. Heat, quantity of seed, and strength of seed or of competing sperm all admitted of more and less – they existed not just in two states but in varying degrees. And though left and right were clearly opposites, seed from opposite sides might be mixed in different proportions. Likewise the womb, which had a left side and a right side, might house a fetus somewhere in between. Using this sense of range and permutations, medieval authors took the subject of sex determination not only beyond the simple distinction between male and female as suggested in Genesis but also beyond the anatomical and functional definitions of sex. The early fifteenth-century scholastic Jacopo of Forlì, for example, in insisting on the centrality of complexion – the mix and balance of qualities, elements, and humors in the body – was choosing a criterion of sex identification less decisive and less susceptible to dichotomy than, say, the presence or absence of a uterus. Furthermore, for Jacopo complexion was only the most important of the three main categories in which males and females differ, the other two being disposition and physique. A fetus (and presumably an adult) might be masculine or feminine with respect to all these categories or might embody some combination. He said, for example, that a fetus might be masculine as regards the reproductive organ (which has, as we have seen, been generated by the organism's complexion) and be feminine with respect to behavior, color, build, ways of moving (*motus operationes*), etc.[119] Or, according to another author, if the virile sperm gets the best of the woman's sperm and develops in the left side of the womb, the result will be a female with certain virile traits, especially a beard and a way of speaking.[120] The existence of hermaphrodites, accounted for by the same sorts of natural causes, likewise suggested that sex definitions and their attendant gender implications might admit of degrees, thus disclosing an apparent tension, to which we shall turn shortly, between scientific principles, on the one hand, and Christian concerns and lay perspectives, on the other. Even when represented benignly (the exception rather than the rule), hermaphrodites posed a challenge to medieval gender dichotomies that reached beyond science and medicine.[121] There was, for example, a certain Saint Wilgefortis, who was one of septuplets. According to the doctrine of the seven-celled uterus, she would have had three brothers, who had developed in the cells on the right side of their mother's womb, and three sisters, who had developed in the cells on the left: Wilgefortis is clearly presumed to have occupied the middle cell. She resisted the marriage arrangement her father had made for her, because she wished to devote herself to a religious life.

119 Jacobus Forliviensis, *De generatione embrionis*, fol. 9vb.
120 *Secreta mulierum minor*, Cambridge University, Trinity, MS O.2.5, fol. 132ra.
121 See Lorraine Daston and Katharine Park, "Hermaphrodites in Renaissance France," *Critical Matrix* 1/5 (1985).

After her betrothal, with the help of God (and perhaps puberty), she grew a mustache and a beard and was able to forestall the unwanted marriage.[122]

Occasionally the sources are explicit in associating character and behavioral as well as physical traits with individuals of one sex or the other. More revealing, however, is the identification of masculine and feminine characteristics embedded in allusions to masculine females and feminine males. Cumulatively these references suggest what "feminine" and "masculine" meant and disclose the values associated with the terms. But they do more. First, they demonstrate the extent to which those gender constructs had been abstracted in the later Middle Ages, creating the explicit possibility of dividing and speaking of the world in terms of gender. Second, to the extent that these references are accompanied by naturalistic explanations, they show a certain cultural discomfort with that same process of abstraction – a desire to anchor properties, whether physical or behavioral, in ordinary natural processes. The eclectic, flexible, and ambiguous approaches available at the confluence of medical and natural philosophical traditions gave writers of the later Middle Ages room to apply gender terms and constructs broadly while sustaining links to the workings of nature.

A compendium of predominantly Aristotelian natural history observes not only that males are larger than females (except among bears and leopards) but also that females are easier to train, shed tears more easily, are more pious, and are more given to envy and lying.[123] A series of chapters on physiognomy characterizes the masculine soul as active, not easily subdued when roused to anger, generous, studious, and controlled by virtue.[124] The same work describes the feminine man in such feminine terms as tenderhearted, envious, easily giving in to passions, intolerant of physical work, bitter, deceitful, and timid.[125] How can we recognize a feminine man? He has less body hair than a masculine man, a trait he shares with eunuchs, who are in turn often said to be feminine,[126] and he exhibits (unspecified) feminine behaviors.[127] A man whose hairline starts high on his neck is womanly, shy, slow, and irascible;[128] and a man with straight eyebrows is feminine, malicious, and flexible.[129] Certain types of men may have one or more

---

122 Vern L. Bullough, "Sex Education in Medieval Christianity," *Journal of Sex Research*, 13 (1977): 190. Versions of this story occur throughout western Europe; Bullough mentions other "bearded" and "transvestite" female saints.

123 *Propositiones de animalibus*, Cambridge University Library, MS Dd.3.16, fols. 74vb–75ra.

124 [Ps.-]Albertus Magnus, *Physionomia*, in *Extractiones*, Bibliothèque Nationale, MS lat. 6524, fol. 79v.

125 Ibid.

126 Constantinus, *De coitu*, ch. 5, p. 98; [Thomas Cantimpratensis], *De proprietatibus et natura rerum*, Bayerische Staatsbibliothek, MS CLM 3206, fol. 136ra.

127 *Secreta mulierum minor*, Cambridge University, Trinity MSS O.2.5, fol. 132va, and R.14.45, fol. 26v.

128 Albertus Magnus, *De animalibus*, bk. I, tr. ii, ch. 2, §134, p. 48.

129 *Propositiones de animalibus*, Cambridge University Library, MS Dd.3.16, fol. 73ra.

feminine characteristics. Hildegard of Bingen, who divides both men and women into groups according to their general constitutions and temperaments (which may be supposed in turn to have derived from the conditions of their birth), held that phlegmatic men have womanly flesh and color, and sanguine men have the prudence and continence of women.[130] The sexual incontinence typical of men is shared by phlegmatic women, who also have facial hair and somewhat virile minds.[131] According to other sources, a bearded woman is lustful and manly;[132] a virile woman's right hand and foot are larger than her left.[133]

Descriptions of this kind take us well beyond the realm of reproductive sexual characteristics into the realm of disposition and social behavior. Some of the traits may have different values, depending on the sex of the person they adorn. Continence may, for some of these authors, be less of a virtue in a man than in a woman, and being difficult to calm once roused to hatred may not be so much of a vice in a man as irascibility is in a woman. The feminine is associated with a few positive qualities (several named by Hildegard, the only woman quoted), such as piety and prudence. These are certainly virtues, and whether or not they were directly borrowed from Christian vocabulary, they are consonant with Christian values. But the feminine is also associated with weaknesses, such as slowness and a limited capacity for work, and with vices, such as envy and deceitfulness. Masculine virtues seem more secular – studiousness, for example, and liberality – and masculine vices are fewer.

Medieval scientific and medical texts do not, however, portray men as more virtuous than women. Rather, the evidence suggests that individuals of either sex may partake of any of these properties – that women may be "masculine" and men may be "feminine." These gender constructs are grounded in the broad notions of sexual differentiation, but they are predicated of the other sex as well as of ostensibly sex-neutral entities. Thus "manly" stands for a set of qualities derived from the notion of an ideal natural man, but applicable to women as well. In particular, the masculine woman, especially when honored with the title "virago," took on the glow of manly virtues, although she was unambiguously on the female side of the anatomical spectrum and thus clearly distinguished from a hermaphrodite.[134] The pagan virago of antiquity, celebrated by Plutarch and others, persisted here and there in the Middle Ages. Isidore of Seville had said that a virago is a woman who has a man's strength and does men's jobs.[135] This sense of "virago" enjoyed a renaissance from the late fourteenth century,

130 Hildegard, *Causae et curae*, bk. II, pp. 75, 73.
131 Ibid., pp. 87–8.
132 Michaelis Scotus, *De secretis naturae*, pt. III, ch. 74, p. 342.
133 Albertus Magnus, *De animalibus*, bk. I, tr. ii, ch. 2, §132, pp. 47–8.
134 Guilhelmus de Mirica, *Physionomia*, Bodleian Library, MS canon. misc. 350, fol. 94v.
135 Isidorus, *Etymologiae*, bk. XI, ch. ii, §22.

starting with Boccaccio's *On Famous Women* and continuing with Christine de Pisan's *Book of the City of Ladies* in 1405.[136] But the Christian virago was a more prominent figure in the late Middle Ages. She too had ancient origins. As Ambrose, archbishop of Milan, had said in the late fourth century, "She who does not believe, is a woman and should be designated by the name of her bodily sex, whereas she who believes progresses to complete manhood."[137] Isidore had mentioned this religious virago too, explaining that the word "virgin" is related to the word "virago" in the sense of incorruptibility and the capacity to resist feminine passion.[138] In the twelfth century, Peter the Venerable, abbot of the great monastery of Cluny, spoke admiringly about the learning of Heloise, leader of a small community of nuns, in a letter in which he alluded repeatedly to woman's weakness. He referred to "virile souls" and said, "You have overcome all women and risen above almost all men."[139] He praised her specifically for turning her powers to holy purposes and her heroism to the defeat of evil. He likened her to Penthesilea, queen of the Amazons and prototype of classical viragos, but with the difference that Heloise's leadership of women is within the army of the Lord.[140]

The tradition of praise for men with feminine qualities is not as long or as strong as that of praise for women with masculine characteristics, but it is significant and serves to fill out the notion of the feminine in the late Middle Ages. Caroline Walker Bynum has shown that the feminine properties of God, and in particular of Jesus, became an important motif in religious imagery from the twelfth century on.[141] Language describing Jesus, and earthly authorities ranging from the Apostles Peter and Paul to medieval abbots and bishops, as "mother" projected specific and evolving notions of the generative, tender, and nurturing feminine principles. During the twelfth century, especially among Cistercian monks, the emphasis was on the union between mother/God and dependent soul as represented by gestation and by the breast milk; later the emphasis was on the suffering and sacrifice of the mother/God as represented by the birth pangs and on the eucharistic aspect of the blood from Jesus' side, which is the food of salvation.[142] Other images of the feminine enrich religious language at this time,

---

136 See also Davis, "Women on Top."
137 Ambrose (Patrologia Latina, vol. 15, col. 1844) cited (in translation) in Joyce E. Salisbury, "The Latin Doctors of the Church on Sexuality" (paper presented at the annual meeting of the American Historical Association, December, 1985), p. 4.
138 Isidorus, *Etymologiae*, bk. XI, ch. ii, §21.
139 Petrus Venerabilis, "Ad Eloysam abbatissam," in *The Letters of Peter the Venerable*, ed. Giles Constable, 2 vols., Harvard Historical Studies 78 (Cambridge: Harvard University Press, 1967), vol. 1, letter 115, p. 304.
140 Ibid., p. 305.
141 Caroline Walker Bynum, *Jesus as Mother: Studies in the Spirituality of the High Middle Ages* (Berkeley and Los Angeles: University of California Press, 1982), ch. 4.
142 Bynum, *Holy Feast and Holy Fast*.

such as that of the Christian soul as the bride of Christ (a metaphor especially popular in the rhetoric of nuns in the late Middle Ages, when marriage was gaining greater religious respectability). As Bynum points out,
the positive uses of these feminine qualities indicate neither that the qualities
were regarded as positive per se in this period nor that women (as distinguished from the more abstract "feminine") were positively valued. Feminine tenderness was a double-edged sword, aimed at once at the promotion
of filial devotion through a love which transcends logic and law and at the
chastisement of passionate and unreasonable women. And when monks
asserted their humility by declaring themselves as weak as women, they
were making a virtue of investing themselves with a failing despised by the
world.[143] Thus, gendered characteristics were interpreted and applied in
more than one way. In the realm of earthly women, feminine unreason
usually meant the inability of the higher faculties to control the passions of
the flesh; in the realm of spiritual transcendence, it was associated with
unfathomable mysteries of faith and grace.

The same gender attributes, encompassing both notions of sex difference
and social expectations, operated not only in those areas of concrete and
common experience but also in more rarified and inaccessible domains. The
difference between these two applications is not a difference between positive and negative or between achieved and unachieved ideals, for "virility"
bears a positive value in both worldly and spiritual language. It is, at least in
part, a difference of levels of abstraction, which occurs not only in religious
but also in scientific language. Species of animals, kinds of plants, and
astrological signs were known as masculine or feminine. For example, one
system of physiognomy mentioned (though not favored) by medieval authors describes human types by the animals they resemble. The animals are
in turn taken to embody certain properties, among which the feminine and
the masculine are prominent. Panthers (except for their legs, which are
strong) represent the feminine. Their faces are small, their mouths are large,
and their necks are long and thin. As a whole they are disjointed and ill-
proportioned. More important for the pursuit of the science of physiognomy is the nature of their souls – small, furtive, and deceitful. Lions, on
the other hand, are emblematic of the masculine.[144]

Similarly, astrological language included, in addition to the specific determination of nativities, the general characterization of cosmic forces. Not
only did astrologers concern themselves with predicting the birth of male
and female children (the attribution of the adjectives "feminine" and "masculine" to the planets sometimes refers simply to their power to contribute to
the production of children of that sex),[145] but they also spoke of the influ-

---

143 Bynum, *Jesus as Mother*, p. 144.
144 Foerster, *De translatione Latina* Physiognomonicorum, p. 11.
145 Alkindrinus, British Library, MS Harley 5402, fol. 31r.

ences of the planets under which children of both sexes were born as masculine and feminine in an extended sense – in the sense of a set of qualities and
values projected by the planets of each gender. The extent to which these
influences are distinct from more literal notions of sex is illustrated by the
fact that Saturn, named after a male god and father of other gods, is nevertheless a feminine planet, associated, not surprisingly, with cold. In alchemy
too the concepts of "masculine" and "feminine" operated at several levels.
The allegory of generating a new substance (often involving talk of a chemi-
cal marriage, a father, a mother, a womb, a birth) drew upon the literal and
concrete notions of sex as involved in reproduction. In this respect, alchemy
seems to employ a clear sexual duality.[146] But alchemy also involves the
cross-attribution of traits that becomes possible when gender concepts go
beyond sexual literalism: the father in labor, giving birth to a son, which is
Philosopher's Stone.[147] The Philosopher's Stone itself was often represented
as the Hermaphrodite or Hermetic Androgyn, a symbolic union of opposites.[148] And, on a level of greater abstraction, alchemy invokes the feminine
aspect of divinity in the form of Wisdom.[149] (See Figure 6.)

These diverse manifestations of gender constructs suggest several conclusions. First, gender in general and nature-linked gender in particular served as
one way of describing both the spiritual and the physical world. Whether
applied to persons and animals without regard to their sex or to entities
(ranging from deity to planets) not thought of in terms of sexual reproduction, notions of "masculine" and "feminine" projected a set of traits and
values. Second, these traits and values, although they constituted a fairly
coherent vision of gender, were not rigidly understood and employed. Positive and negative attributions, literal and metaphorical attributions, and essential and accidental attributions of "feminine" and "masculine" all coexisted in
the later Middle Ages. Although the female principles center on moral and
physical weakness, bearing pejorative connotations, and the male principles
center on moral and physical strength, bearing positive connotations, devia-
tions from such dichotomous usage are significant, if not frequent, and many
various traits cluster around the central ones. Third, this flexibility derives
from the diverse rules and structures of the domains to which the gender
concepts apply – from social virtue to Christian theology – and from the
diverse rules and structures of the domains from which they are borrowed.
Ideas drawn from anatomy, physiology, alchemy, physiognomy, embryol-

---

146 See Boswell, *Christianity, Social Tolerance, and Homosexuality,* p. 308.
147 See Allison Coudert, *Alchemy: The Philosopher's Stone* (Boulder, Colo.: Shambahala,
    1980), pp. 136–7.
148 Ibid., pp. 132–3; E. John Holmyard, *Alchemy* (Harmondsworth: Penguin, 1957), pl. 34.
149 E.g., Marie-Louise von Franz, ed. and comm., *Aurora consurgens: A Document Attributed to
    Thomas Aquinas on the Problem of Opposites in Alchemy,* trans. R. F. C. Hull and A. S. B.
    Glover, Bollingen Series 77 (New York: Random House, Pantheon Books, 1966), esp. chs.
    1, 2, 12, and commentary.

ogy, and astrology, not to speak of Genesis, converge, producing not a synthesis but a constellation of gender-laden characteristics. Finally, though they do not constitute a single system, many of these contributing traditions tie the traits to explanatory frameworks from medicine and natural philosophy. Four qualities, seven uterine cells, two seeds, seven planets, stand behind both the usual cases – the attribution of specific traits to males and females – and the unusual cases – the attribution of traits typical of one sex to a member of the other. Like the flexibility and variety in the application of gender notions, their grounding in natural processes lent medieval language and culture a set of gender traits that conveyed the sense of duality without being strictly dichotomous.

Neither the flexibility and diversity of application, however, nor particular variations in the specific traits and values associated with "feminine" and "masculine" swamped the duality with which persistent sex distinctions colored gender notions. Although some scientific and medical models implied the existence of a continuum of sexual differentiation (as in the case with the fusion of two seeds) or the existence of a middle term (as in the case of the seven-celled uterus), the characterization of properties, behaviors, and beings did not easily admit of mediation. Physically ambiguous organisms and behaviorally ambiguous individuals did indeed exist in the eyes of medieval writers. But, however plausible the naturalistic explanations for their existence, their ambiguity met with responses that reflected less acceptance than discomfort or even hostility.

Irregular natures within a regular Nature

One striking feature of the abstraction of gender to the levels of symbolism and metaphysics represented in both theological and scientific language is the extent to which it permitted a tolerance of sexual ambiguity and gender mixes – indeed, the alchemical hermaphrodite and mother–Jesus are invested with significant positive value. The open attitude at the level of cultural abstractions did not, however, reflect back down upon the world of concrete biological and social existence. If Jupiter and Ganymede can sleep together, asked the philosopher and poet Alan of Lille in the twelfth century, why are men condemned for sexual relations with each other? Because (he had the character Nature answer) poetry and allegory are not to be taken literally and have entirely different rules from those of everyday life.[150] Here below in the world of mortals, from Alan's perspective, neither the irregular sexual behavior of sodomites nor the ambiguous sexual identity of hermaphrodites should be placed in a positive light. It is true there were occasional exceptions – prudence, as we have seen, could be regarded as a feminine trait

150 Nikolaus M. Häring, "Alan of Lille, *De planctu naturae*," *Studi medievali*, 3d ser., 19 (1978): ch. VIII, [prose 4], ll. 115–54, pp. 836–8.

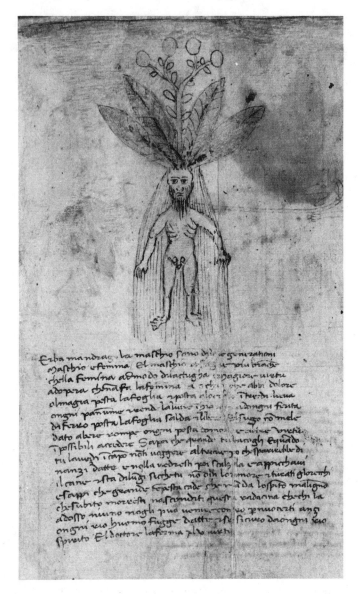

Figure 6. Male (left) and female (right) mandrakes. Plants, like planets and alchemical principles, could reflect the sexual differentiation of nature. Classical herbals distinguished the appearance and medicinal virtues of "male" and "female" forms of this plant. In the Middle Ages the duality was transposed to the representation of the human-shaped roots as sexually differentiated, here seen in a fifteenth-century example. At the same time,

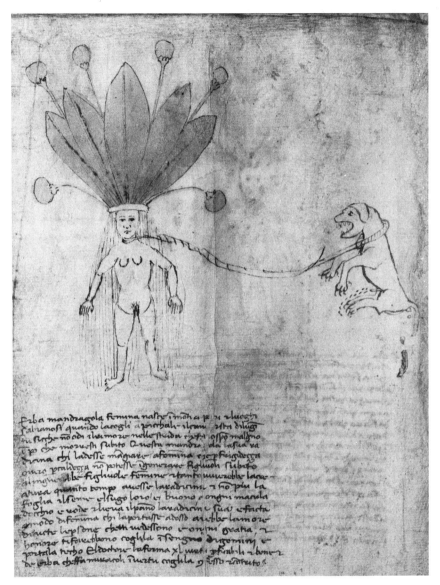

Ezba mandragola femina naf[...] m[...]h a [...] [...] [...]luo[...]
[...]almanoft quando iacogli apenbali iltem [...] [...]tn diligo
[...]ho[...] no ob [...]he moze nelle fu[...]da [...]g[...]a off[...] maligno
[...] [...]ho mozu ch futto [...] nofta mundu da lafaa va
[...]na chi lado[...]e magnau afomina [...][...]f[...]gu[...]u
[...]za [...]ald[...]za no poh[...]f [...][...]mcaue [...]g[...]oh f[...]b[...]
[...]gn[...] [...]h[...] fighuole femone [...]h u[...]e[...] lao[...]
[...][...]ca q[...]nto tempo aue[...]e lacad[...]m [...] [...] pu la
f[...]glia il f[...]m[...] f[...]go loro [...] buono [...] ong[...] ma[...]
[...]o[...]ho [...] [...]te zlu[...]a ilpano lacad[...]m [...] [...] [...]fa[...]a
[...]o [...]f[...]mna chi lap[...]ta[...] ado[...] a[...]tb[...] la m [...]
[...]uto [...]p[...]n[...] ch[...]h u[...]o[...]o [...] ong[...] g[...]a[...] [...]
h[...]z[...] [...][...]o[...]ho [...]ghla [...] [...]g[...] [...]g[...][...]
[...][...]la [...]bo [...][...]o[...] la f[...]ma [...]l[...] [...] [...] [...] b[...]
[...] [...]ba [...]ffa [...]o[...] [...] [...] [...] g [...] [...]o[...]

the association of mandrake with fertility was heightened. Regarded as deadly to harvest, the root was supposed to be pulled up by a rope tied around a dog's neck. (*Erbario,* Rimini, Biblioteca Civica Gambalunga, MS 8, fol. 101r and 101v. Reproduced by permission of the Biblioteca Civica Gambalunga.)

in a man, self-control as a masculine trait in a woman. But neither Joan of Arc, to take a lay example, nor the bearded Saint Wilgefortis, to take a religious one, could be held up as a literal model for ordinary women. Indeed, their exceptional qualities, supernatural in the context of their extraordinary stories, could be potentially disruptive irregularities in more pedestrian circumstances. Joan's enemies gave prominent and successful play to the charge that she dressed as a man.

Albertus Magnus rehearsed Aristotle's view that hermaphrodites are really either male or female but that by the same sort of material accident responsible for certain tumors, they possess secondarily organs of the other sex. The hermaphrodite's true sex and principal genitals are consistent with its underlying complexion. This picture of hermaphrodites would not seem to pose much of a challenge to sex distinctions, but Albertus went beyond Aristotle to point out some of its social implications: in intercourse, a hermaphrodite can be both active and passive, lie on someone or under someone. Furthermore, in keeping with the notion that hot and cold present a continuum, Albertus undermined the Aristotelian reassurance that one can always tell the real sex from the individual's complexion by adding, "however, sometimes even the complexion of the heart is so intermediate that it is scarcely possible to discern which of the sexes should prevail."[151] Such breaches of the ordinary pattern of things commonly elicited two types of response. First, and more generally, hermaphrodites were pejoratively described as rebellious or disruptive. Second, and more subtly, the traits and behaviors of the individuals in question were at once identified and suppressed by attempts to reduce them to permutations of the conventional categories of masculine and feminine. Attributes that did not fit the accepted range known as "feminine" were necessarily "masculine," and vice versa. The reductionism implicit in a language limited to two types had several effects. One was to constrain the ways in which medieval authors spoke about sex and expressed gender. Another was to preclude clear distinctions among various kinds of diversities, differences, and exceptions; hermaphrodite anatomical features, transvestite acts, and homoerotic behavior became associated, even confused, in medieval language.

Even scientific texts, although they provided naturalistic theories for the existence of hermaphrodites, masculine females, and feminine males, expressed a profound discomfort with displaced gender attributes. In addition to the negative quality of many of the characteristics transferred (the lustfulness of masculine women, the maliciousness of feminine men), such persons were open to the charge of fraud: their bodies are misleading and so are their

---

151 Albertus Magnus, *De animalibus*, bk. XVIII, tr. ii, ch. 3, §66, p. 1225: ". . . tamen aliquando etiam complexio cordis ita media est quod vix discerni potest quis sexuum praevaleat."

mores – they are deceitful; they are liars.[152] The accusation of hypocrisy applied alike to the woman with a large right foot and the man with a large left foot, according to scholastic opinion, and to the hyena, a creature of elusive sexual identity, according to the more widely familiar bestiaries:

Its nature is that at one moment it is masculine and at another moment feminine, and hence it is a dirty brute. . . . Since they [hyenas] are neither male nor female, they are neither faithful nor pagan, but are obviously the people concerning whom Solomon said: "A man in double mind is inconstant in all his ways."[153]

Similarly, Tiresias, the classical prophet who changed from male to female and back again, suffers among the sorcerers and soothsayers in the circle of Dante's Hell devoted to the punishment of fraud.[154] Perhaps false prophesy is Tiresias's crime, but all Dante mentions is the story of his unstable sexual identity. The suffering soul next to him, Aronta, may also be tainted by what Dante sees as distorted sexuality. He describes him as the one "who turns his back to [another's] belly."[155] The hostile image is rendered more perverse by the fact that these souls have their heads on backwards.[156] In ancient representations, Tiresias was often pitiable, but not perverse.

Sometimes the deceptiveness has the connotation of an unspecified threat, especially when it has to do with behavior rather than or in addition to physical makeup. One medical source condemns coitus with the woman on top as usurpation,[157] and Hildegard of Bingen placed her condemnation of male and female transvestism between an assertion that women should not say mass and a warning against sexual perversions, including sodomy – "when a man sins with another man in the manner of a woman."[158] A disorder of either sex or sex roles is a disorder in the social fabric (including male hegemony in the family) and in the religious order (including the exclusively male priesthood). It is even possible to see such disruptions as a threat to the political order: the notion of usurpation has legal connotations. (In connection with the early modern period, Natalie Davis has argued that both from the symbolic perspective of a topsy-turvy world in which authority is turned upside down and from the perspective of social unrest in which women and

---

152 E.g., ibid., bk. I, tr. ii, ch. 2, §132, pp. 47–8; *Physionomia*, in *Extractiones*, Bibliothèque Nationale, MS lat. 6524, fol. 79v.
153 White, *Book of Beasts*, pp. 31–2. See also Boswell, *Christianity, Social Tolerance, and Homosexuality*, pp. 304–9. Cf. *Physiologus*, versio Y, xxxvii, p. 129, and versio B, xviii, p. 34.
154 Dante, *Inferno*, canto XX, ll. 40–5.
155 Ibid., l. 46: "quel ch'al ventre li s'atterga."
156 Cf. Dorothy Sayers, trans. and comm., *The Divine Comedy of Dante Alighieri the Florentine*, cantica I, *Hell* (Harmondsworth: Penguin, 1949), canto XX, l. 46.
157 Cartelle, ed., *Liber minor de coitu*, pt. II, ch. 6, p. 98.
158 Hildegard, *Scivias*, pt. II, vis. 6, chs. 76–78, pp. 290–2; and ch. 78, p. 291: ". . . vir secundum modum feminae cum alio viro peccaverit. . . ."

men disguised as women often played a role, women on top and cross-dressing constituted political challenges.)[159]

Thus medical writers might explain the natural origins of sexually ambiguous individuals, and spiritual leaders might make sense of metaphorical gender paradoxes, but physicians and canonists reflecting on unusual anatomy or behavior in ordinary people sounded more hostile. In the extent to which various sectors of society condemned those whose bodies were beyond the borders of clear sex definitions or whose actions were beyond the borders of clear and, for all their variations, binary gender definitions, we have a crude indicator of the late medieval determination to enforce restrictive norms of sex and gender. For the most part, medical and scientific disapprobation was limited to the attribution of negative personality traits – lustfulness and deceitfulness at worst – and were not the subject of extensive comments.

A singular exception to this relative neglect is the discussion of anal intercourse and related subjects in Peter of Abano's commentary on the pseudo-Aristotelian work known as *Problems*, a long series of natural questions on a wide variety of topics.[160] Peter took his cues from this late classical text, but he added considerably to it. He remarked, for example, that "some exercise the wicked act of sodomy by rubbing the penis with the hand; others by rubbing between the thighs of boys, which is what most do these days; and others by making friction around the anus and by putting the penis in it in the same way as it is placed in a woman's sexual part, and it seems Aristotle is speaking more about these."[161] The chapter consists mainly of a long naturalistic explanation why some men derive sexual pleasure from anal stimulation: in some males, the pores and passages that would normally convey the semen – especially its more spiritous, less humid part – to the penis are narrow, blocked, or misdirected. This is the case in eunuchs and in men called "effeminate," in whom the blocked pores and associated cool complexion give rise to womanly nature and behavior. In some men these vessels may terminate at the base of the penis or around the anus, displacing the sensation created by the need to release seed. They cannot ejaculate through the penis, but their slight, often dry seed can be dispersed or emitted by rubbing around the anus. (Other men, in whom

159 Natalie Davis, "Women on Top." Her argument is based on sources from a century or two later than those with which we are concerned, but her general framework is suggestive for the late Middle Ages, and some of the particular traditions to which she refers date back to that period.
160 See Nancy G. Siraisi, "The *Expositio problematum Aristotelis* of Peter of Abano," *Isis* 61 (1970): 321–39.
161 Petrus de Abano, *Expositio problematum Aristotelis*, pt. IV, probl. 26, fols. [70]vb–[71]ra: "Notandum est quod illud nephandum opus sodomiticum quidam exercent manu fricando virgam. Alii puerorum inter cossas confricatione, quod et plurimi agunt hodie. Alii autem fricationem faciendo circa anum et virgam in ipsum imponendo sicut in vulvam imponitur et de talibus videntur esse sermo Aristotelis magis."

some passages lead to the anus and some to the penis, can experience emission and pleasure in both places, a situation discussed by Avicenna.[162])

Although Peter distinguished such anal emissions from "natural intercourse," he considered it natural *for these individuals*, in the sense that the disposition of their pores and vessels is innate. He applied to them the familiar sexual economy – the desire to emit seed caused by the pressure of superfluity is reinforced by the memory of the pleasure of previous emissions – and compared the dry emissions with their attendant pleasure to those of boys just reaching puberty and to those of men who are suffering from inflamations or fevers.[163] The anatomical nature of the condition leads Peter to consider the possibility of a surgical remedy for the ill formed pores, which might be carefully opened with a knife. But this proceedure could result in death from a corruption of the pores or in other undesireable consequences: "Also, if it were done, he who was a man at first might change into a woman, and thus would be changed into something worse. . . . (This is not, however, to be taken to mean that the man would change into a woman in an essential sense, but rather in an accidental sense, by acquiring womanly attributes and behavior.)"[164] Peter referred to Avicenna, who "said those men who want to cure them are stupid."[165] He clearly disagreed with and therefore did not reiterate Avicenna's reason, namely, that "the origin of their illness is spiritual, not natural,"[166] but he elaborated on the medical authority's suggestion that an indirect approach might help: the pressures which give rise to desire might be alleviated by redistributing the moisture within the body, using diet and medicine. Reducing desire was apparently a serious issue, for these men could become insatiable like women (especially young women), always seeking to be rubbed, since, having little moisture, they expel little and thus feel desire again right away.

Up to this point, Peter's account has been strikingly naturalistic. Although he clearly believed there was something wrong with such men, their condition was comprehensible and comparable to other natural situations. He applied negative terms to them, such as "womanly" and "insatiable," but did not treat them as blameworthy or even apply the word "sodomite" to them. But, following the text on which he had been commenting, he identified a second group of men with the sexual sensibilities and appetites he has been describing: those who are not born that way but who come to it

162 Avicenna, *Liber canonis*, bk. III, tr. ii, fen 20, ch. 42, fol. 358ra.

163 Petrus de Abano, *Expositio problematum Aristotelis*, pt. IV, probl. 26, fols. [69]va–[70]ra.

164 Ibid., fol. [70]rb: "Item si fieret qui vir erat primo, mutaretur in mulierem et sic mutaretur in peius. . . . Non tamen intelligendum quod vir essentialiter mutetur in mulierem sed potius accidentaliter, acquirendo actus et mores muliebres."

165 Petrus de Abano, *Expositio problematum Aristotelis*, pt. IV, probl. 26, fol. [70]rb: "Unde Avicenna 20ª tertii [Canonis] . . . dicit quod stulti sunt homines qui volunt eos curare. . . ."

166 Avicenna, *Liber canonis*, bk. III, tr. ii, fen 20, ch. 43, fol. 358ra: "Nam initium egritudinis eorum meditativum est non naturale."

"on account of depraved and filthy habit – such are sodomites."[167] Although Peter took the trouble to explain how such a practice could become a habit starting from the innocent experience of seeking to release seed and explained in physiological terms why adolescent boys were susceptible (hence, many nations prohibit intercourse with children) and even how the habit gives rise to what is, in a sense, a new nature, still he spoke of this group as "those who are damned by the polluted sodomite vice."[168] To them Avicenna's opinion on the spiritual origin of the disorder applies. They are twice blameworthy. First, by their own actions they have perverted their original natural inclinations (to release seed, to engage in reproductive intercourse), investing themselves with new inclinations and, in that sense, a new nature. Second, they give in to these new inclinations by practicing the various forms of sodomy mentioned earlier. What is at issue here is not an accident of birth, though astrological influences may come into play, but rather a perversion of the soul as Peter understood it from Aristotle's ethics.

Although Peter's account is exceptional in many respects, its two parts represent two dimensions of medieval attitudes – an accepting if not approving understanding and a moralistic condemnation. In part, the relative mildness of the former outlook reflected the confidence that although many perceived aberrations might stretch the boundaries of "feminine" and "masculine," they did not break them. Indeed, being contained, they demonstrated the fundamental strength of the categories. The men Peter described might have womanly attributes, but they were still essentially men. In part, too, the mildness was due to the understanding that nature itself was prodigious and not narrowly constrained. The regular patterns of the world below the moon, the world subject to change, consisted in the realization of forms in accordance with their final causes, but their courses were often deflected by accidents and material necessities, not to speak of magic and supernatural intervention. Some of these deflections, such as the birth of daughters, had an order, purpose, and pattern of their own. Others, such as the males whose seminal passages stopped at their anus, were more unusual and sometimes called "monsters" and had no such place. They were, nevertheless, products of nature in the largest sense. In this respect, the mores, like the stature and build, of hermaphrodites, masculine men, and feminine women, were innate and not subject to fundamental change by the intervention of natural philosophy or medicine. Medieval naturalists were not, however, materialists or determinists. On the contrary, they took pains to convey the belief that innate or acquired disabilities could and should be overcome, that the inclinations of humans

---

167 Ibid., fol. [70]va: ". . . propter pravam consuetudinem obscenam advenit, quales sunt sodomite."
168 Ibid.: ". . . qui scelerato vicio sodomitico sunt dampnati." He names Avicenna as his authority for the laws of nations (fol. [70]vb).

were not imperatives like the downward fall of a stone. But they saw the sources of change or resistance as moral or spiritual – precisely beyond the control, if not the concern, of their sciences. A story told about the ancient physiognomer Philemon in a widely circulated pseudo-Aristotelian letter illustrates their perspective:

The disciples of the wise Hippocrates painted a picture of him on parchment and took it to Philemon, saying, "Study this face and point out to us its qualities and complexions." Inspecting the compositions and arrangements of the face, he compared [the man's] parts to each other, saying, "This man is lustful, a betrayer who loves sex." On account of this [the students] wanted to kill [Philemon], saying, "You idiot! This is the face of one of the worthiest and best men in the world." But Philemon calmed them and set them straight, saying, "This is the face of the wise Hippocrates. What you asked of me regarding my science and what its opinion is, this have I shown you." So when they came to Hippocrates, they told him what they had done, and what Philemon had answered to them and his judgment [of Hippocrates]. Hippocrates said to them, "Surely Philemon has said what is true, nor has he let one detail escape. However, from this I recognized these shameful things and considered [they] ought to be condemned. I made my soul queen over them, and withdrew her from them, and I triumphed over my desire's resistance."[169]

The distinction made in this story between the operations of natural conditions, inclinations, and forces, and the human ability to exercise spiritual power and free will was a commonplace of medieval natural philosophy, often rehearsed in the context of astrological doctrines. The stars, according to Dante, *initiate* some terrestrial effects, but these can be entirely overridden by the tireless efforts of a healthy will.[170] The primacy of the will does not negate the integration of disposition and patterns of behavior with constitution and build; character and mores remain among the proper concerns of medicine and natural philosophy. Naturalists as well as moralists, however, distinguished the given of a person's constitution and disposition from the actions to which that person is thereby inclined. Perhaps for this

169 Eduard Taube, ed. *Aristoteles de arte physiognomonica ad Alexandrum scriptor*, Programm königlichen katholischen Gymnasiums zu Gleiwitz (Gleiwitz: Gustav Neumann, 1866), pp. 5–6: "Discipuli enim Ypocratis sapientis pinxerunt formam ejus in pergameno et portaverunt eam Philemoni dicentes: Considera hanc figuram et indica nobis qualitates et complexiones ejus. Qui respiciens compositiones et dispositiones figurae comparavit partes ejus ad partes dicens: Iste homo est luxuriosus, deceptor, amans coitum. Ob quam rem voluerunt eum interficere dicentes: O stulte, haec est figura dignioris et melioris hominis, qui sit in hoc mundo. Philemon autem pacificavit eos et correxit eos dicens: Haec est figura sapientis Ypocratis; quod vos quaesivistis a me de mea scientia, hoc ostendi vobis et quod inde sentio secundum ipsam. Quando ergo pervenerunt ad Ypocratem, dixerunt ei, quod fecerant et quod respondit eis Philemon et judicium ejus. Quibus dixit Ypocras: Certe verum dixit Philemon nec praetermisit unam litteram; veruntamen ex quo perspexi et consideravi haec turpia esse reprobanda, constitui animam meam reginam super ipsam et retraxi eam ab eis et trumphavi super retentionem concupiscentiae meae."

170 Dante, *Purgatorio*, canto xvi, ll. 65–78; see also Nicole Oresme, in G. W. Coopland, *Nicole Oresme and the Astrologers: A Study of His* Le Livre des Divinacions (Liverpool, University of Liverpool Press, 1952), pp. 56, 68, 90.

reason, naturalists and physicians rarely mentioned same-sex sexual relations, which they may have regarded as possible but not necessary consequences of an individual's makeup. In a rare reference to sodomy, Albertus
Magnus, citing a case from the literature, reports that a man with, among
other features, "a feminine voice, womanly words, and all his organs and
limbs lacking in strength, . . . because of his inability to withstand desires,
committed all shameful acts and also was subjected by others contrary to
nature."[171] As Philemon knew, there were transcendent considerations beyond the realm of natural causes, and there was consequently a system of
beliefs, especially concerning behavior, which was independent of natural
knowledge and with which it interacted.

Gendered natures: Ecclesiastical and social orders

Thus, although medical texts and works of natural philosophy often took a
negative tone, they did not contain the pattern of invective against what was
regarded as deviant sexual behavior that developed in the religious and to
some extent in the secular literature of the later Middle Ages. Furthermore,
although medical writers were frequently concerned with sexual conduct in
the context of particular health problems such as sterility, they did not (with
certain notable exceptions) express views about the morality or propriety of
sexual states or habits unless they had a bearing upon health. And they did not
often represent either anatomical variations like hermaphroditism or behavioral variations like anal intercourse as essentially unhealthy. It is largely
beyond science and medicine that the strongest rhetoric for the enforcement
of sex definitions as gender constructs occurs, although this rhetoric sometimes draws upon the language of nature. When the thirteenth-century
encyclopedist Vincent of Beauvais declared "sodomy" (by which he meant
the emission of semen in an inappropriate place) to be unnatural, he did so not
in the *Speculum naturale*, his summary of natural knowledge, but rather in the
Speculum doctrinale, where he gave an outline of orthodox Christian doctrine.[172] Similarly, in his theological writings Albertus Magnus fiercely condemned sodomy (in this case, in a narrower sense) as "a sin against nature,
male with male and female with female,"[173] which is more heinous than
adultery, but in his more naturalistic work, *On Animals*, he just called it a fault

---

171 Albertus Magnus, *De animalibus*, bk. I, tr. ii, ch. 3, §159, p. 57: "Dicit enim hunc
habuisse . . . vocem femineam, verba muliebria, membra et omnes artus sine vigore . . . :
impatientia libidinum turpia fecisse omnia et passum esse ab aliis etiam contra naturam."
172 Boswell, *Christianity, Social Tolerance, and Homosexuality*, p. 316, n. 48. Giles of Rome,
who also wrote on both natural philosophy and theology, takes up the subject in a biblical
commentary (ibid., p. 323, n. 69).
173 Albertus Magnus, *Summa theologica* (Borgnet, vol. 33, p. 400), cited in Boswell, *Christianity, Social Tolerance, and Homosexuality*, p. 316, n. 51.

and mentioned a remedy for it, probably from an Arabic source: apply ash of hyena fur mixed with pitch to the man's anus.[174]

The distinction between natural and unnatural sexual acts was not elaborated in medieval writings on nature per se but rather in the canon law and in the broad, synthetic theology which flourished from the midthirteenth century on. Condemnations of sexual acts between men, although frequent, were part of a larger shift toward the control of sexual behavior in general, including coital positions and clerical celibacy (discussed later in the contexts of sterility and abstinence respectively). For example, charges of misusing semen and circumventing the reproductive intent of Nature and God were leveled against those who masturbated and those who engaged in contraceptive practices. Indeed, this was the period during which the position of the Church on contraception was clearly established, elaborated, and given legal and theoretical underpinnings.[175]

A number of elements in the climate of the later Middle Ages contributed to the articulation of a sexual orthodoxy. First, successive waves of ecclesiastical reform and the simultaneous evolution of marriage into a sacrament focused interest on the meaning of chastity in various circumstances – clerical celibacy and abstinence, marital fidelity and restraint. In all situations, chastity did not permit the pursuit of sexual pleasure for its own sake, a prohibition that covered marital intercourse as well as sexual interaction between persons of the same sex. Second, the rise and endemic persistence of heresies from the twelfth century on presented a challenge to ecclesiastical doctrine and attitudes concerning sexual impulses and acts. Movements like the Cathar, or Albigensian, heresy subscribed to a radical dualism which in principle rejected the body and the natural world as essentially evil instruments of the enemy of the soul, the good, and God. Pressed to defend the relationship of the Creator to Nature, the advocates and enforcers of orthodoxy needed to tread lightly in their condemnations of the pleasures of the flesh, lest they seemed to be condemnations of the flesh itself.[176] The Cathars' position against earthly marriage not only added impetus to the Catholic promotion of marriage as a sacrament but probably also fueled rumors that heretics engaged in coitus interruptus, homosexual practices, and other nonreproductive sexual acts. The association of these behaviors with heretics in turn heightened the aura of spiritual contamination surrounding them. The records of an ecclesiastical court report the testimony of one heretic who said, "I believe neither in sin nor in the redeeming power of good works; in my opinion, incest with mother, daughter, sister, or first

---

174 Albertus Magnus, *De animalibus*, bk. XXII, tr. ii, ch. 1, §23, p. 1360. See Boswell, *Christianity, Social Tolerance, and Homosexuality*, p. 317, n. 54.
175 Noonan, *Contraception*.
176 Ibid., p. 230.

cousin is not even a sin; incest is merely a shameful act."[177] Balancing between the advocacy of restraint (evident in the campaigns to suppress the practice of clerical marriage and to codify and enforce the rules of lay marriage) and the resistance to radical, heretical asceticism (evident in the repeated affirmation of marriage and procreation), canonists and theologians worked out in detail the general position that sexuality and sexual acts were acceptable *under appropriate circumstances.*

If sexual regulation in the institutions of marriage and holy orders and the challenge of heresies played a role in the formulation of the religious definitions of acceptable and unacceptable sexual behavior, the enforcement of gender roles was also a significant factor in this process. The insistence that men should be masculine and that women should be feminine cannot explain some of the emerging prohibitions, such as the censure of (usually male) masturbation in the penitentials: there is no sign that masturbation was regarded as effeminate behavior in the late Middle Ages, as it sometimes has been in modern times. However, descriptions of homosexual acts, between women and between men, were commonly put in terms of role reversals, bearing the implication that there is something inherently feminine about taking what was construed as a passive role in intercourse and something inherently masculine about having sex with a woman. Early penitentials had used language that reflected these assumptions, and it turned up with some regularity later, both within and beyond ecclesiastical documents.[178] We find Hildegard of Bingen saying, "But if any layman has committed fornication in a sodomite fashion, that is, has sinned with a man as with a woman. . . ." She similarly condemned sodomy in which "a man has sinned with another man in a feminine manner."[179] Like the prohibition of transvestism, which is associated, among other things, with preventing women from celebrating the mass,[180] the ecclesiastical position against sexual acts between persons of the same sex carries the message of role differentiation, and like the tone of the medical and physiognomic texts which derogate masculine traits in women and feminine traits in men by calling them deceptions and hypocrisies, it communicates firm moral disapprobation. Although the danger that women might pass themselves off as priests was troublesome, most of the concern centered on men. The emphasis may have been due in part to the fact that the authors and policymakers were almost all men, often products (if not residents) of male monastic communities. It may also reflect a greater anxiety about the degradation of the sex on

---

177 Emmanuel Le Roy Ladurie, *Montaillou: The Promised Land of Error*, trans. Barbara Bray (New York: Random House, 1978), pp. 327–8.

178 Pierre J. Payer, *Sex and the Penitentials: The Development of a Sexual Code, 550–1150* (Toronto: University of Toronto Press, 1984), pp. 40–4, 135–9.

179 Hildegard, *Scivias*, pt. II, vis. vi, ch. 78, p. 291:"Vir qui secundum modum feminae cum alio uiro peccauerit. . . ."

180 Ibid., ch. 77, p. 291.

which so much of the ecclesiastical and social order depended. Yet in the spiritual as in the natural world, the very extension and enforcement of distinctions between the feminine and the masculine dilute the categories themselves. To be sure, the presumption that couples accused of sodomy consisted of a passive feminine member and an active masculine member reinforces dualistic gender constructs by implying their universality. On the other hand, the emphasis upon specific acts in which individuals engage and for which they are responsible renders the application of "masculine" and "feminine" transitory and mutable. Albertus Magnus's "remedy" for sodomy, a topical application, and Peter of Abano's suggestion about diet and medicines were clearly not aimed at changing the patient's essence, but rather at changing his behavior.

Those dealing with the natural world, and particularly with an individual's inborn constitution, were concerned with the challenge to duality presented by ambiguous or intermediate constitutions, such as hermaphrodites or masculine women. They gave only scant attention to sexual acts of women with women or, with the exception of Peter of Abano, men with men. Those dealing with the spiritual world, and particularly with an individual's soul and will, were concerned with the challenge to duality presented by spiritual transgressions such as sodomy. But they invoked the order of nature both in condemning sin and in affirming the orthodox meaning of Creation. There were other ways, secular, if still Christian, in which medieval writers approached the double threat of sexual and gender disruption that they perceived especially in sexual relations between men. Two examples will illustrate some of the contexts in which these concerns were manifested, though they cannot be said to represent a coherent cultural perspective. Once again, the ordinary rules of nature form an ideological backdrop, and once again situations, individuals, and behavior that we would call "lesbian" or "gay," insofar as they are acknowledged, are discussed in other terms, including those of the bipartite division of gender.

One source which condemned the sexual transgressions of men with men in terms of a binary ideal of the sexes is Alan of Lille's polemical *Complaint of Nature*. Like Peter of Abano's commentary, this work is exceptional in the content and extent of its attention to this subject, and so, although it is indicative of certain attitudes, it is not in any sense typical. Alan, an opinionated polymath writing in the second half of the twelfth century, presented sodomy as emblematic of what was wrong with the world. Furthermore, although learned in theology, in this work he represented the acts that he attacked more as failures of nature than as failures of will. In accordance with a Neoplatonic view of how perfection can preside over imperfection, Alan's Goddess Nature, who rules over the order of Creation, has placed too much trust in her deputy, Venus, with the result that her human subjects have disobeyed her laws, especially those governing sexual conduct. In the course of the work, which deals with how this sad state of affairs came to be and how it is to be remedied, Alan alluded frequently to sexual misconduct, especially to sexual acts between men. One of Alan's most persistent images represents human decadence in terms of grammatical disorder. In particular, confusion and corruption of grammatical gender – masculine and feminine nouns, pronouns, and adjectives – and confusion and corruption of human gender are expressed simultaneously in elaborate plays on words. In the opening lines, for example, the persona of the author complains that because Venus is at war with herself, she changes *ille* (a pronoun which can stand for "he" or for any masculine noun) into *illa* (a pronoun which can stand for "she" or for any feminine noun).[181]

Our modern cultural assumptions would lead us to believe that when sex and grammar are being compared, sex is the real issue. This is not necessarily the case in the twelfth century, when the seven liberal arts in general and grammar in particular were at the foundation not only of a new curriculum and a new approach to learning but also of a new way of reading nature and Scripture. The age was fascinated by the significance of the Word and the role of language in human dignity – as when Adam named the animals – and in human failing – as when the serpent beguiled not simply by appeal to the senses but by false argument. So Alan of Lille's concern about the degradation of language is a serious one, not a witty stand-in for his condemnation of sexual degradation.[182] Rather than diluting the significance of Alan's concern with sexual decadence, his preoccupation with language and his connection of language with fundamental contemporary social values serve to give the disorder of the sexes broad moral and metaphysical weight. These are not merely examples of human frailty but symptoms of the incursion of chaos into the divinely ordered cosmos and society.

Alan frequently expressed his objections to the disruptions represented by sexual disorder in terms that reflect anxiety about the maintenance of gender roles. In particular, he wished to uphold the masculinity of the male, which he saw undermined by (among other things) effeminacy, sexual activities with other men, and masturbation. Even before Nature has appeared on the scene, the narrator complains that "the sex of the active type degenerates into the passive type," that "Venus's art of magic hermaphroditizes" men.[183] In spite of the superior beauty of women, men are not attracted to them. (Here the narrator proclaims his sexual rectitude: he would not eschew all

---

181 Alanus de Insulis, in Häring, "Alan of Lille, *De planctu*," ch. I, meter 1, ll. 5–6, p. 806: ". . . illos facit illas."

182 This argument underlies Jan Ziolkowski's study, *Alan of Lille's Grammar of Sex: The Meaning of Grammar to a Twelfth-Century Intellectual*, Speculum Anniversary Monographs 10 (Cambridge, Mass.: Medieval Academy of America, 1985).

183 Alanus de Insulis, in Häring, "Alan of Lille, *De planctu*," ch. I, meter 1, ll. 15–18, p. 806: "Activi generis sexus se turpiter horret / sic in passiuum degenerare genus. . . . Ars magice Veneris hermaphroditat eum."

those sweet kisses or, he implies, their reproductive consequences.)[184] Nature complains that human beings alone of all creatures disobey her laws, and in this she alludes to the framework of responsibility and will. She, like the character of the narrator, emphasizes sexual abominations. The acts and practices in question are here represented as transgressions because they are unnatural: Nature, exercising a certain rhetorical delicacy, refers to these breaches in the grammar of natural intercourse by alluding to figures in classical mythology guilty of them. Helen of Troy's adultery, Queen Pasiphae's lust for a bull, and Myrrha's incest with her father (the crime is hers, not his) are all evoked; and Narcissus's self-love is given a physical connotation. Both men and women are implicated, and in many of the incidents gender roles do not play a conspicuous part. In other cases, however, they do. Tiresias is, once again, blamed for having been turned into a woman by Venus. And Medea's infanticide, although not explicitly sexual, is condemned among the sexual abuses because it shows she is an unnatural mother, a mother who forgets the name of mother, betraying her role.[185] Alan applies the language of role betrayal most persistently to unmanly men. Subjects should not act as predicates, hammers should not act as anvils, he insists, using his favorite metaphors for the active masculine and the passive feminine role.[186] It is being out of place, out of character that is wrong; and it is men being out of place that concerns him above all.

Alan does not, however, spare women whose minds are afflicted by the madness of sexual desire.[187] Here, those whom Nature created passive, become active and dangerous. This is one of the few moments in the work when Alan seems worried about women getting out of hand, and the ill effects are slightly different from those of men's transgressions. Women's disobedience of Nature's laws comes primarily in forms that attack the integrity of the family, rather than in forms that attack the proper regulation of sexual intercourse. Adultery, incest, and the murder of parents, husbands, and children undermine not so much the gender roles associated with sexual expression as the gender roles associated with social integration – "In place of fidelity there are deceptions; in place of dutifulness there is guile."[188]

Sexual contact between women is nowhere at issue in this work, in spite of the prominent condemnations of sexual contact between men. (This same imbalance obtained in earlier penitentials.)[189] Once again, the disparity may in part be attributable to male authorship and to a predominantly male audience, but the asymmetry of gender values must also play a role. In spite

184 Ibid.
185 Ibid., ch. VIII, [prose 4], ll. 68–76, p. 835; ch. IX, meter 5, ll. 45–50, p. 844.
186 These images are persistent in *De planctu*. See Ziolkowski, *Alan of Lille's Grammar of Sex*, esp. ch. 1.
187 Alanus de Insulis, in Häring, "Alan of Lille, *De planctu*," ll. 37–8, p. 843.
188 Ibid., l. 46, p. 844: "Inque fide fraudes, in pietate dolum."
189 Payer, *Sex and the Penitentials*, esp. pp. 137–8.

of the impetus to control female sexuality in the interests of the family in
particular and society in general (interests expressed in medieval views on
sterility and abstinence, for example), the passive sexual and reproductive
roles attributed to women and the lesser value placed upon the feminine are
likely to have led to a relative lack of concern about women betraying their
gender roles within the domain of sexual relations. But women making love
to women *were* sometimes seen as behaving "like men" and *were* prosecuted
by lay authorities in the late Middle Ages. Such cases, which surface only
toward the end of the period, reflect the expanding role of secular government in the regulation of morals and social life and represent gender enforcement at a very different level from Alan of Lille's esoteric invective. A
French royal register of 1405 mentions an appeal for pardon on the part of a
sixteen-year-old married woman named Laurence. She and Jehanne, her
work companion in the fields and vineyards, had had a number of sexual
encounters (perhaps an extended relationship), for which they were apparently both prosecuted. For purposes of her application for a royal pardon,
Laurence, who is in prison, represents Jehanne as the manlike aggressor in a
series of sexual incidents: "she climbed on her as a man does on a woman,
and the said Jehanne began to move her hips and do as a man does to a
woman."[190] Many arguments against such acts (for example, that they involve pleasure without procreation and are unnatural) apply equally to men
and women. Some late medieval commentators on Scripture and Roman
law made sure to condemn sexual acts between women, sometimes with
and sometimes without good textual authority. Repeated transgression
could become a capital crime for both women and men, but fewer women
were executed than men.[191] Whatever parity existed on the basis of the
dominant rationales for condemning comparable acts was moderated to
women's advantage by the lesser dignity of the female and the passive and
secondary roles attributed to her in sex and reproduction.

The views of Alan of Lille and the story of Laurence and Jehanne underscore the binary character of medieval gender categories to which medicine
and science contributed, and the consequent practice of labeling the masculine and the feminine. Both imply the existence of masculine behaviors
which belong properly to men and feminine behaviors which belong properly to women and seek to enforce them, whether by a learned polemic or
by a legal system. At the same time, both reflect the dissonance which arose
as a result of attempts to label persons and behaviors which did not seem to

190 Cited in Charles du Fresne du Cange, *Glossarium mediae et infimae Latinitatis* (Niort and
London: L. Favre and David Nutt, 1882–7), vol. 4, p. 202, s.v. "hermaphroditus": ". . . et
adonc icelle Jehanne rebrassa laditte Laurence et monta sur elle, comme un homme fait sur
une femme, et commencà icelle Jehanne a remuer ses reins et faire en la maniere que un
homme fait à femme. . . ." Jehanne's fate is not mentioned.
191 Louis Crompton, "The Myth of Lesbian Impunity: Capital Laws from 1270–1791," *Journal of Homosexuality* 6 (1980/81): 11–25.

fit properly. If men simply *were* male and masculine, if women simply *were* female and feminine, there would be no need for oxymorons. But, as things were, men who were seen as "submitting" sexually to other men were characterized as feminine and, for official purposes, Jehanne was called a manlike woman. The designations simultaneously reassert a commitment to the ideal of a two-termed system and identify the troublemakers – those whose transgressive behavior earns them paradoxical or unstable labels. Alan's treatment of the possibility of a third gender makes the commitment to duality even clearer. Latin grammar, the basis of his polemic, has three fully functioning genders – masculine, feminine, and neuter – and Alan even entertained briefly the idea of placing nonreproductive males (sodomites, who are effectively sterile, and eunuchs) within the domain of the third.[192] Rather than undermine the rules of sex and their implications for gender, however, Alan chose to dismantle the rules of grammar by declaring that nature and grammar have just two genders and that neuter is a different type of form, a negative and confused category.[193] Although "neuter" presented an opportunity to construct a grammatical category corresponding to "homosexuals," Alan declined to make use of it and thus accorded individuals engaged in stigmatized acts no natural category, no ontological status. In labeling Jehanne's behavior "manlike," the legal system insisted that all nouns and adjectives must belong to either the masculine or the feminine gender. The inclusiveness of this duality strengthened gender distinctions by making them universally applicable, yet at the same time it muddied the clarity of each definition and the contrast between them. Or, to put it another way, the socially construed adjectives became at least partially dissociated from the socially construed nouns. The words "woman" and "man" each encompassed a range of dispositions and behaviors, and a "masculine" man might share traits with a "masculine" woman.

Besides distancing them from whatever advantages or disadvantages might follow from a separate definition and identity, the namelessness of those who engaged in sexual activities with members of the same sex reinforced the effects of a rather fluid sexual vocabulary. Those who were in various ways not *simply* masculine or feminine were not fully distinguishable from each other. The word "hermaphrodite" applied to eunuchs and to men who engaged in sex with men; the word "sodomy" covered a multitude of sins. Women called "masculine" and men called "feminine" might be expected to transgress norms either within or beyond heterosexual boundaries. Daston and Park have remarked on the links among notions of hermaphroditism, transvestism, and homosexuality in early modern society,[194] and some of the same associations existed in late medieval culture. At

192 Alanus de Insulis, in Häring, "Alan of Lille, *De planctu*," ch. X, [prose 5], ll. 43–9, p. 846.
193 See Ziolkowski, *Alan of Lille's Grammar of Sex*, pp. 21–2, 35.
194 Daston and Park, "Hermaphrodites in Renaissance France."

the center of the constellation were anxieties about same-sex relations. Unlike hermaphrodites, eunuchs, and members of one sex possessing traits of the other, homosexuals and homosexuality had neither a name nor a natural explanation. Scientific and medical learning confirmed this exclusion by its relative silence. The comments of Avicenna, the Arabic authority whose work was widely read in the West, had excluded it from the business of medicine, and the subject was almost unmentioned in Latin scientific and medical literature, with the exception of Peter of Abano's discussion and Albertus Magnus's limited remedy.[195]

Both in the exposition of gender traits and in the isolation of gender problems, the notion of the natural played a critical but not a comprehensive role. Natural philosophy and medicine, among the authoritative arbiters of what was natural, were therefore participants in the construction of the concepts of the feminine and the masculine, in the enforcement of the duality which they implied, and in the disapprobation of what was therefore seen as deviant. Underlying and organizing medical and scientific specifications of female and male traits was a set of theories, some of which had been carefully elaborated and refined by scholastic debates. Ideas about seeds, heat, complexions, and uterine cells were candidates for a firm and consistent system of gender. However, because the differences between the theories, though debated, were never definitively resolved, and because the texts proffered a rich array of specific traits, the contribution of medicine and science to medieval conceptions of gender came less in the form of a specific ideology than in the form of a smorgasbord of concrete details collected in and given authenticity by a wide variety of writings about nature, health, and related topics. The choices were not so open as to allow all possible constructions of gender. Women were undoubtedly cooler, weaker, and less intelligent. But the diversity of this body of knowledge and the eclecticism of many of the texts within it left open the way for the coordination and calibration of ideas from those sources with others, especially those reflecting the ecclesiastical and lay norms.

These converging perspectives assumed or argued that appearance, anatomy, constitution, temperament, habits, and social relations were all essentially related to each other. The specific attributes to which they alluded depended upon the subject at hand – the development of the embryo, the adjudication of marriage disputes, the condemnation of women enjoying each other, or the treatment of an illness. The diversity of options did not necessarily weaken or dilute medieval gender constructs. On the contrary, the flexibility of language and concept allowed "feminine" and "masculine" to be frequently invoked in widely divergent conditions and contexts. The

195 Jacquart and Thomasset, *Sexuality and Medicine*, pp. 155–61.

plant pennyroyal has masculine (white) and feminine (red or purple) varieties, both of which have admirable and virile medicinal power,[196] and
mandrake roots were shaped like a man's or a woman's body. (See Figure 6.)
The case studies of sterility and abstinence that follow provide examples of
choices and applications of feminine and masculine traits in other, more
human situations.

196 [*Materia medica*], Bibliothèque Nationale, MS lat. 820, fol. 165ra.

5

Sterility: The pursuit of progeny and the failure of reproductive function

Modern concepts of childhood, motherhood, and fatherhood, modern conditions of Western industrial society, and modern scientific developments in reproductive theory and technology have all contributed to radical alterations in our understanding of fertility and infertility. The impact and meaning of having children and not having children are influenced by such considerations as our life expectancy, our standard of living, our sense of control over nature, and our beliefs about marriage. All these factors and many others related to ideas about fertility and sterility have been transformed since the fifteenth century. For their own reasons and on their own terms, authors of the later Middle Ages sustained an interest in and concern about aids and impediments to childbearing. The context, content, and meaning of the causes and remedies of sterility as understood by medieval natural philosophers and medical authors are the subject of this chapter. Like sexual abstinence, the topic encompasses a constellation of beliefs and practices that engage both the ideas of medical theorists and natural philosophers and elements of the wider social and cultural milieu.

John of Gaddesden's *Rosa Anglica*, a derivative and popular early fourteenth-century medical survey of standard topics from fevers to surgery, includes a chapter on sterility. The introduction to his treatment of the subject begins thus:

Sterility is the failure to reproduce in a man and a woman, so that in a man it may be said to be a failure to act and produce a fetus, and in a woman a failure to conceive. And sterility is spoken of as defeating offspring; or sterility is spoken of as stopping, since it stops, that is, it comes to nothing or does nothing; or it is spoken of as harming, that is, impeding the fetus. Its definition is: sterility is a certain ill disposition by reason of which a man may not generate or a woman may not conceive.[1]

---

1 Johannes Anglicus, *Rosa Anglica*, bk. II, ch. xvii, fol. 74va: "Sterilitas est defectus generandi in viro et muliere, ut in viro dicatur defectus agendi et fetus producendi, et in femina defectus concipiendi. Et dicitur sterilitas quasi sternens prolem vel dicitur sterilitas quasi stans, quia

These comments are illustrative of the late medieval medical outlook on infertility in several respects. First, they are indicative of an active interest. John's own exposition of the problem, its causes, signs, and cures, is fairly lengthy, given the comprehensive and concise character of his work. More than a dozen separate treatises and innumerable *consilia*, or brief exemplary cases, come down to us from the thirteenth through the fifteenth century.[2] Virtually all general works on medicine included the topic, often according it substantial space; few major recipe collections failed to provide multiple instructions for diagnosis and treatment. Second, in its rather obscure enumeration of the senses of "sterility," the *Rosa Anglica* suggests the broad medieval understanding of the term. The concept included everything from the permanent inability to reproduce to temporary circumstantial impediments to conception, sometimes blending in with general recommendations on conception, regimen, or gynecology. (The titles "On Sterility" and "On Impregnation" are essentially equivalent.)[3] It also extended beyond conception to the fetus's survival and development, sometimes blending in with general recommendations on obstetrics. Third, John's definitions unambiguously point to the involvement of both sexes, using the words "man" and "woman" three times each. Although the classical sense of the word *sterilitas* referred predominantly to barren women or female animals, secondarily to plants, and occasionally to males (usually castrated males), the medieval medical position was persistent and unambiguous in its inclusiveness. Finally, in spite of the parallels established between infertility in men and women, John's introduction reveals a significant distinction between the natures of male and female failure. Although his specific phrasing is not standard, the association of men's deficiencies with acting, producing, and generating and of women's deficiencies with conceiving is one way in which late medieval authors dismantled the symmetry they themselves had constructed. The man's responsibility for erection and ejaculation and the woman's responsibility for gestation and birth, not mentioned here by John, constituted another axis of differentiation between male and female sterility. This chapter will explore the elements of John of Gaddesden's definitions as they were embodied in the natural philosophy and medicine of the twelfth through the fourteenth century, and as they related to the larger social and cultural climate.

stat, id est deficit vel quiescit, vel dicitur quasi fetum ledens, id est impediens, cuius definitio est: Sterilitas est quedam dispositio mala in viro vel muliere ratione cuius vir non generat vel mulier non concipiat."

2 See Lynn Thorndike and Pearl Kibre, *A Catalogue of Incipits of Mediaeval Scientific Writings in Latin*, rev. ed., Mediaeval Academy of America 29 (Cambridge: Mediaeval Academy of America, 1963).

3 One manuscript, Bibliothèque Nationale, lat. 7066, brings together a handful of works with the titles *De impregnatione mulieris*, *De preparatione mulierum ad conceptum*, *De impregnatione mulieris*, *De iuvantibus mulieres ad impregnandum*, *Regimen de conceptione*, and *De sterilitate mulierum*.

From the early Middle Ages, a pattern of concern about fertility had been established: philosophers had discussed sterility as a way of approaching general questions about the reproductive process; physicians had discussed sterility as a disorder to be remedied. Isidore of Seville, in a chapter on the human body, explained the process of human generation, including the roles of semen and menstrual blood. Both fluids must be in good condition for generation to take place. The semen or the blood may be too thick or too thin, causing the male or female to be sterile.[4] Isidore used the existence of sterility informally as a way of illustrating and confirming the principles of reproduction in the context of a larger discussion of human physiology. This way of dealing with the subject was to be carried on and formalized by scholastic philosophers, who employed the facts of sterility as elements in highly structured arguments about generation. Likewise, later medical writers built on the interest expressed in fragmentary texts on gynecology, some of which survive in an eighth- to ninth-century manuscript. In these texts, the word "sterility" is not used, but numerous recipes and instructions explicitly designed to facilitate conception appear. For example, for a woman to conceive and give birth to a son, both the man and the woman should drink a potion made with the sexual organs of a female wolf.[5]

In some respects, the absence of the word "sterility" in many early medical texts is not surprising. Works of this sort seldom dealt in abstractions. Although they occasionally named a condition, such as "suffocation of the womb," that was closely associated with barrenness, they more frequently just gave instructions: how to achieve an effect (for example, to prevent facial hair), what to do in a certain situation (if, for example, a woman has postpartum pain), or how to tell if something is the case (whether a girl is a virgin, for example). Thus, in early medical texts written with a practical orientation, a construct such as "sterility" would have been superfluous, if not entirely out of place. In another sense, this small matter of terminology is significant, because it is indicative of some differences between philosophical and medical assignments of meaning and emphasis. Later medical writers, influenced by the concepts and vocabulary of learned medicine, especially as developed in the universities, came to employ the term and to acknowledge its theoretical implications, but their concerns, like those of their early predecessors, remained tied to the practical challenges of infertility.

Although natural philosophers and medical authors were not always dealing with precisely the same subject when they wrote about sterility, both groups were certainly directly concerned with it and presented it as a topic worthy of a chapter or a *questio* or even a treatise. The status of sterility may be contrasted with that of contraception in this regard, for although instruc-

4 Isidorus, *Etymologiae*, bk. XI, ch. 1, §139–42.
5 *Liber de muliebria causa*, in Egert, *Gynäkologische Fragmente*, 7, p. 25.

tions and recipes for preventing conception are scattered throughout the medical literature on sexual and reproductive subjects, "contraceptives" does not appear to be an independently defined category deemed worthy of its own tracts or chapters. This difference reinforces the observation that sterility was a marked concern of medical and philosophical authors, and it touched in a variety of ways upon sex difference. For example, reproductive capability was sometimes part of the very definition of female health.[6] In addition, the discussions of reproductive disabilities were sometimes personal in nature and projected an urgency at least as great as discussions of, say, painful chronic illnesses. Some of the reasons for the importance attributed to infertility lie within the theoretical constructs which explained it, but understanding of the urgency of the subject depends in part on a consideration of the social and economic concerns with which fertility and infertility were connected.

A 1326 court case from Provence illustrates how medical expertise responded to (or, in this instance, capitalized on) cultural norms.[7] A certain Master Antoni Imbert was accused of offering fraudulent, diabolical, and expensive cures to sterile women and impotent men. A parade of witnesses testified against him. Rissenda, Jacoba Grossa, and Alaxia paid Imbert for various medical potions and magical charms that he promised would make them conceive and keep them from miscarrying. Ricorda brought in her daughter Jacoba for the same purpose and paid a considerable sum. He told her the young woman would get pregnant and would get along with her husband. Bertranda, wife of P. Gasqui, also brought in her daughter and seems to have paid even more for the doctor's services. He told the daughter that she would conceive if she followed his directions and "that he would make it so that she would be restored to her husband's love . . . [and there would be] renewed love and affection between them."[8] The case illustrates a number of social and cultural aspects of the medical problem of sterility. First, there was clearly a strong market for what Master Antoni had to offer: people would pay well for the assurance of fertility. Second, although the general charge accuses him of defrauding men as well, all of the patients who testified (and probably most of the patients he treated) were women: in spite of medieval attributions of sterility to men as well as women, there was differential responsibility for fertility. Third, mothers brought in their daughters, not only confirming that reproduction was, in a social sense, women's work but also suggesting the significant stake that families had in

6 Bernardus de Gordonio, *Lilium*, pt. VII, ch. xiv, fol. 192ra.
7 Joseph Shatzmiller, *Médicine et justice en Provence: Documents de Manosque, 1262–1348* (Aix-en-Provence: Publications de l'Université de Provence, 1989), 56, pp. 176–83.
8 Ibid., p. 180: ". . . quod feceret ut ipsa reduceretur in amorem dicti viri sui. . . . noviter amor et dilectio inter eos."

the marriages and progeny of their kin. Finally, in several cases, the production of children is linked to domestic affection and tranquillity: a fertile household was a functioning household.

Honest practitioners as well as charlatans and opportunists operated in this kind of environment, and though not all offered love potions, many tried to help patients like Imbert's. The medical literature also reflects a growing concern for the survival, health, and welfare of children. Evidence of the intensity of interest resides, for example, in the fact that the number of childhood diseases discussed in the Latin medical literature is considerably greater than the number found in the written sources upon which the authors drew, doubling in the period from the twelfth to the fifteenth century.[9] Those who dealt with such subjects were conscious of the religious, economic, and social senses in which children were valued.

The reasons put forward by physicians and natural philosophers for the existence of sexual differentiation, appetite, and pleasure resonate with the religious formulations of medieval sexual teleology: in nature, everything exists for some purpose, and sex exists so that living things, which are subject to decay and death as individuals, can achieve perpetual existence as species; in the divine plan, everything exists for some purpose, and sex exists so that God's creatures can fulfill the commandment, "Be fruitful and multiply." Thus a child's birth is not just a local event; it is a metaphysical phenomenon. The theological and naturalistic formulations of this position did not, as a rule, compete with one another. On the contrary, the Aristotelian position formed a part of the Christian argument in Aquinas's *Summa theologiae*: woman was made as a helpmate to man in the work of generation.[10] Bernard of Gordon explicitly integrated contemporary Christian moral teaching into his treatment of sexual hygiene, saying that intercourse should be between married couples and only for the purpose of children.[11] Similarly, at the same time as the medical literature on children's health was expanding, there was a rising concern within the Church and among Christians in general for the psychological and spiritual well-being of children.[12]

---

9 Luke Demaitre, "The Idea of Childhood and Child Care in Medical Writings of the Middle Ages," *Journal of Psychohistory* 4 (1977): 462–5 and 476–7.

10 Thomas Aquinas, *Summa theologiae*, bk. I, q. 92, art. 1, p. 654.

11 Bernardus de Gordonio, *De regimine vii etatum* [= *De regimine sanitatis*], ch. 14, Cambridge University, Gonville and Caius, MS 593, fol. 42vb. The chapter on intercourse opens, "Coitus non est licitus nisi gratia prolis," and later gives advice to those "quibus autem licentia ex lege data est coiendi [*sic*] coeant gratia prolis. . . ."

12 Mary Martin McLaughlin, "Survivors and Surrogates: Children and Parents from the Ninth to the Thirteenth Centuries," in Lloyd deMause, ed., *The History of Childhood* (New York: Psychohistory Press, 1974), pp. 101–81. This study is accompanied by extensive notes which amount to a bibliographical essay on sources and scholarship. See Philippe Ariès, *Centuries of Childhood: A Social History of Family Life*, trans. Robert Baldick (New York: Random House, 1962). John Boswell, *The Kindness of Strangers: The Abandonment of Children in Western Europe from Late Antiquity to the Renaissance* (London: Allen Lane, Penguin Press, 1989 [c. 1988]), treats oblation (and likewise the placement of children in other

In the thirteenth and fourteenth centuries, baptism soon after birth became the common practice, replacing the custom of performing baptisms only twice a year and thus securing access to salvation for innumerable infant souls.[13] The otherworldly fate of the many infants who died soon after birth was the concern not only of Church officials but also of bereaved parents. There is poignant evidence in the testimony of women accused of causing the deaths of their children that they took care to baptize the infants first,[14] and governments took an interest in the baptism of foundlings.[15]

There was a great deal of variety in the socioeconomic position of children in the Latin West during the later Middle Ages. Well-to-do families in towns, for example, may have had fewer children than those in the country: Sylvia Thrupp reports that wealthy merchants in London from the late thirteenth century to the early sixteenth century were likely to have only one son living at the time of their death.[16] The practice of primogeniture, which developed in some rural areas of Europe in the late Middle Ages, put considerable pressure on landholding families among the nobility and the peasantry; in other areas the survival of more than one son is attested in the division of the father's land.[17] In spite of the many variations, a few discernible patterns illuminate what children were good for in the late Middle Ages. Some of these patterns have to do with the preservation, consolidation, or extension of family wealth and status. The most obvious examples of the role played by progeny in these processes come from the ranks of the nobility. (This is, of course, also a sector of the population with access to learned medical practitioners.) Among families controlling significant land and power, the matrimonial placement of children was, among other things, a business affair of economic, social, and political interest to the extended families of both bride and groom. A marriage included significant property transactions: not only the immediate transfer of wealth between the families and from one generation to the other (for example, in the form of a dowry) but also long-term arrangements regarding the future disposi-

families) as a form of "abandonment," but does acknowledge ecclesiastical concern (e.g., pp. 264–5).

13 John Douglas Close Fisher, *Christian Initiation: Baptism in the Medieval West, a Study in the Disintegration of the Primitive Rite of Initiation* (London: S. P. C. K., 1965), pp. 110–12.

14 Y.-B. Brissaud, "L'infanticide à la fin du Moyen Age: Ses motivations psychologiques et sa répression," *Revue historique de droit français et étranger* 50 (1972): 240–3. Brissaud's evidence, from legal appeals, is likely to contain some false claims of baptism.

15 Boswell, *Kindness of Strangers*, pp. 322–5.

16 Sylvia L. Thrupp, *The Merchant Class of Medieval London (1300–1500)* (Chicago: University of Chicago Press, 1948), pp. 199–200. "With sinister uniformity the figures hover close to the figure one," from 1200 to 1527.

17 This practice was made possible in many cases by changes in agricultural technique that considerably raised the productivity of cultivated lands. Georges Duby, *L'économie rurale et la vie des campagnes dans l'occident médiéval (France, Angleterre, Empire, IXᵉ-XVᵉ siècles): Essai de synthèse et perspectives de recherches*, 2 vols., Collection historique (Paris: Aubier, Editions Montaigne, 1962), vol. 1, pp. 215–19.

tion of the property and affairs of the two families, the couple, and the couple's anticipated children. A sermon prepared in the thirteenth century for the meeting at which a marriage contract was to be negotiated stressed the importance of the meeting: "Again, many conditions and agreements concerning the dowry and things of this kind are normally made at it, and unless they are foreseen and taken care of by a careful discussion they give occasion for many evils in the future."[18] Another sermon written for the festivities following a wedding not only called upon the guests not to overdo the carousing but also reminded them, perhaps with the possibility of family and factional rivalries lurking in the background, that the gathering's purpose was to promote friendship between the party of the bride and the party of the groom.[19] Even though, from the twelfth century on, there emerged a new sensibility that placed a greater value on the couple's mutual regard and a new articulation of religious doctrine that placed emphasis on the individual's consent in marriage, matrimony involved family members as interested parties, and children thereby constituted not merely a social asset but, in a sense, a vehicle for social action.

In a general way, this pattern held for other levels of society as well. Among townsfolk, landed peasants, and even landless laborers, marriages involved transactions undertaken by the families of the bride and groom, at least in the case of first marriages, although when there was less property involved, the arrangements were less complex and less likely to involve long-term arrangements such as ongoing commercial ties. For most families, having too many children might pose economic problems. The placement of a child in a marriage, in a religious house, in an apprenticeship, in a profession, or in a political position normally involved a capital outlay of some consequence. The difficulties faced by surplus sons and daughters without dowries were significant. But the childless couple, although exempt from these problems, was cut off from the economic and social advantages and opportunities afforded the family as a whole by well-placed children. The content and meaning of these advantages varied from one social group to another. For a merchant family, an important expansion of business might be involved; a peasant household might hope only that family and marital ties with other households would yield a marginal increase in their ability to survive a famine. If poorer families had less chance of advancing their economic position through children, they had greater direct need for their offspring's labor. Indeed it was precisely the poorest families who had the greatest need, since, in the absence of land or capital, labor was their

---

18 Humbertus de Romanis, *De eruditione praedicatorum* (Venice, 1603), L, pars secunda, p. 66, quoted and translated in d'Avray and Tausche, "Marriage Sermons" p. 84: "Item multae conditiones, & pacta, pro dote, & huiusmodi, in eo solent fieri, que nisi per diligentem tractatum praevideantur, et expediantur, dant occasionem multorum malorum in futuro."
19 D'Avray and Tausche, "Marriage Sermons," pp. 84–5.

livelihood. In general the family was the locus and basic unit of almost every level of existence, from the material to the affective.

Children played a role in the creation and perpetuation of social bonds, as well as in the promotion of a family's economic interests. Within the family, they reaffirmed the ties between the parents and their relatives. Children's placement could also initiate or reaffirm social connections between families. Marriage of children was only one of the ways in which these links were effected. One family might place a young child in the household of another as a servant, as an apprentice, or (among the nobility) as a hostage. The result might be the strengthening of a local pattern of allegiances, the transmission of a heresy, or the affirmation of a patron–client relationship.

Late medieval ideas (philosophical, medical, social, religious) about the production of offspring existed against a background of radical demographic changes. Unprecedented economic prosperity in the twelfth and thirteenth centuries improved living standards, especially nutrition, contributing to a rise in the overall fertility rate and to a dramatic increase in population. By the decades around the turn of the fourteenth century, however, a series of economic and agricultural crises (due in part to the expanded population and the extension of cultivation to marginal lands) led to an overall downturn in prosperity and population and introduced a period of instability that culminated at midcentury with the Black Death. Some evidence suggests a new sense of infertility as a general problem and as a medical concern in the fourteenth century,[20] that is, at the moment when Europe's experience of expansion was at first undermined and then reversed, but interest in the problem was not limited to hard times. At the local and family level, times were never so good that fertility and the survival of children ceased to be a problem. During the period of growth, for example, the unsanitary conditions in towns suddenly overpopulated by the unchecked influx of immigrants from the countryside would not have contributed to the production of large numbers of healthy children – and many medical authors lived in such towns. Thus the presence and visibility of infertile couples and infant mortality were never insignificant, even though they might be subject to fluctuations.

The religious, economic, and social advantages of children do not constitute a cause for the desire of couples to produce offspring or, therefore, for the considerable number of treatises on sterility and the ubiquity of advice about aids to conception. They do, however, indicate some characteristically medieval ways in which the desire for children was experienced and framed.

20 Luis García-Ballester, Michael R. McVaugh, and Agustín Rubio-Vela, *Medical Licensing and Learning in Fourteenth-Century Valencia*, Transactions of the American Philosophical Society 79/6 (Philadelphia: American Philosophical Society, 1989), p. 21; Jacquart and Thomasset, *Sexuality and Medicine*, p. 170.

IMPEDIMENTS TO FERTILITY

Sterility in the conceptual networks of medicine and natural philosophy

Heat or cold; the waning of the moon; an imbalanced constitution or an imbalanced pattern of behavior; incompatible anatomies or incompatible substantial forms: these are among the reasons medieval authors gave for infertility. There are works, especially the terse recipe books, that pay no mind to causes and give no hint of theoretical underpinnings. For the most part, however, even the works most oriented toward practice reflect at least occasional, if sometimes only implicit, connections with theories of conception. Some make reference to causes in titles and headings; some allude to properties of drugs linked to principles of physiology, such as hot or cold; some emphasize a particular anatomical part or sexual function, implying its centrality. Thus, although notions about infertility – especially those aimed at remedying the problem – were by no means mere corollaries of academic theories of reproduction, the ideas of the learned philosophers and physicians had a significant bearing upon the ways in which sterility was viewed, even in nonsystematic works.

Certain differences between the medical and philosophical approaches demand acknowledgment. Although the abstract term "sterility" appeared with some frequency in the titles and texts of medical chapters and opuscula, the medical concept retained its relationship to the specific problems of individuals which the authors, or at least the readers, might encounter and treat. And, more specifically, whereas natural philosophers sometimes construed "sterility" narrowly, applying it to the essential and therefore permanent constitutional inability to produce offspring, medical writers concerned themselves with a diverse cluster of problems, including accidental or temporary impediments to conception, the incompatibility of individually fertile partners, and the occurrence of miscarriages and stillbirths. Isidore's brief characterization of physiologically based sterility and a later scholastic treatise on the essential sterility of mules (the subject of a long disquisition in Aristotle's *Generation of Animals*) illustrate a natural philosophical view that represents sterility more as a state of affairs to be explained than as a condition to be dealt with.[21] This difference was significantly mitigated by the translation of Avicenna's *Canon*, which included brief but rich chapters on sterility, its signs, and its cures,[22] and also by the general development of theoretical and academic medicine in the thirteenth and fourteenth centuries. Yet, in spite of the strong theoretical underpinnings of Avicenna's work, it shares a more problem-oriented approach with the early collections of recipes. Likewise,

---

21 Magister Paulus, *De causa sterilitatis mulorum*, Bibliothèque Nationale, MS lat. 16133, fols. 83ra–86rb, based on Aristotle, *Generation of Animals*, II, viii.
22 Avicenna, *Liber canonis*, bk. III, tr. i, fen 21, chs. 8–10.

even those later Latin medical works which incorporate explanations empha-size concrete measures to encourage conception and prevent miscarriages.

In the fourteenth century several works by authors associated with the medical faculty at the university of Montpellier included under the heading of sterility a wide variety of disorders, which they explained and categorized and for which they offered remedies. One author mentioned intractable sterility only briefly. He assured his reader that his recipes and instructions would work unless the man or woman was sterile *by nature* – that is, presum-ably, by innate and immutable structure or constitution.[23] He also referred to the classic example of irremediable (but not innate) sterility: "If some-thing which is a cause of permanent sterility should happen externally to a man, such as when the veins which are behind the ears are cut, through which the spermatic fluid mainly descends from the brain to the kidneys and genitals, the defect has no remedy, unless God makes it through a mira-cle."[24] (The repeated references to this condition as a cause of sterility consti-tute a sobering warning about using texts of this kind to make epidemio-logical inferences about the period.) By contrast, Albertus Magnus, who considered sterility within the larger subject of the body's natural functions, did not emphasize the distinction between innate and disease-induced causes of sterility.[25] Medical authors had little reason to go on at length about conditions that were beyond the reach of their art. Therefore, what they called "sterility" (when they did employ the word) was a cluster of prob-lems ranging from short-term failure to conceive to long-term child-lessness. The same Montpellier treatise boasts of success in one case in which conception had not occurred in thirteen years and in another in which there had been no sign of conception for nine years.[26]

---

23 *De impedimentis conceptionis* (Pagel, "Raymundus de Molieriis," p. 536). The text edited by Pagel, *De impedimentis conceptionis ex parte viri,* is the second part of a treatise *De impedimentis conceptionis,* or *De sterilitate,* attributed in two of the ten manuscripts in which it is found to Raymond of Moliere. The first part was published by Arlt in *Schule von Montpellier.* Paul Diepgen argues the work is by Raymond's colleague in early fourteenth-century Montpel-lier, Arnald of Villanova: "Studien zu Arnald von Villanova: Zweite Folge," *Archiv für Geschichte der Medizin* 6 (1913): 380–91. Juan A. Paniagua rejects the attribution to Arnald, inclining instead toward Raymond: *El Maestro Arnau de Vilanova médico,* Cuadernos valen-cianos de historia de la medicina y de la ciencia, ser. A, 8 (Valencia: Catedra e Instituto de la Historia de la Medicina, 1969), p. 59. In any case it is undoubtedly a product of Montpellier in the first half of the fourteenth century. It is referred to hereafter as *De impedimentis conceptionis.*

24 *De impedimentis conceptionis* (Pagel, "Raymundus de Moleriis," p. 533): "Si accidat viro extrinsece aliquid quod est causa sterilitatis perpetue ut quando vene que sunt retro aures sunt rupte per quas principaliter descendit humiditas spermatica a cerebro ad renes et membra genitalia, iste defectus non habet remedium nisi tantum Deus per miraculum facit." The idea persisted through the centuries, e.g.: Nemesius, *De natura hominis,* ch. XXIV, p. 109; Constantinus, *De coitu,* in *Opera omnia,* p. 299; Johannes Anglicus, *Rosa Anglica,* bk. II, ch. xvii, fol. 74va.

25 Albertus Magnus, *De animalibus,* bk. II, tr. i, ch. 1.

26 *De impedimentis conceptionis* (Pagel, "Raymundus de Moleriis," pp. 536–7).

One of the results of this broadly construed concept of sterility within the medical tradition is its shading off into "impediments to conception" and thence, on the one hand, to prescriptions for ideal conditions for conception and, on the other hand, to problems such as menstrual retention and suffocation of the womb. Many gynecological and obstetrical matters were regularly discussed in close proximity to chapters on sterility. One reason for this association is the common practice of organizing general medical works from head to foot, so that all genital problems are clustered together. But this organizational fact is not sufficient to explain the integration of infertility and female complaints into the same specialized works, such as treatises called *On the Diseases of Women*, or into the same chapter, such as John of Gaddesden's in *Rosa Anglica*. For medical authors, at least, the distinction between the two classes of information was not meaningful.

The contrast between medical and philosophical perspectives on the subject is by no means a sharp one. Medical scholastics like Jacopo of Forlì often operated on a plane of abstraction far removed from the immediate needs and experiences of their patients, and natural philosophers, especially those, like Albertus Magnus, who were influenced by medical ideas, sometimes compromised theoretical consistency (or at least clarity) in the face of the imperatives of experience.[27] A treatise on the sterility of mules by a certain "Master Paul," though dominated by theoretical arguments about absolute sterility, nevertheless mentions a contingent factor, the partners' difference in size, which he applies to humans: "And on account of this difference, Alanus of Spain cannot breed with Canicula of Norway or Blanceta of France, even though they are of the same species."[28] The debates about reproductive theory illustrate how both medical and philosophical authors engaged in scholastic disputations and how university education in the two fields shared many goals, approaches, and assumptions. Similarly, unsystematic compilations and handbooks, whether they derived mainly from Aristotelian or medical sources, often had much in common.

Yet, especially in compilations of remedies and in specialized works on the diseases of women or on sterility, there is a variety that raises questions about the seriousness of the authors' or compilers' theoretical allegiances. The theory is not always explicit, and it is also not always consistent: the assumption or assertion of an apparently one-seed explanation may exist side by side with the assumption or assertion of an apparently two-seed explanation, for example. Even more common is a mixing or juxtaposition of levels and categories of analysis. Authors and compilers dealt with the problem of sterility on the levels of physiological constitution, anatomical

27 Jacquart and Thomasset, "Albert le Grand."
28 Paulus, *De causa sterilitatis mulorum*, Bibiliothèque Nationale, MS lat. 16133, fol. 83rb: "Et ideo propter istam differentiam Alanus de Hyspania cum Canicula de Norveya vel cum Blanceta de Francia misceri non potest licet sint eiusdem genus."

structure, dietary habits, medical astrology, and sexual behavior. The multiplicity of approaches, especially in the medical literature, is indicative of the extent to which sterility was a personal and social problem at least as much as it was a scientific problem. Thus, texts take a pragmatic, instrumental posture, identifying the problem in specific and local terms and applying one or, more typically, several ad hoc procedures aimed at the symptoms or at their immediate causes. For example, cures for a prolapsed uterus might include mechanical manipulations to push the womb back and acrid suffumigations to chase the womb back.

Some such works project a sense of immediacy and concreteness about cases of infertility. Not only medical *consilia*, which ordinarily contain anecdotes about real or fictional cases of all kinds, but also more impersonal forms of presentation allude to the experiences of individuals. In a fourteenth-century manuscript, a certain William of Wheatley addressed a little treatise *On the Prognostic Signs of Sterility* to his lord and relative, Helius of Wheatley. Full of poetry, piety, and Plato, as well as material about complexions, it has, nonetheless, a personal and immediate tone.[29]

Theories of infertility

Medieval scientific and medical theories about the nature and causes of sterility ranged from the metaphysical to the mundane, from notions of substantial form to views about drunkenness. Some regarded the phenomenon as complicated. According to Albertus Magnus: "Since there are many things which cause coitus, there must be many circumstances promoting and impeding generation, for whatever has a part in the causes also has a part in those causes' circumstances, which impede and promote [the causes'] operations."[30] Albertus recommends that naturalists "inquire into the multitude of causes," barring only the impossible task of pursuing an infinite causal chain.[31] Others propose or imply a much simpler view of sterility. Recipe books, in particular, are likely not only to omit speculation about causes but also to offer only a narrow range of measures to be taken: applying wool soaked in ass's milk to the woman's navel, for example, or having her bathe and drink a potion.[32] In the works of systematic, academic authors there is, of course, more discussion of general principles than in eclectic and

---

29 Wilielmus de Wethelay, *De signis pronosticis sterilitatis*, Oxford, New College, MS 264, fols. 253ra–264rb. On William's view about sexuality see Michael Johnson, "Science and Discipline."
30 Albertus Magnus, *De animalibus*, bk. X, tr. i, ch. 2, §25, p. 740: ". . . cum enim multa sint quae causant coitum, oportet etiam esse multa accidentia promoventia et impedientia generationem: quaecumque enim communicant in causis, communicant etiam in accidentibus causarum illarum impedientibus et promoventibus operationes ipsarum."
31 Ibid.
32 [Remedies], British Library, MS Sloane 430, fol. 51v.

pragmatic texts. A scholarly treatise of the early fourteenth century presents an elegantly organized array of perspectives from which sterility can be viewed: sterility may reside in the woman or the man; its cause in either case may be intrinsic or extrinsic; intrinsic causes, enumerated for each sex, include various anatomical and physiological disorders; the extrinsic include bad habits and injuries; and finally, sterility may reside in the couple, in such forms as physical incompatibility or insufficient mutual attraction.[33] This was to be a popular organization for discussions of sterility among medical writers.[34] Aristotelians dealt with the subject at the highest level of abstraction when they applied their scientific method to mules' infertility.[35]

Whatever their differences, however, most authors writing on the subject during the late Middle Ages agreed that the causes of a couple's infertility might reside with the female or the male or both. Considering the fuss about who was the primary cause of successful reproduction, this general agreement on the burden of unsuccessful reproduction may be a little surprising. If the male's role in generation is not only the dominant but the most difficult one, demanding the ability to refine blood into semen and to communicate form to the fetus, it would seem to allow the greater opportunity for failure, and its failure would seem to have decisive significance. In his question "Whether the Impediment to Generation Is Due More to the Father than to the Mother," Albertus Magnus presented the argument (which he rejected later in the *questio*) in favor of male responsibility: "To the extent that a thing is more noble, more things are required for its operation. And male is nobler than female; therefore, more things are required for its action. But that for which more things are required can be impeded by more things."[36] Nevertheless, especially in medical sources, the male role is not given primacy.

We can account for this apparent symmetry of responsibility for sterility by observing, first, that the force of common experience is considerable in this area. Among other things, people in this period often had more than one spouse in the course of their reproductive years. Albertus Magnus pointed out matter-of-factly that if a man has produced children with another woman, and he and his present partner cannot have children, she may be presumed to be the infertile one.[37] Second, authors writing from different

---

33 *De impedimentis conceptionis* (Pagel, "Raymundus de Moleriis"; Arlt, *Schule von Montpellier*).

34 See, e.g., Bernardus de Gordonio, *Lilium*, pt. VII, ch. xiv; and Johannes Anglicus, *Rosa Anglica*, bk. II, ch. xvii.

35 Aristotle, *Generation of Animals*, II, viii, 747a23–749a6, pp. 248–61. The subject is engaged not only by commentators on the *De animalibus* but also in a separate treatise: Paulus, *De causa sterilitatis mulorum*, Bibliothèque Nationale, MS lat. 16133, fols. 83ra–86rb.

36 Albertus Magnus, *Quaestiones de animalibus*, bk. x, q. 1, p. 214: "Quia quanto res est nobilior, tanto plura requiruntur ad eius operationem; sed mas nobilior est femina, ergo plura requiruntur ad eius actionem; sed illud ad quod plura requiruntur, ex pluribus potest impediri. . . ."

37 Albertus Magnus, *De animalibus*, bk. X, tr. i, ch. 2, §19, p. 738.

theoretical orientations could and did present different rationales for this apparent parity. The text *On the Diseases of Women*, usually attributed to the female practitioner "Trotula," uses a common phrase in declaring that the failure to conceive may occur "as much by the fault of the man as by the fault of the woman." But the reasons for sterility in the woman are not analogous to the reasons for sterility in the man, the former having to do mainly with defects of the womb, the latter with defects in the seed or its delivery.[38] The Montpellier treatise likewise finds that the cause of a couple's childlessness may lie with either partner, but its formulation, as suggested above, is more symmetrical: either partner may be too hot or too cold; the woman's uterus may be fallen or the man's penis may be too long.[39] Though the notion that the cause of sterility may reside in either partner is not consistently applied, even by those who assert it explicitly, most texts concerned with the causes of infertility give some consideration to each partner.

Causes: Men, women, and couples

Texts that discuss the causes of sterility illustrate both the conceptualization of sterility in a way that places at least some importance on female–male parallels and, at the same time, the fragility of that conceptualization. The formulaic "as much the fault of the man as the fault of the woman" is as much a rubric for pragmatism and flexibility as it is a theoretical position about the reproductive contributions of the sexes. Late medieval accounts of the causes of sterility present patterns of symmetry, punctuated not infrequently with lapses and contradictions. The significance of the patterns lies both in their persistence and in their failures.

The most fundamental of the causes widely addressed was the set of physiological conditions arising from the interaction of the four qualities (hot, cold, moist, and dry) in the body of the individual. The doctrine of the four qualities was accepted by medical and philosophical authors and found expression in general, unsystematic tracts, lists, and compilations as well as in more formal or systematized works. Closely tied to the idea of complexions, these concepts were specific enough and flexible enough to be applied easily to almost any particular theoretical or empirical conditions. Every healthy animal or person sustained a balance among these qualities, each of which had an important role to play in the normal operations of the body, and each of which, in excess, could be the source of ill health or even death.

---

38 [Ps.-]Trotula, *De passionibus mulierum*, Cambridge University Library, MS Dd.11.45, fols. 67r–68v. For a discussion of who Trotula is and what she wrote, see John F. Benton, "Trotula," pp. 30–53. Monica H. Green is preparing a study, edition, and translation of this text.

39 *De impedimentis conceptionis* (Arlt, *Schule von Montpellier*, pp. 18, 24–5; Pagel, "Raymundus de Moleriis," pp. 531–2).

This was true of males and females alike, though, as we have seen, woman's natural complexion was understood to be colder than man's. Fertility, like the other normal operations of the body, required an adequately, though not perfectly, balanced mixture. Thus, sterility could arise in either sex as a result of a defective overall temperament, especially one too hot or too cold. Petrus Gallegus, a thirteenth-century translator, put it succinctly when, citing his Arabic source, he asserted that "some do not reproduce because of heat, some because of cold."[40] The effects of imbalance might be general, or they might take a specific physiological or mechanical form: too much humidity, for example, can cause a man's semen to be watery and weak or a woman's uterus to be slippery.[41] Failure of the reproductive process might also occur as the result of a qualitative imbalance in some part of the body, especially in the reproductive parts. In men, the testes were a commonly identified locus, causing either a failure to produce sperm or the production of deficient sperm.[42] In women, the uterus was frequently thought to suffer from an excess of some quality, causing it to be either inhospitable to the sperm or incapable of sustaining the growth of the embryo.[43]

Fertility problems arising from specific organs might be anatomical as well as qualitative. A man's penis might be too long in absolute terms (the seed would cool too much while traveling the distance) or in relative terms (a bad structural match between partners could prevent conception).[44] A woman might have any number of anatomical problems. Her vagina might be too narrow for intercourse or too wide to promote pleasure or retain seed.[45] Her womb might be badly shaped or badly positioned, result-ing in either the failure of conception or some impediment to the normal growth of the child.[46] Sometimes the structural causes of infertility were attributable to specific stresses or systemic weaknesses. Albertus Magnus suggests at one point that childbirth can dry, wrinkle, and close a woman's womb[47] and at another point that the shortness of a man's penis might be the result of the excess demands made upon his flesh (otherwise destined to extend his penis) by his fat.[48] And all these disabilities – both the ana-

---

40 Excerpts from his *De animalibus*, in August Pelzer, "Un traducteur inconnu," p. 442: "Et ab hoc dixit abenfarag [Aboulfaradj ibn at-Tayib], orientalis philosophus, circa materiam, in qua sumus, quod quidam non generant propter calorem, quidam propter frigus."
41 Bernardus de Gordonio, *Lilium*, pt. VII, ch. i, fol. 87va; Albertus Magnus, *De animalibus*, bk. X, tr. i, ch. 1, §12, p. 735.
42 [Ps.-]Trotula, *De passionibus mulierum*, Cambridge University Library, MS Dd.11.45, fols. 67r–68v, especially 67v.
43 Ibid.; Albertus Magnus, *De animalibus*, bk. X, tr. i, ch. 1, §14, pp. 735–6.
44 Bernardus de Gordonio, *Lilium*, pt. VII, ch. i, fol. 87rb-va; *De impedimentis conceptionis* (Pagel, "Raymundus de Moleriis," p. 532); see also Lemay, "William of Saliceto," pp. 173–5.
45 [Ps.-]Trotula, *De passionibus mulierum*, Cambridge University Library, MS Dd.11.45, fol. 73r–v; British Library, MS Sloane 1124, fol. 175rb-vb.
46 Albertus Magnus, *De animalibus*, bk. X, tr. 1, ch. 1, §3, p. 731, and §9, pp. 733–4.
47 Ibid., tr. 2, ch. 1, §18, p. 737.
48 Ibid., §44, p. 748.

tomical and the physiological – could be either innate or the result of an illness or accident. Childbirth itself, for example, might cause sterility by producing a fallen womb or a stretched vulva.[49]

The acquisition of a reproductive disability is often related in turn to behavior, for the actions of each partner and of the couple together have a bearing on the success or failure of procreation. Where actions for which individuals are responsible are directly related to their fertility, the possibility of resonances between notions of natural sex differences and sociocultural values is especially strong. As in the case of the severed ear-vein, so in the case of medical prescriptions and proscriptions, we cannot simply assume that people did what they were told or that if someone was telling people *not* to do something, it was because they were busy doing it. We can, however, look for instances in which outlooks and attitudes of which we have independent evidence from other sources correspond to those projected by philosophical and medical texts. Sometimes it is difficult to place a cultural interpretation upon a medical instruction. Women are urged, for example, not to move around or – heaven forbid – jump after intercourse.[50] Sometimes it is less difficult. A commentator on the treatise *On the Secrets of Women* believed the women should lie still *during* intercourse.[51] In both cases the scientific reasoning is the same – the seed will be dislodged by the motion – but in the latter case female sexual pleasure and activity are at issue as well.[52]

The largest group of recommendations comes under the heading of regimen: there are dozens of areas of diet, hygiene, and habit subsumed under this rubric, and they are generally governed by the principle that excess is unhealthy and moderation is healthy. The pattern of thought in these cases is analogous to but developed independently of the system of qualities and complexions. Of course, too little coitus might be a cause of infertility,[53] but so might too much coitus.[54] Moderate frequency of intercourse is a principle involved in medical views about abstinence treated in the next chapter; prescriptions regarding several other areas of behavior merit consideration here. Conception will be impaired if the man or the woman has eaten too much or is too hungry and if either is too fat or too thin.[55] There are specific medical or philosophical rationales for such injunctions. For example, a fat person or animal uses for fat the blood which would otherwise be involved in the production of sperm.[56] The systematic promotion of moderation in

---

49 Albertus Magnus, *De animalibus*, bk. X, tr. i, ch. 1, §18, p. 737, and tr. ii, ch. 1, §43, p. 748.
50 *De impedimentis conceptionis* (Arlt, *Schule von Montpellier*, p. 14).
51 Cited in Lemay, "William of Saliceto," p. 171.
52 Brundage, *Law, Sex, and Christian Society*, pp. 452–3; idem, "Let Me Count the Ways" (unpublished paper).
53 Bernardus de Gordonio, *Lilium*, pt. VII, ch. i, fol. 87ra–b.
54 Ferckel, "Johannes de Ketham," pp. 208–9.
55 *De impedimentis conceptionis* (Arlt, *Schule von Montpellier*, p. 14).
56 *Propositiones de animalibus*, Cambridge University Library, MS Dd.3.16, fol. 76ra.

physiological theory and medical regimen supported and was supported by a network of cultural and intellectual strands. Perhaps the strongest of these were the related traditions of classical natural philosophy, Stoic ethics, and Christian theology, in each of which is visible the imprint of the past upon the Middle Ages and, at the same time, the mold the Middle Ages impressed upon these enduring ideas. Balance and harmony had played an important role in the ancient Greeks' view of the world. Using a vocabulary borrowed in part from the language of social order, they had emphasized the proportion and moderation of the macrocosm and the microcosm.[57] In the formulation of Patristic Christianity, in the influential works of Boethius and others, and in the ancient and Arabic works translated in the twelfth and thirteenth centuries, elements of this outlook flowed into the Latin West.

Disharmony and imbalance suggest unruliness, a deviation from the normal and normative in both nature and society. Thus, many failures of moderation possess simultaneously a scientific and a moral tone. Too much drink or too much sex could be unhealthy in general and impediments to conception in particular. At the same time, these excesses represented violations of upright behavior, whether this was understood in terms of the direct insistence on moderation in ethics or in terms of the Aristotelian insistence on the fulfillment of rationality. Gluttony and lust were enemies of both health and virtue. They were also *sins*. The principles of balance imply the condemnation of radical asceticism as well as of overindulgence. Both miserliness and profligacy are improper. Similarly, one can err by refusing food as well as by overeating. Women who are too thin are especially prone to miscarriage,[58] and overzealous fasting can be a form of pride. The complicity and tensions among science, ethics, and religion on the subject of asceticism were at the center of medieval views on sexual abstinence. They are relevant here to the extent that, at the very least, common standards of conduct were consonant with medical opinion in prescribing neither too much nor too little food, drink, sex, work, sleep, exercise, and bathing.

The condemnation of immoderation thus constituted an important link between the medical and scientific domains, on the one hand, and the moral and religious, on the other. Marital chastity, which set standards for the quantity and quality of marital intercourse and was consonant with certain medical recommendations, was a form of moral moderation. Other pro-

---

57 This was the case, in different ways, for the Hippocratic writers, Plato, Aristotle, the Pythagoreans, and the Stoics; it was even so for some Epicureans. The sense of order, harmony, and proportion manifested itself in a variety of ways in medieval science and medicine. See, e.g., John E. Murdoch, *Album of Science: Antiquity and the Middle Ages*, Albums of Science (New York: Charles Scribner's Sons, 1984), pp. 52–61; Dales, ed., *Marius;* the *De philosophia* edited in Cadden, "*De elementis;*" Arnaldus de Villanova, *Aphorismi de gradibus*, pp. 223–8.

58 Albertus Magnus, *De animalibus*, bk. X, tr. ii, ch. 2, §54, p. 752.

scriptions and prescriptions in relation to infertility illustrate the inextricable links between medical and social regulation, supporting but going beyond the principles of balance. The excessive youth of one of the partners, for example, could be an impediment to conception. Such coupling might simply be a case of medical or moral intemperance, but it also represented a disregard for physical and ethical maturity. Naturalists held that puberty, though it entailed the actualization of generative capacity, was by no means the age at which the ability to reproduce was perfected.[59] This view supported the increasingly prominent position of the Church against the marriage of children, who had certainly come into possession of some level of rational and spiritual competence but had not yet developed the full capacity to consent.[60]

Among the instances of correspondence between medical opinions on fertility and broader medieval interests in controlling behavior, perhaps the most striking example is the concern to regulate coital position, which carries certain gender implications. Albertus Magnus gave purely mechanical reasons for insisting that for conception to occur intercourse must take place with the woman on her back; breaking this rule could result in infertility. If the man enters from the rear, for example, his sperm will not be deposited close enough to the mouth of the uterus to effect conception; if the woman is standing the sperm will fall downward, away from the womb; when the woman is on top, her womb is turned over (*revoluta*).[61] (The same mechanical reasoning is behind the admonition that under no circumstances should a woman jump after intercourse.) Almost all the instructions are phrased in terms of constraints on what the woman may do, and when an ancient source on which Albertus is commenting asserts that "women can conceive in any of the positions," he simply skips over the passage.[62] This stance is, not coincidentally, congruent with the moral view of the matter which Albertus takes in his theological writing.[63] William of Saliceto gives his version of the *right* way (typically phrasing it in terms of the woman's position): she should be on her back with her head lowered, her left thigh raised with her foot under it, and her right leg extended.[64] Any other position might be generally harmful, especially to the man. One text warns of the danger to very young, very old, or convalescent men when the woman "usurps" the man's position.[65] There is circumstantial evidence that the sociopolitical implications of the wording

59 Jacquart and Thomasset, "Albert le Grand," pp. 85–7; Demaitre, "Idea of Childhood," pp. 466–7.

60 McLaughlin, "Survivors and Surrogates," pp. 125–6, esp. n. 143.

61 Albertus Magnus, *De animalibus*, bk. X, tr. ii, ch. 1, §45, p. 748.

62 Aristotle, *History of Animals* (*Works*, Barnes, X, ii, 634b36–40, vol. 1, p. 986); Albertus Magnus, *De animalibus*, bk. X, tr. i, ch. 1, pp. 730–7.

63 Brundage, *Law, Sex, and Christian Society*, pp. 452–3; idem, "Let Me Count the Ways" (unpublished paper).

64 Lemay, "William of Saliceto," p. 170.

65 Cartelle, ed., *Liber minor de coitu*, bk. II, ch. vi, p. 98.

were taken seriously,[66] just as there were specific reasons that breaking the rules could result in infertility. The condemnation of what were taken to be unnatural coital positions by religious authorities was related to what they understood to be the function of sexual intercourse and sexual pleasure. Their purpose, procreation, might be subverted by improper positions.[67] Thomas Aquinas tied his condemnation of any but the standard position to Aristotelian natural philosophy's assignment of roles in reproduction. The woman on her back was appropriately passive; the man on top appropriately active.[68] But from at least the early thirteenth century canonists and then theologians also rejected intercourse with the woman facing away from the man as unnatural on grounds not directly related to procreation: either because it was associated with sodomy or because it was thought to be the animal (i.e., inhuman) position.[69]

If concern about coital positions constituted an important point of convergence for medicine, natural philosophy, canon law, and theology, and thus illustrates the way in which scientific understanding reinforced and was reinforced by other aspects of medieval culture, it also constituted a point of divergence. The sources and goals of the scientific authors were not always consonant with those of religious authorities, and neither group had sufficient power to prevail over the other – though the sides were by no means evenly matched. The unspoken disagreement was not over the propriety or impropriety of specific positions, nor even about the general principles upon which proscriptions were based. (The principles were different but they were not in direct conflict.) Rather, it was over the specific preoccupations and goals of those seeking to regulate coital positions. Many canonists and theologians were especially concerned to place limits on sexual pleasure, even within marriage. Sexual intercourse was an essential (or, at the very least, usual) characteristic of marriage, according to canon law. The marriage debt of each partner to the other was so solemn that it had to be paid upon demand, even on those days when intercourse was prohibited by the Church.[70] According to a thirteenth-century writer of model sermons, in such a case the acceding, though not the demanding, partner was judged to be free from sin.[71] But the concept of the marriage debt, though it involved affection as well as procreation, by no means included a right to sexual

66 Davis, "Women on Top," pp. 124–51.
67 Noonan, *Contraception*, pp. 163–4.
68 Brundage, "Let Me Count the Ways" (unpublished paper), p. 11.
69 Ibid.
70 Brundage, *Law, Sex, and Christian Society*, pp. 278–88; R. H. Helmholz, *Marriage Litigation in Medieval England*, Cambridge Studies in English Legal History (London: Cambridge University Press, 1974), esp. pp. 87–90; Elizabeth M. Makowsky, "The Conjugal Debt and Medieval Canon Law," *Journal of Medieval History* 3 (1977): 99–114. These subjects are discussed further in chapter 6.
71 D'Avray and Tausche, "Marriage Sermons," pp. 96–7.

pleasure. Medieval churchmen quoted Jerome, holding that marital relations should not be governed by passion or impelled by desire for pleasure;
and they quoted Augustine, holding that unnatural acts between wife and
husband were worse than between a man and a prostitute.[72] It is difficult to
guess what practices the Fathers of the Church had in mind, but at least
some authors in the thirteenth century revealed that the association of unusual positions with lasciviousness and excessive pleasure was a central
feature of their condemnation of those positions. A penitential and a theological commentary might disagree about whether intercourse in a certain
position was a mortal sin or merely a moral fault, but they agreed the
problem was the pursuit of pleasure.[73] Deviation from the norm was, apparently, too much fun.

Or was it too little fun? Medical and scientific authors, who were preoccupied with the prevention or cure of reproductive failures, rather than the
prevention of moral failures, often condemned the same acts for different
reasons. In addition to pointing out the general health hazards and the
mechanical impediments to conception created by unorthodox positions,
they warned that these eccentricities might result in *less* pleasure. After
listing the ills that may result from the woman-on-top or lateral positions,
(including sores on the penis, hernias, and gout) a twelfth-century treatise
On Intercourse suggested: "Whoever desires a safe and natural practice
should arrange that she lie on her back with her thighs higher than her
head, and so that it will be more pleasing to both."[74] The author may
simply have intended the promise of greater pleasure as an inducement to
healthy behavior or may have had in mind the connections between pleasure and fertility. In spite of the subtleties of the scholastic analyses, which
somewhat dissociated pleasure (especially female pleasure) from conception, late medieval authors concerned with solving fertility problems
recommended that both partners have pleasure in intercourse and even
recommended that they experience pleasure simultaneously. In the early
fourteenth century, John of Gaddesden summarized his view of the theoretical issue and then went on to state the practical problem: "It is surely
not necessary that the sperm of the man and the woman meet, but conception occurs easily and properly if they do meet. For the woman's sperm is

---

72 Ibid., pp. 99–100; Brundage, "Let Me Count the Ways" (unpublished paper), pp. 2, 7. See
   also James A. Brundage, "Carnal Delight: Canonistic Theories of Sexuality," *Proceedings of
   the Fifth International Congress of Medieval Canon Law, Salamanca, 21–25 September 1976* (Vatican
   City: Biblioteca Apostolica Vaticana, 1980), pp. 361–85; and Payer, *Sex and the Penitentials*.
73 William of Rennes and Albertus Magnus, in Brundage, "Let Me Count the Ways" (unpublished paper), pp. 10–11.
74 [*De coitu*], New York Academy of Medicine, MS "Collection of Surgical and Gynecological
   Texts," fol. 88ra: "Qui autem tutum et naturalem appetit usum, faciat ut mulier supina
   iaceat et femora capite alteriora porrigat, et ut quia magis delectet utrumque." Cf. Cartelle,
   ed., *Liber minor de coitu*, bk. II, ch. vi, p. 98.

not true sperm, but a certain watery, whitened menstruum. . . . Here, however, it is noted that men sometimes ejaculate too fast and the woman slowly, on account of her coldness."[75] For the man, John recommends dry mint, which works against the unrestrained flow of seed, or an ointment containing a little camphor (an anaphrodisiac) to be applied over the kidneys. "And he should touch the woman with his hand on her genitals and breasts, and kiss her; then know her. And this works as a cure."[76] (Here medieval expertise is being applied to mitigate constitutional and sexual differences between men and women.) In these cases, the goal of the prescriptions – the enhancement of pleasure – is the opposite of the canonists', even though their substance – curing sterility – is concordant. Some theologians seem to have perceived the tension between the two perspectives, and a few even authorized practices consonant with the medical view, because they produced better children.[77]

The interplay of scientific and religious opinion on the relationship between pleasure and deviant coital positions illustrates both the convergence and the divergence of the several forces operating to shape behavioral norms. In the case of issues surrounding sterility (as in the case of issues surrounding sexual abstinence), medicine and theology offered overlapping but not congruent ideologies. On the one hand, there was a correspondence between the two domains in their attempt to restrict specific sexual behaviors – a correspondence based at least in part on a mutual interest in promoting fertility. On the other hand, the different and sometimes mutually contradictory rationales they put forth reveal differences not only in the traditions and strategies upon which they drew but also in the assumptions on which they were founded. In contrast, the way in which ideas about the causes and treatments of sterility participated in notions about sex difference, and particularly the medical contributions to the preference for male children, created little in the way of tension or ambiguity. However, both the measures against sterility and the methods for producing sons exhibited a marked independence from the general emphases of more theoretical discussions of reproduction and sex determination and took full advantage of the practical implications of academic eclecticism.

75 Johannes Anglicus, *Rosa Anglica*, bk. II, ch. xvii, fol. 75ra: "Et ideo non est necessarium quod concurrat sperma viri et mulieris adinvicem, sed conceptio fit facilis et idonea si concurrant, quia sperma mulieris non est verum sperma, sed quoddam menstruum aquosum dealbatum. . . . Hic tamen notandum quod viri aliquando nimis cito emittunt sperma et tarde mulier propter frigiditatem suam."

76 Ibid., fol. 75ra–b: "Et debet tangere mulierem cum manu contra muliebria et mamillas, et osculari eam. Deinde cognoscere eam. Et hoc valet in cura. . . ."

77 Jean-Louis Flandrin, "Sex in Married Life in the Early Middle Ages: The Church's Teaching and Behavioral Reality," in *Western Sexuality: Practice and Precept in Past and Present Times*, ed. Philippe Ariès and André Béjin, trans. Anthony Forster (Oxford: Basil Blackwell, 1985), p. 119.

STERILITY, FERTILITY, AND SEX DIFFERENCE

"As much the fault of the man as the fault of the woman"?

Because of the importance of a roughly parallel view of the sexes in many medical texts, because of the unsystematic and eclectic character of so many handbooks and compilations, and because of the frequent occasions for observation, the cause of a couple's infertility was understood to inhere in either sex or (among more complete and sophisticated authors) in the couple together. In spite of these apparently egalitarian indications, the texts that dealt with sterility tended in the aggregate to place the burden upon the woman. There may be several reasons for this emphasis. One, surely, is the likelihood of a woman's suffering injury or infection as a result of child-birth, especially repeated childbirth. Another may be the frequency of ovulatory failure due to malnutrition, a condition endemic, if unevenly distributed, in medieval Europe. A third reason is undoubtedly literary: the legacy from antiquity included a genre of medical writing, gynecology, which had no male counterpart and which provided the basis for commentaries and collections, as well as the precedent for new works. Finally, reproduction was conceptualized as work that women did: it was a major socioeconomic function and, in spite of theories of male activity and female passivity, could be viewed as an active and affirmative responsibility. (See Figure 4.) Conversely, the concept of barrenness and, indeed, the word "sterility" itself, when used outside medicine and philosophy, applied to women, not to men.

Medicine and natural philosophy, even while repeating the commonplace "as much the fault of the man as of the woman," underscored the emphasis on the woman in cases of reproductive failure. Furthermore, like the sex differences which permeated the discussions of sexual pleasure, those related to infertility are not simply differences of more and less. They are not as clearly articulated nor does a consistent pattern emerge, for the distinction is not the subject of much direct comment. Nevertheless, they too participate in the construction of the masculine and the feminine.

Some of the evidence cited in connection with the causes of sterility indicates the separate characteristics of male and female difficulties. The amount of attention devoted to the problems of each sex is a first crude indicator of the difference in emphasis. Constantine the African's brief treatise *On Coitus* and another work by the same name written more than a century later, around 1200, dealt almost exclusively with male sexual and reproductive issues, but they are exceptional and, furthermore, they are not aimed at procreation per se. Most works centered on questions of fertility have much more to say about women than about men. The quantitative difference has qualitative implications: women's fertility and women's health are bound closely together, especially around the condition of the womb and the state of the menses. The specialized work commonly ascribed to "Trotula," *On the Diseases of Women*, and John of Gaddesden's broad survey of medical and surgical information both reflect the Galenic tendency to associate female reproductive capacity with female health. (See Figure 1.) In both sexes, of course, constitutional disorders can give rise to infertility. In men, however, "gonorrhea" (the continuous flow of sperm), mentioned regularly in tracts on sterility and in general medical works, did not have larger significance for the individual's health. Female complaints, on the contrary, are bivalent, constituting not only limited problems in and of themselves but also broader problems for the women. One author suggested treating sterile women as if they had hectic fever.[78] Menstrual retention is the most prominently featured cause of sterility among women: the same author put it first in his list of ten intrinsic causes. Yet, as medical attitudes toward sexual abstinence will show, menstrual retention was also harmful to women in itself.

In the context of sterility, men and women were distinguished not only by the extent to which their physical well-being was linked to their reproductive functions but also by the way in which those reproductive functions were conceptualized. Whereas the scholastic interest in the question of the female seed had focused attention on the moment of conception, both philosophical and medical writers took a wider view of the process of generation when they addressed sterility and fertility. In particular, while the male role was limited to the proper conception of the fetus, the female role included in addition proper gestation and parturition. Thus, miscarriages, stillbirths, and, for the most part, unhealthy or deformed children were posted to the woman's account. In a passage which recalls ideas about the plurality of female pleasures, Albertus Magnus explained that women have all the same occasions for failure as men, and then some:

Hence there can be many causes on the part of the man for non-impregnation: either from failure of the seed; or from his excessive heat or fluidity or cold; or from a defect of the generative members – a long or short penis or [one that] cannot become erect, or cold testicles. And there can be equivalent causes on the part of the woman, and yet several more, since she not only furnishes seed but also conserves it, and there can be failure in the conserving.[79]

Once again, the "fault" residing with the woman is not only greater but also more diverse. Of one recipe listed under the heading of menstrual retention,

78 *De impedimentis conceptionis* (Arlt, *Schule von Montpellier*, p. 14).
79 Albertus Magnus, *Quaestiones de animalibus*, bk. X, q. 1, pp. 214–15: "Unde multae causae non-impraegnationis possunt esse ex parte viri: vel ex defectu seminis vel ex nimia caliditate eius vel liquiditate vel frigiditate vel ex defectu membrorum generativorum, quia virga longa vel curta, vel quia non potest surgere vel quia testiculi frigidi. Et consimiles causae possunt esse ex parte feminae, et adhuc plures, quia ipsa non solum semen ministrat, sed etiam conservat ipsum et defectus potest esse in conservando. . . ."

an early fourteenth-century physician boasted, "This not only provokes [menstruation] but also aids the embryo and cleanses the womb."[80] The breadth of female responsibilities affects the proportions and emphases within the lists of causes and recipes in medieval works. For this reason and others already discussed in connection with pleasure, sections about men's sterility devote a higher proportion of their content to what we might regard as sexual dysfunction than sections on women's sterility. Even setting aside the considerable space regularly allocated to menstrual retention, sections on women's sterility place great emphasis upon the condition of the womb. Although not the subject of much academic speculation or debate in the late Middle Ages, the centrality of the womb in the characterization of the female had persisted since antiquity and manifested itself especially in medical and (to a lesser extent) in natural philosophical discussions of sterility. Even the most positive view of the uterus emphasized its vulnerability. "The womb is truly a noble organ and thus is more prone to harm."[81] Although some works may suggest parallels between the womb and the testicles or the penis (as when *On the Diseases of Women* introduces the subject of sterility with references to women's wombs and men's testicles), these are formal extensions of the general principle "as much the fault of the man as the fault of the woman" and have little bearing on the texts' substance.[82]

Placing the burden of responsibility for infertility upon women had two consequences. First, it constituted a socially significant domain of feminine weakness and incapacity. As a practical matter, a man might find a way to replace a wife, if the couple were childless, but not vice versa. Second, it implicitly accorded women responsibility for fertility. The medical texts, especially compilations of advice and remedies, offer concrete evidence of this perspective. Many aspects of sexual conduct, as described in these texts, involve actions and decisions taken by men (for example, choosing a fertile wife or choosing the conditions for intercourse);[83] some instructions for overcoming sterility involve actions by midwives and doctors; but in significant numbers of cases, the women themselves are called upon to solve the problem. In cases of incompatibility of physiological temperament, the man can get a new wife, but the woman can also change her diet.[84] A specialized tract on sterility suggests that long-term remedies, such as a moderate regimen, be undertaken by the woman and the man, and also describes cures in

---

80 *De impedimentis conceptionis* (Arlt, *Schule von Montpellier*, p. 21): ". . . et hoc non solum provocat ymo etiam juvat conceptum et matricem mundificat."
81 Albertus Magnus, *Quaestiones de animalibus*, bk. X, q. 1, p. 214: "Matrix vero membrum nobile est, et ideo laesioni est pronior. . . ."
82 [Ps.-]Trotula, *De passionibus mulierum*, Cambridge University Library, MS Dd.11.45, fols. 67r–68v; British Library, MS Sloane 1124, fols. 176vb–178rb.
83 [Elections], British Library, MS Cotton. App. VI, fol. 13vb; Hildegard, *Causae et curae*, bk. I, p. 18.
84 Lemay, "William of Saliceto," p. 174.

which the woman is to make sexual advances, as well as some in which the man is to do so. Even in cases in which the "fault" was understood to lie with the man, the woman might provide the solution: if the man's penis is too short, the woman should see to it that his seed falls in the bottom of the womb.[85]

The treatments and cures suggested in medical works reinforce the impression of women's responsibility and fault. Men and women alike were advised about their habits regarding eating, drinking, sleeping, phlebotomies, and purges and about the times and circumstances for sexual intercourse; men and women alike were prescribed various oral medicines or ointments, according to the specific characteristics of their conditions. Some recipes are for aphrodisiacs, intended to increase desire or enhance pleasure in women and men, or, more specifically, to encourage men's erections. These recipes are not always distinguishable from stimulation by foreplay, since some are salves applied to the genitals by rubbing. Yet in spite of these commonalities, remedies for the two sexes clearly differ in a number of ways. First, once again, the volume of advice aimed at women is greater. Second, in addition to the types they share with men, women's prescriptions include pessaries and suffumigations – the latter a procedure for directing vapors or smokes through the vagina and into the womb. These correspond to the emphasis placed upon the uterus in the analysis of the causes and nature of infertility. Third, there seems to be more emphasis on foreplay for the sexual arousal of women than of men, though this is hard to measure. A medical author of the early fourteenth century may have been the source of John of Gaddesden's instructions, quoted earlier, for the encouragement of simultaneous emission: he recommends that the husband "smoothly stroke his lady, breasts and belly, and excite [her] for having intercourse."[86] They are probably following Avicenna on this point, but the advice is widely repeated, appearing not only in works on sterility but also in a commentary on the pseudo–Albertus Magnus *On the Secrets of Women*.[87] Nor is the point simply to achieve simultaneous emission, for women's pleasure had generally positive effects on fertility. Bernard of Gordon, a medical professor at Montpellier, numbered a woman's sexual appetite among the things upon which her ability to conceive might depend.[88] These instructions seem inconsistent with the frequent association of women with sexual appetite. Finally, and perhaps most significantly, medical works of various genres are far

---

85 *De impedimentis conceptionis* (Pagel, "Raymundus de Moleriis," pp. 532 and 536). Cf. Lemay, "William of Saliceto," p. 169.

86 *De impedimentis conceptionis* (Pagel, "Raymundus de Moleriis," p. 536): ". . . maritus . . . debet dominam suaviter palpare mamillas et ventrem et excitare ad coytum. . . ."

87 Avicenna, *Liber canonis*, bk. III, fen xxi, tr. 1, ch. 10, fol. 363vb; see Lemay, "William of Saliceto," pp. 169–70.

88 Bernardus de Gordonio, *De regimine vii etatum*, Cambridge University, Gonville and Caius, MS 593, fol. 40vb.

more likely to represent the woman as the patient. The works that collected real or hypothetical case histories typically featured women in their stories about curing infertility. General works and collections of recipes are less likely to speak of individuals, but when they do, they most often speak of women. At the end of his treatise on sterility, having just covered problems attributable to couples rather than to one partner, one author touted his cures by boasting about two cases he has successfully treated. One woman had been with her husband for thirteen years with no sign of pregnancy. He treated her with an herbal preparation, and within two months she had conceived. She gave birth to a healthy son. The second woman had been married for nine years to a knight in the household of a viscount, likewise with no sign of conception. After a purgation (presumably of the retained menses), she also conceived a son. He ends the treatise by mentioning "certain other women," all of whom became pregnant.[89]

These last examples illustrate some of the ways in which sex differences enter into medieval thinking about sterility. The emphasis upon the female partner is consistent with and reinforces the academic theories of reproduction and the more general cultural presumptions that represented women as weak, incapacitated, and, in some sense, unhealthy. These links and associations are not, however, either obvious or simple. Reproductive action, according to scholarly analyses, resided mainly with the male, so although female passivity and female responsibility could be reconciled by pointing to the unsuitability or intractability of the female matter or the female receptacle, they did not follow logically from any scholastic version of reproduction. Similarly, the commonplace framework and organization for writing about sterility called for consideration of men's problems, women's problems, and couples' problems, offering no apparent reason for placing more weight on one sex or the other. Yet the actual emphasis on women agrees with the mutually reinforcing tendencies of society and medicine – the former to see the production of offspring as a central, if not defining, female role; the latter to deal with fertility as a domain reaching from preconditions through conception and gestation to parturition. As the proudly reported cases illustrate, the problem of fertility was not just the problem of impregnation but rather the problem of bringing forth a healthy child, preferably a son. The social and medical promotion of sons is thus another area in which medieval ideas about fertility intersect with medieval ideas about sex difference.

"So that a woman may conceive a male"

"A woman complained to us about sterility and especially for the generation of males. . . ." Thus begins a series of medical cases composed by Taddeo

---

89 *De impedimentis conceptionis* (Pagel, "Raymundus de Moleriis," pp. 536–7).

Alderotti.[90] The late medieval preference for sons is one area in which the literature of medicine and, to a lesser extent, philosophy responded to social norms. To be sure, there was a firm classical tradition to draw on, but medieval instructions for conceiving and bearing male children and, especially, for guessing the sex of a fetus are too frequent and too varied to be attributed solely to respect for ancient authorities on the subject. The Aristotelian view of sex determination emphasized the relative vigor of the (male) seed and intractability of the (female) material, whereas the medical authorities, especially Galen, emphasized the relative strengths of the male and female contributions. Both traditions, however, incorporated the opinion that left (testicle or side of the womb) was the origin of the female and right (testicle or side of the womb) was the origin of the male. Like discussions of and recommendations for sterility in general, practical suggestions about having or detecting sons showed little interest in the hierarchies of causation constructed in theoretical works. Essential and accidental features of the process of sex determination played indifferently into the recommended techniques, with variations on the left–right distinction taking a leading role.

Medieval texts offered many reassertions of these principles and added others. Works on natural philosophy of the less formalized and academic sort, whether predating or contemporary with the more structured academic genres, offered ample and amply flexible explanations for the process of sex determination. For example, the notion that the child's sex depends on which way the penis is twisted in intercourse refers apparently to the principle that sex is determined by whether the fetus develops on the left or right side of the womb.[91] Hildegard of Bingen's system explained the sex and character of the offspring based on the strength of the father's semen and on the degree of love between the parents.[92] A treatise found in fourteenth-century manuscripts invokes the left–right principle among others: having said earlier that coarse sperm makes sons and subtle sperm makes daughters, the author of this compilation gives the reasons why sperm that falls in the right portion of the womb will develop into a male child and sperm that falls in the left portion will develop into a female. If, he continues, the sperm of a weak man lands on the right side and joins the sperm of a stronger woman, the child will still be a male, but a womanly one, having womanly behavior. Indeed the man's sperm may be so weak that the child will be both sexes. Similarly, if the male sperm is dominant and the child develops on the left side, a girl with certain virile traits, such as

90 Thadeus [Florentinus], *Experimenta*, Bibliothèque Nationale, MS lat. 6964, fol. 100ra: "Conquesta est nobis mulier de sterilitate et precipue ad masculorum generationem. . . ." On the nature and uses of collections of *experimenta* and *consilia*, see Siraisi, *Taddeo*, pp. 270–302.
91 [Ps.-]Albertus Magnus, *Anathomia*, Bibliothèque Nationale, MS lat. 7349, fol. 19r–v.
92 Hildegard, *Causae et curae*, bk. II, pp. 35–6.

masculine speech and a beard, results. Again, in the extreme case, the child will be of both sexes.[93] Ideas of this kind formed the basis of strategies for predicting and attempting to control the sex of a child.

Discussions of the general patterns of sex determination like the preceding one often have a certain symmetry to them. Borrowing from theories of reproduction and extending them into the notions about fertility and infertility, they do not exhibit a particular interest in one sex or the other, but this seeming neutrality is undermined by the value laden language of the explanations. Right, after all, is better than left; strength better than weakness. (The unusual association of male with coarse and female with subtle runs counter to physiological concepts of coction and refinement and may reflect a more popular and less esoteric sense that boys are robust and girls are fragile.) The appearance of symmetry is abandoned almost entirely when the texts offer their innumerable instructions for guessing the sex of a fetus. Certain signs are suggested over and over. If the woman has milk (whether detected by swelling or secretions is not clear) in the right breast first, the child will be a boy; if in the left breast, a girl. Several other common tests have to do with left and right: if a pregnant woman swells on the right side or, when asked to walk, puts her right foot forward, the child is a boy. Some methods are not widely repeated: if the mother's eye has good color, the child is a boy.[94] In these passages, in contrast to those concerned with the general causes of female and male offspring, the specific interest in males becomes apparent. Although some do give the signs for both sexes, many do not bother with girls and indicate only how to tell if the child will be a boy.

The focus on the male is even more emphatic in passages which give instructions for ensuring a child of the desired sex, for even Albertus Magnus, a philosopher with an appreciation of the ultimate causes of sex determination, was ready to affirm that the art of medicine could affect the child's sex.[95] The methods mention girls – but only secondarily. An early medieval gynecological text supplies two recipes to produce sons and one to produce daughters – all three involving parts of a hare.[96] A late medieval tract gave high praise to a recipe that was, above all others, efficacious in promoting generation. It included among other ingredients "the right testicles of cocks, . . . the left ones if you want to have a girl."[97] Here, as elsewhere,

---

93 *Secreta mulierum minor*, Cambridge University, Trinity, MSS O.2.5, fols. 131ra and 132rb–va; and R.14.45, fols. 25r–v and 27r.
94 *Secreta mulierum minor*, Cambridge University, Trinity, MS O.2.5, fol. 131rb and R.14.45, fol. 25v.
95 Albertus Magnus, *Quaestiones de animalibus*, bk. IX, q. 18, pp. 210–11.
96 *Liber de muliebra causa*, 7–9 (Egert, *Gynäkologische Fragmente*, p. 25).
97 *De impedimentis conceptionis* (Pagel, "Raymundus de Moleriis," p. 533): "Deinde utatur ista medicina divinitus revelata que super omnes alias valet ad generandum. Rp. vitella cruda ovorum VI butiri re(centis?) seri caprini ana quart. 1 priapi thauri satirion zedarii zingiberis conditi mente testiculorum dextrorum gallorum mutonis et ferris, si vis habere feminam sinistrorum. . . ."

preference for a boy is the default position; medical authors, like queens with daughters, were aware of the premium placed on the male child.

What does this preference for boys mean? It may in part reflect the new vigor of literary traditions of misogyny in the later Middle Ages. From the often crude representations of the French fabliaux to the clerkish tone of Andreas Capellanus, the elaboration of popular and Patristic invectives against women was rich and important from the twelfth century to the early fifteenth-century debate about *The Romance of the Rose*, in which Christine de Pisan defended women's honor. The image of woman as ruled by her appetite was an element in the preference for sons, as well as in the discussions of the sexes' reproductive roles and sexual pleasure.

Beyond such cultural and intellectual traditions lie general socioeconomic conditions, some of which may, in turn, be related to other factors, such as infant mortality sex ratios.[98] It is the rule rather than the exception for agricultural societies to favor high fertility and male children: in a family economy, large families are – or are perceived to be – preferable, and boys are – or are perceived to be – more productive. Furthermore, in many cultures, sons are more likely to maintain close economic and social ties to their parents' household, while daughters become linked to their husbands' families. These conditions obtained in the late Middle Ages, where even in the growing towns agricultural values has not yet been replaced. And even in the areas of Europe where practices of primogeniture did not apply (and these were many), privileges, properties, and trades were as a rule passed from fathers to sons and sometimes barred to daughters, while at the same time daughters often required dowries for marriage and sons, thereby, acquired possessions. Such social and economic constraints were both effects and causes of the value placed on sons. They may help to explain not only the frequent medical formulas for producing sons but also what appear to be high proportions of males in the population (which might be attributable to female infanticide or to treatment producing differential infant survival rates)[99] and the high proportion of girls among abandoned children.[100]

In pursuing this subject as formulated in the medical and scientific literature or as reflected in the social realities of the time, we need not exclude the possibility that mothers (and fathers) cherished their daughters or that women recognized and even resisted the misogyny inherent in the prefer-

---

98 Lauris McKee, "Sex Differential in Survivorship and the Customary Treatment of Infants and Children," *Medical Anthropology* 8 (1984): 92–3, summarizes the cross-cultural literature on the sex mortality differential.

99 Emily Coleman has presented indirect evidence from the ninth century in "L'infanticide dans le Haut Moyen Age," *Annales: Economies, sociétés, civilisations* 29 (1974): 315–35, translated with some additional references in *Women in Medieval Society*, ed. Susan Mosher Stuard ([Philadelphia]: University of Pennsylvania Press, 1976), pp. 47–70. See, however, Brissaud, "L'infanticide," which emphasizes illegitimacy, without regard to the child's sex.

100 R. Trexler, "Foundlings of Florence," *History of Childhood Quarterly* 1 (1973): 259–75.

ence for sons.[101] Nevertheless, the way in which fertility and infertility were conceptualized in the later Middle Ages incorporated the value placed upon bearing sons, and perhaps even some general sense of reproductive control: "So that a woman may conceive a male: let her take and eat the testicles of a cock. However, if a woman wishes not to become pregnant, she should have with her something from the members of two crows."[102]

The subject of sterility has, then, offered an opportunity to explore the diversity of medieval medical and natural philosophical ideas about sex difference and reproduction in the context of aspects of the culture within and beyond arts faculties and medical schools. The importance of childbearing in the economic and social systems and in the religious ideology of the period received theoretical support from the natural philosophers' conviction that reproduction was an essential feature of living nature; it received concrete support from the observations and prescriptions of the medical profession, which, although not holding to an explicitly pronatalist position, nevertheless devoted countless folios to practices designed to promote fertility.

With respect to the applications of medical and philosophical ideas, the case of sterility reinforces the impression made by the analysis of gender notions in the preceding chapter that the elaborate theories and subtle debates of scholastic medicine and natural philosophy did indeed enter into the language and concepts operating at the borders between the elite intellectual traditions and the broader social norms. They operated at these points of intersection, not as well integrated machines forming and enforcing some clear ideological agenda, but rather as repositories of used parts, some suitable, some unsuitable for the flexible, piecemeal, multifunctional construction that mediated among the different and not always compatible dimensions of medieval culture. In the case of sterility, the selective and ad hoc character of the ideas resulted in no small part from the practical nature of the problems facing physicians (and recognized by some natural philosophers).

The quantity of material written about sterility is not in itself evidence of its larger social and cultural significance. Many tracts were written about kidney stones, and almost every survey of medical knowledge contained a chapter on the subject, yet kidney stones do not play a significant role in medieval life and thought. But sterility does not cause pain like kidney stones, it is not life-threatening like the plague, and it does not manifest

---

101 There is evidence that such resistance occurred in other societies: see Daniel Scott Smith, "Family Limitation, Sexual Control, and Domestic Feminism in Victorian America," in Mary S. Hartman and Lois Banner, eds., *Clio's Consciousness Raised: New Perspectives on the History of Women*, Harper Colophon Books (New York: Harper and Row, 1974), pp. 119–36.

102 *Experimenta*, Vienna, Nationalbibliothek, MS CVP 2532, fol. 28v: "Ut mulier masculum concipiat. Gallorum accipiat et comedat, tamen si mulier nolit gravida fieri aliquid de membris duorum corvorum secum habeat."

dramatic symptoms like fevers. That medical attention to fertility does have a larger meaning is suggested not only by its recurrence in the medical literature but also by its appearance in works on natural philosophy and, more important, by attitudes about children and their socioeconomic functions. From the perspective of these interests, the promotion of childbearing was a widely shared goal, although there were some points of disagreement about acceptable or effective means, and although, as the next chapter will show, respect for sexual abstinence brought new issues into play.

Physicians and natural philosophers located sterility within the framework of widely accepted views of physiology and health, invoking ideas of balance and regime, for example. In addition, they drew on more specific concepts about male and female reproductive contributions, about sex determination, and about pleasure, which were being debated in the faculties of arts and medicine. Yet on these matters, those concerned with sterility, even when, like Bernard of Gordon or Albertus Magnus, they were participants in the learned systematic conversations, tended to be pragmatic and opportunistic, taking an approach that belonged more to the eclectic and ad hoc habits of mind characteristic of an earlier time and of a less rarified and more practical context.

The flexibility inherent in that approach precluded the transfer of any formulaic relation between the sexes from academic theories to medical practice. Indeed, we have already seen that no such formula existed. But the flexibility did not result in a meaningless jumble of assertions and prescriptions; rather, it was sufficiently stable to constitute the basis for a certain congruence of medical and social understandings. Choosing from the array of available tools and materials, medical writers crafted a set of beliefs and recommended practices which accommodated the preference for sons and negotiated the delicate business of according women the main responsibility for childlessness without giving them credit for full reproductive activity.

6

Is sex necessary? The problem of sexual abstinence

The case of sterility has illustrated the harmonious, if ambiguous, interaction of science and society in the later Middle Ages; the case of sexual abstinence will reveal a more ambivalent relationship among medical, natural philosophical, social, and religious agendas. When medieval families wished to have children, the medical community was ready to assist. The conviction that sterility was a problem was a corollary at once of the social desirability of offspring, of the philosophical view that reproduction was the means by which creatures were supposed to attain general (if not individual) immortality, and of the medical assumption that reproduction was the purpose and normal function of certain bodily parts and processes. In addition, the existence of theoretical disputes about the respective roles of females and males in the reproductive process left the medical community with room for flexibility. Thus medicine and social values were easily accommodated. True, their agreement was not always based on the same assumptions or the same reasoning, but they reinforced one another anyway. Medical texts, for example, seldom mention marriage, whereas legitimately constituted families were the locus of the social interest in fertility, but from a practical point of view, medical remedies for sterility were intended for and employed by married couples. To the extent that religious beliefs were involved, they also favored the promotion of fertility in appropriate circumstances, though doctrine more strongly *opposed* contraception than it *promoted* childbearing. The dynamics of medieval opinion on sexual abstinence are more complicated, and the relations among natural philosophy, medicine, society, and religion more strained.

The subject of sexual abstinence holds up a mirror to medieval views about sex by posing the question, "What happens without it?" It reflects the various cultural forces regulating sexual activity and the place sexual impulses and acts held in the medieval constellation of meaning. Certain assumptions, interests, doctrines, and circumstances created pressure to ab-

stain from sexual activities; others created pressure to engage in them. The
tension between reasons for and against abstinence forms the field upon
which religious, social, and medical concerns met and in the process uncov-
ers differences between the sexes.

THE REINS OF RESTRAINT: VARIETIES OF ABSTINENCE

Virginity was the crowning jewel of sexual continence. Although in the
later Middle Ages it had lost some of the ideological and magical force it had
possessed earlier in the history of the Latin West, it retained both literal and
symbolic importance. The notion of virginity had a place in both religious
and secular values, and the protection of virginity was sometimes an issue in
saints' lives and in marriage arrangements. Medical authorities thus saw fit
to comment on the subject as a condition occasionally if not frequently
encountered among adults.

The religious value of virginity was composite. In its most literal form it
was the absence of the experience of intercourse. In its most heroic form it
was a source of Christian martyrdom. It was an active expression of the
love of God, a vehicle of humility, a token of the rejection of the world,
and a representation of mystical purity.[1] Although frequently contrasted
with marriage – the low road away from fornication and toward salvation – virginity was not inconsistent with the married state. Saint Alexis is
the married virgin best known to medievalists, because an eleventh-
century French poem about him is one of the earliest surviving works in
that language.[2] The story is told and retold in medieval European vernacu-
lars from Middle English to Portuguese. Married in obedience to his father's wishes, Alexis approaches his wife on their wedding night only to
preach to her of the celestial life and announce his intention to undertake a
pilgrimage. For decades his pious parents and wife mourn his absence, but
when he returns he is so changed by poverty they fail to recognize the
beggar to whom they give alms. He lives by their charity until, at his
death, his identity is revealed.

As the case of Alexis suggests, the Christian concept of virginity could be
applied to men as well as to women, and the word *virgo*, although it was
usually feminine in classical Latin, had a masculine form disseminated by

1 Some of these dimensions are discussed in John Bugge, *Virginitas: An Essay in the History of a
Medieval Ideal*, International Archives of the History of Ideas, ser. min., 17 (The Hague:
Martinus Nijhoff, 1975); and Clarissa W. Atkinson, " 'Precious Balsam in a Fragile Glass': The
Ideology of Virginity in the Later Middle Ages," *Journal of Family History* 8 (1983): 131–43.
2 Gaston Paris, ed., *La vie de saint Alexis: Poème du XIᵉ siècle*, Les classiques français du Moyen
Age (Paris: Librairie Ancienne Honoré Champion, 1911). See also Jean Leclercq, *Monks on
Marriage: A Twelfth-Century View* (New York: Seabury Press, 1982), pp. 43–8; Atkinson,
" 'Precious Balsam,' " pp. 135–6.

Patristic writers[3] and employed by late medieval authors.[4] Male virginity was a theme in the development of monastic ideals, and although both new formulations of the ideals and an expansion of opportunities for the expression of women's piety feminized the construct in the later Middle Ages, this form of spiritual purity maintained a degree of gender neutrality.[5] The persistence of the male ideal and the increasing frequency of female application gave rise to a paradoxical situation in which a virtue characterized as masculine enabled individuals, especially women, to transcend their sexual and thereby their gender identity. The almost magical powers of female virgins were a staple of late medieval saints' lives and unicorn stories. (See Figure 7.)

Church practices shared some gender symmetries with Church teachings and tended, in the later Middle Ages, to deemphasize virginity for ordinary people of both sexes. The Church's efforts to encourage couples to have their marriages sanctified, for example, would have been significantly hampered by requiring bride and groom to be virgins, and of course no such requirement existed. In fact a curious turn of canon law, developed in the thirteenth century and abandoned by the sixteenth, led ecclesiastical courts to treat prior fornication as a legitimate condition in a marriage contract in certain cases.[6] Nor was it required for either a woman or a man who wished to enter a monastic community or take religious vows. On this point, however, a gender asymmetry is introduced, for although men might occupy any position in the Church without claiming to be virgins, women who were not virgins sometimes could not aspire to the title of "nun" (as distinguished from "sister").[7]

The social value of virginity in the later Middle Ages resided mainly with females, and women's sexuality was subject to greater social control. Families that guarded the purity of their daughters celebrated the sexual exploits

---

3 Lewis and Short, *A Latin Dictionary* (Oxford: Oxford University Press, 1879), s.v. *virgo*, cite Tertullian, Jerome, and Paulinus for the masculine form. It also appears in a classical inscription: P. G. W. Glare, *Oxford Latin Dictionary* (Oxford: Oxford University Press, Clarendon Press, 1982), s.v. *virgo*. Atkinson, although concerned exclusively with women's virginity, cites Patristic opinions which could and in some cases did apply to men as well, (" 'Precious Balsam,' " see esp. pp. 132–5).

4 E.g., Humbert de Romans, cited in Alexander Murray, "Religion among the Poor in Thirteenth-Century France: The Testimony of Humbert de Romans," *Traditio* 30 (1974): 314.

5 Bugge, *Virginitas*, esp. chs. 3–5.

6 Helmholz, *Marriage Litigation*, pp. 172–80.

7 Bugge, *Virginitas*, pp. 115–22, explains one set of reasons why virginity became what he calls "deontologized." Eleanor Commo McLaughlin, in emphasizing the momentousness of a woman's loss of virginity, remarks on "certain rigorist religious orders" that would accept no woman not a virgin: "Equality of Souls, Inequality of Sexes: Women in Medieval Theology," in Rosemary Radford Ruether, ed., *Religion and Sexism: Images of Women in the Jewish and Christian Traditions* (New York: Simon and Schuster, 1974), p. 223.

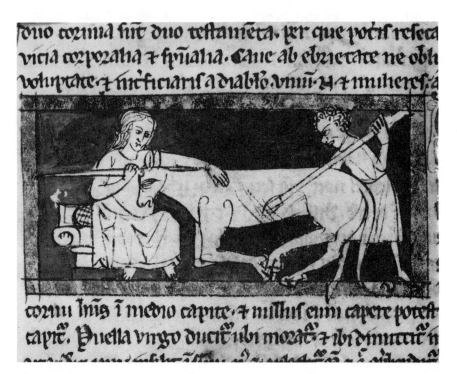

Figure 7. Unicorn and virgin. The bestiary tradition invoked the quasi-magical powers of female virginity in its account of the unicorn, which could not be caught or (as in this thirteenth-century example) killed by hunters unless first lured and tamed by a virgin. The unicorn was interpreted as representing Christ and the virgin as representing Mary. (Oxford, Bodleian, MS Douce 88, fol. 7v. Reproduced by permission of the Bodleian Library, Oxford.)

of their sons.[8] Bernard of Gordon was a prominent professor of medicine at the university at Montpellier, which, like Padua and Bologna, was a famous international center of medical learning.[9] Writing on the subject of child rearing in a general work on regimen, he placed chastity tenth on a list of things a tutor should teach a young man and first on the list of traits to be

8 Georges Duby, *Medieval Marriage: Two Models from the Twelfth Century*, trans. Elborg Forster (Baltimore and London: Johns Hopkins University Press, 1978), pp. 92–6. For a case in which civil authorities uphold the legitimacy of female virginity as a condition in a marriage contract, see Jean-Philippe Levy, "Officialité de Paris et les questions familiales à la fin du XIVᵉ siècle," in *Etudes d'histoire du droit canonique dediées à Gabriel Le Bras*, Ouvrage publié avec le concours du Centre national de la recherche scientifique, (Paris: Sirey, 1965), vol. 2, p. 1274.
9 On Bernard and his works see Luke Demaitre, *Doctor Bernard de Gordon: Professor and Practitioner* (Toronto: Pontifical Institute of Mediaeval Studies, 1980).

encouraged in young women.[10] (The virtue of chastity limited sexual acts to forms and circumstances deemed appropriate and prescribed a modest and restrained attitude toward those acts; it was thus equivalent to virginity in some situations and not in others.) By giving such instructions in a medical work, Bernard reinforced not only general values concerning proper sexual conduct but also the specific emphasis on the sexual conduct of women. The basis for the social value of female virginity was the security of legitimacy for children born in a subsequent marriage. In the late Middle Ages, the force of social concern for legitimacy can be seen in the regularity with which courts discovered the motive for infanticide to be the desire to hide an illegitimate birth. The evidence reveals a profound sense of shame in the country as well as in the towns, among the poor as well as among the rich.[11] Virginity was not, of course, the only means of avoiding illegitimacy, but it was the most reliable, if also the most severe. Noble families especially went to considerable length to preserve the virginity (and thereby the marriage value) of their daughters.[12]

Health practitioners assisted in the elevation of female virginity by providing certification of a woman's purity. Usually this office would be performed by a midwife, that is to say, a woman with obstetrical experience and knowledge, who would make a visual inspection. One very frequently copied and quoted source from the thirteenth century asserts that one can tell from a urine sample: a virgin's urine is clear; that of a *corrupta*, cloudy.[13] By providing the means to support social norms, physicians demonstrated their willingness to participate in and advance social goals. In addition to testing for virginity, they offered other means of guaranteeing legitimacy as well, such as recipes for preventing a woman from committing adultery.[14] Medical texts offer no such methods for the detection of male purity and fidelity.

Medical authors were not, however, simply apologists for or enforcers of social norms. Some, at least, were also willing to meet what were conceived of as less than respectable social needs. A tract on cosmetics which included some gynecological sections and was widely circulated in medical manuscripts gave instructions for counterfeiting virginity, including the use of a pessary filled with animal blood which would rupture during intercourse. The fact that some versions of the text omit these instructions, declaring that they have presented all the information that can decently be discussed,

10 Bernardus de Gordonio, *De regimine vii etatum* [= *De regimine sanitatis* = *De conservatione vite humane*, bk. IV], Cambridge, Gonville and Caius, MS 593, fols. 35vb–36ra.
11 Brissaud, "L'infanticide."
12 Duby, *Medieval Marriage*, pp. 92–3.
13 [Ps.-]Albertus Magnus, *De secretis mulierum*, ch. ix, p. 111. For a different urine test for virginity, see *Experimenta*, Vienna, Nationalbibliothek, MS CVP 2532, fol. 96v.
14 *Experimenta*, Vienna, MS CVP 2532, fols. 71r, 113r. See also [Ps.-]Albertus Magnus, *De secretis mulierum*, ch. x, p. 112.

underscores their acknowledged immorality.[15] Thus, in the case of virginity, medicine sometimes upheld the prevailing values and sometimes responded to social circumstances that failed to conform with those values. Medicine's complicity with the insistence on virginity is compromised by its role in a conspiracy to replace the substance of virginity with a mere shadow. Yet medicine is by no means at war with the value it evades, since the very act of counterfeiting (and the social circumstances that require it) must be based on the recognition of virginity as the true currency. Furthermore, in their attention solely to female virginity, medical texts reveal involvement with secular interests rather than with the increasingly tenuous gender neutrality of ecclesiastical values.

In spite of earlier Christian interest in male self-control, religious precepts and social opinion on virginity were in some respects easily accommodated to each other in the later Middle Ages. Virginity ensured freedom from the sin as well as from the social consequences of unchastity or illegitimate birth. Was this mutual support a true union or a marriage of convenience? There were important social and religious interests in limiting sexual activity. But in this as in all virtues, religion exacted not only material but also mental and spiritual compliance. Blamelessness of thought and intention were needed to meet the religious but not the secular requirements. In theological terms, physical virginity might be unchaste, if it involved uncontrolled thoughts and desires; and the essence of virginal purity might exist in spite of the absence of physical virginity, as might happen in cases of saved prostitutes. This non-physical model of virginity came to prevail in the Christian rhetoric of the late Middle Ages.[16] Jacques de Vitry, a prominent preacher of the early thirteenth century, asserted in a sermon on the married state that virginity is not lost in marriage but is retained in marital chastity.[17] This spiritual perspective diverged in two ways from that of socially construed virginity. First, in secular terms physical virginity was the primary concern, although moral decency was not insignificant. Natural philosophers endorsed this more physical, secular concept when they entertained the view that virgins might have especially great sexual appetite, thus embracing the distinction between acts and intentions and assigning primacy to the former in the definition of virginity.[18] The second, and consequent, divergence between the religious and secular views is that the religious formulation encouraged greater parity between female and male virginity not only doctrinally but by deemphasizing

15 *De ornatu mulierum*, Munich, Bayerische Staatsbibliothek, MS CLM 444, fol. 210rb; Bibliothèque Nationale, MS lat. 16089, fol. 115rb; Oxford, Exeter College, MS 35, fol. 230ra; Oxford, Bodleian, Digby 79, fol. 111v; and [Ps.-]Trotula, *De passionibus mulierum*, Cambridge University Library, MS Dd.11.45, fol. 73r–v; British Library, MS Sloane 1124, fol. 175rb–va. See Cadden, "Questions of Propriety."
16 Atkinson, " 'Precious Balsam.' "
17 D'Avray and Tausche, "Marriage Sermons," p. 88.
18 *De secretis mulierum*, Bibliothèque Nationale, MS lat. 7106, fol. 21r.

the observable anatomical aspect of the virtue, the unbroken hymen, to which sex difference was most relevant. On the other hand, the views of medical authorities were closer to the religious perspective on this point, for though they understood virginity in physical terms, they were not primarily interested in anatomy. But whereas religious writers displaced anatomical concerns with spiritual, medical writers and natural philosophers displaced anatomical concerns with physiological.

The strongest form of sexual abstinence in the Middle Ages was the vow of permanent sexual continence associated with full membership in religious orders. The number of men and women who took vows of chastity as members of religious communities was not negligible. Such vows were required not only of priests, monks, and nuns but were also a common element in many of the heresies and loosely organized confraternities in which lay piety often expressed itself in the late medieval and early modern period. Sexual restraint was an element of social order in the lives of those devoted to religious service, and the enforcement of restraint was an important aspect in the administration of Church institutions. One frequently mentioned manifestation of the unruliness of monks was sexual misconduct, and the imposition of celibacy and continence became a significant aspect of the perennial efforts at ecclesiastical reform. Colorful exceptions to the contrary notwithstanding, both monks and nuns took their vows of chastity seriously in at least one diocese in the midthirteenth century: on the basis of a register of hundreds of visits by Bishop Eudes de Rigaud to religious houses, Penny Johnson estimates that fewer than 5 percent of monks and nuns were guilty of breaching them.[19]

In certain respects, vows of chastity and their enforcement constituted an aspect of the larger social order as well. They regulated in a significant way the interaction of that community with the rest of society. Furthermore, the religious life offered the laity a life for surplus sons and daughters that was respectable and, perhaps more important, nonreproductive, and thus guaranteed not to produce still more heirs. This practice did not affect men and women in the same way, since for sons of propertied families the Church offered numerous opportunities for advancement, most of which were closed to women, and since as the medical recipes for having sons suggested, daughters, who had fewer choices in any case, were more likely to be sent off in hard times or when local conditions created the need for large dowries.

The congruence of religious and social interest with respect to the vows of religious life had its limits. Considerable family control over the marriage of children continued to exist and was widely considered appropriate.[20] For

---

19 Presentation by Penny Johnson to the Invitational Workshop in Honor of Mary Martin McLaughlin, New York, February 23, 1990.
20 At least among families of property, a powerful competing model of marriage – as a set of social, economic, or political opportunities – placed constraints on most daughters and

young people, especially young women, withholding consent might be effective in postponing marriage or in vetoing a particular marriage, but often in practice they were left with few real choices. In these situations, a vow of chastity might be an attractive alternative, even a way of exercising power. The story of Christina of Markyate, the daughter of an aristocratic family in twelfth-century England, as told by a religious follower at the end of her exemplary life, illustrates some of the problems that might surround the commitment to sexual abstinence.[21] At an early age Christina makes vows to devote herself to a religious life, and when her family presents her with a husband, she refuses to marry. Her parents subject her to bribery, torture, and solitary confinement, to no avail. They authorize her intended, who has been accused of being rendered effeminate by her behavior, to rape her. He does not succeed, and she makes a heroic escape. Throughout the story, both parties press their claims with religious authorities, some of whom act on the basis of their obligation to protect a religious vocation and others of whom act on the basis of their obligation to uphold contracts and the legitimate power of parents over children. In other words, the Church's own interests were divided between protecting virginity, on the one hand, and, on the other hand, enforcing the sacrament of marriage and preserving a modus vivendi with the laity. For Christina, the solution was to win the consent of the man to whom she had been promised. In the course of the later Middle Ages, pious women devised an increasing number of ways to enact and embody militant spirituality, with female abstinence assuming a special place in medieval religious sensibilities.[22] At a more general level, the solution was the accommodation of religious and secular interests through the evolution of a set of ideals for the lay Christian that advanced secular interests while incorporating religious values and practices, such as marital chastity and prescribed patterns of fasting and sexual abstinence.

Virginity and permanent vows, although they were the subject of a good deal of discussion and held an important symbolic place, were rarer than less absolute forms of sexual abstinence in the Middle Ages. The most common reason for deliberate (if perhaps imperfect) abstinence was the postponement of marriage. The population of Europe, especially in the wake of the demographic boom of the twelfth century and the subsequent exhaustion of avail-

---

some sons who did not and could not expect, as individuals, to control much property or power. David Herlihy, "The Making of the Medieval Family: Symmetry, Structure and Sentiment," *Journal of Family History* 3 (1983): 116–30. Families of less substance often had the same concerns on a smaller scale. Duby, *Economie rurale*, vol. 1, pp. 215–16; Shulamit Shahar, *The Fourth Estate: A History of Women in the Middle Ages,* trans. Chaya Galai (London and New York: Methuen, 1983), pp. 223–6.

21 Charles H. Talbot, ed. and trans., *The Life of Christina of Markyate, a Twelfth Century Recluse* (Oxford: Clarendon Press, 1959), pp. 34–118.
22 See Bynum, *Holy Feast and Holy Fast.*

able new lands, began to marry rather late.[23] Although important differences in laws, customs, and conditions led to considerable variation in practices from time to time and from place to place, limited statistical information suggests that the average interval between puberty and marriage was on the order of ten years for men and five years for women.[24] The coexistence of late marriage and a low illegitimacy rate would suggest that abstinence, nonreproductive sexual practices, or some combination was very common. It would be useful and fun to know what unmarried people actually did in the late Middle Ages, but evidence and methods are difficult to come by.[25] Medical sources suggest, as we shall see, that abstinence was perceived as a problem and that nonreproductive sexual practices – especially masturbation – were among the solutions entertained.

Other, less radical and more temporary renunciations of sexual activity were demanded of medieval populations. During Lent, for example, married Christians were called upon to refrain from sexual intercourse, just as soldiers were to stop fighting, all were to place restrictions on their diet, and houses of prostitution were to close (at least during Holy Week).[26] Fast days and feast days were opportunities for the Church to make its messages and its institutional power felt in the lay community. These religious demands were not as problematic as permanent religious vows, for they offered no fundamental challenge to lay morality or secular interests. Yet they strained common assumptions about marital relations and were subject to exceptions.

23 David Herlihy, "The Generation in Medieval History," *Viator* 5 (1974): 346–64, esp. pp. 355–60.

24 Jean-Louis Flandrin, *Families in Former Times: Kinship, Household and Sexuality*, trans. Richard Southern (Cambridge: Cambridge University Press, 1976), pp. 184–7; Duby, *Economie rurale*, vol. I, pp. 208–19; Herlihy, "Generation"; Shahar, *Fourth Estate*, pp. 228–29. Herlihy ("Making of the Medieval Family," p. 126) holds that in elite families, women married earlier in this period, in which case the greatest weight of the premarital sexual burden in the upper classes would have been borne by the young men. Perhaps we have here an explanation for the numerous recipes for anaphrodisiacs apparently intended for men, as well as for widespread and institutionally well developed prostitution.

25 These questions are the subject of considerable controversy among historians of early modern Europe. Jean-Louis Flandrin, "Contraception, mariage et relations amoureuses dans l'occident chrétien," *Annales: Economies, sociétés, civilisations* 24 (1969): 1370–90; idem, "Mariage tardif et vie sexuelle: Discussions et hypothèses de recherche," *Annales: Economies, sociétés, civilisations* 27 (1972): 1351–78 (including extensive use of late medieval sources); André Burguière, "De Malthus à Max Weber: Le mariage tardif et l'esprit d'entreprise," *Annales: Economies, sociétés, civilisations* 31 (1972): 1128–38; J. Depauw, "Amour illégitime et société à Nantes au XVIIIᵉ siècle," *Annales: Economies, sociétés, civilisations* 31 (1972): 1155–82; and John M. Riddle, "Oral Contraceptives and Early-Term Abortifacients during Classical Antiquity and the Middle Ages," *Past and Present* 132 (1991): 3–32.

26 See Jean-Louis Flandrin, *Un temps pour embrasser: Aux origines de la morale sexuelle occidentale (VIᵉ–IXᵉ siècle)*, L'univers historique (Paris: Editions du Seuil, 1983); Jacques Rossiaud, "Prostitution, jeunesse et société dans les villes du Sud-Est au XVᵉ siècle," *Annales: Economies, sociétés, civilisations* 31 (1976), pp. 291, 314, n. 13; Leah L. Otis, *Prostitution in Medieval Society: The History of an Urban Institution in Languedoc*, Women in Western Culture and Society (Chicago: University of Chicago Press, 1985), pp. 85–8.

Perhaps because it corresponded to more widely and strongly held taboos, religious opinion upheld without exception the duty of a woman to refuse her husband during her menstrual period.[27] The Old Testament warnings were grave, and popular beliefs included the expectation that children conceived during menstruation would be born with leprosy or epilepsy.[28] Medical and scientific texts, silent on the subject of abstinence on feast days, support the opposition to intercourse during menstruation. Very simply, according to one source, if conception occurs, the child will be monstrous or weak.[29] Whether or not conception occurs, the man's health is endangered. Men with cold constitutions are especially likely to suffer ill effects (as they do when they have intercourse with prenubile girls),[30] and intercourse with menstruating women can cause male sterility, as well as leprosy and cankers.[31] The implied mechanism for the harm done to offspring and to men is the association of menstrual blood with cold; life-sustaining heat will be insufficiently communicated to the fetus and may be drained from the man. This particular imperative for abstinence harks back to the special place menstruation held in female physiology. It was essential and salutary, because it purged the woman of potentially harmful superfluities. Once released from the woman's body, the menses no longer endanger her, but medical and more colloquial opinion agreed in regarding them as dangerous to others.

Medical authors and natural philosophers also supported the religious prohibition of intercourse during pregnancy, as their views on sterility suggested. And, as observed in connection with the problem of pleasure, they followed Aristotle, who believed that women and mares are the only females that will copulate when they are pregnant.[32] Though one thirteenth-century text does mention that intercourse during pregnancy induces labor,[33] physical harm to woman, man or fetus was not a prominent concern. Rather, the emphasis even in medical writings was upon the moral implications of woman's unrestrained sexual appetite. We have already encountered, in connection with the nonreproductive indulgence in sexual pleasure, the medical report of the woman who "gave birth to a lovely child who resembled her husband and a few days later gave birth to an ugly child

27 D'Avray and Tausche, "Marriage Sermons," p. 97. For more on the theology and natural philosophy of menstruation, see Wood, "Doctors' Dilemma."
28 Erikson, *Medieval Vision*, p. 195.
29 *Secreta mulierum minor*, Cambridge University, Trinity MSS O.2.5, fol. 130va–vb, and R.14.45, fol. 24v.
30 [*De coitu*], New York Academy of Medicine, MS "Collection of Surgical and Gynecological Texts," fol. 87vb.
31 Bernardus de Gordonio, *Lilium*, pt. VII, ch. i, fol. 87rb; commentary on [Ps.-]Albertus Magnus, *De secretis mulierum*, Prologue [II], p. 5. See Jacquart and Thomasset, *Sexuality and Medicine*, pp. 177–93.
32 Aristotle, *Generation of Animals*, IV, v, 773b25–26.
33 *Propositiones de animalibus*, Cambridge University Library, MS Dd.3.16, fol. 75rb.

who resembled her ugly lover."[34] Against the background of prescribed abstinence, the adultery underscores the dangers created by women's sexual appetite. Similarly, the widely disseminated treatise *On the Secrets of Women*, although based mainly on natural philosophical and medical sources, concerned itself not with the health consequences of intercourse during pregnancy but with the evidence it provided of women's sexual insatiability.[35] Women, according to scientific authorities, want pleasure as well as offspring. This double desire distinguishes them from female animals and shifts the issue of sexual appetite from the domain of nature to the domain of the will, hence to an area in which self-control in general and sexual abstinence in particular ought to be exercised.[36] The moral tone of medical and scientific writing on the subject of abstinence during pregnancy is related to the scholastic fascination with the plurality of women's pleasure and attests the integration of natural and moral discourse on this point, as does the invocation of health and nature in religious writings.[37]

The arguments against intercourse during pregnancy are related to those being developed in this period against other forms of nonreproductive sexual activity and bear forcefully the implication that continence is the favored, if not the required, behavior in a wide range of circumstances. Although canonists and theologians rendered these arguments more systematic and more general from the twelfth century on, coordinating their positions against contraception, abortion, and sodomy, the support of medical writers, apparent in the cases of intercourse during menstruation and pregnancy, was not similarly extended. There is, for example, very little medical disapprobation of contraception or homosexual behavior. In this respect natural philosophy and medicine did not produce a program for the control of sexuality in the way theology did.[38] In addition to those instances in which medical interests explicitly coincided with other cultural forces, the medical literature occasionally offered acknowledgment and indirect support to religiously or morally mandated abstinence. The extremely well circulated obstetrical treatise

---

34 Bernardus de Gordonio, *Lilium*, pt. VII, ch. ii, fol. 88rb: "Ideo accidit quod quedam mulier peperit unum filium pulchrum qui assimilabatur viro suo, et post paucos dies peperit unum turpem qui assimilabatur amassio suo turpi." Cf. *Propositiones de animalibus*, Cambridge University Library, MS Dd.3.16, fol. 75rb: "Quedam mulier post impregnationem fornicata fuit et peperit duos filios quorum unus assimilabatur coniungi et alter fornicatori."

35 *De secretis mulierum*, Munich, Bayerische Staatsbibliothek, MS CLM 3875, fol. 216vb.

36 Bernardus de Gordonio, *Lilium*, pt. VII, ch. ii, fol. 88rb; Nemesius, *De natura hominis*, ch. XXIV, p. 100.

37 Hildegard, *Scivias*, pt. I, vis. ii, ch. 22, pp. 28–9; D'Avray and Tausche, "Marriage Sermons," pp. 99, 107. Aquinas is unusual in taking a more generous position on intercourse during pregnancy. See Michel Riquet, "Christianity and Population," in Orest Ranum and Patricia Ranum, eds., *Popular Attitudes toward Birth Control in Pre-industrial France and England* (New York: Harper and Row, 1972), p. 38 (trans. from "Christianisme et population," *Population* 4 [1949]: 615–30).

38 See, e.g., Noonan, *Contraception*; and Boswell, *Christianity, Social Tolerance, and Homosexuality*.

known as *On the Diseases of Women,* or "Trotula," prefaces discussion of the ill effects of abstinence with the matter-of-fact observation that coitus is forbidden for some women – because of a vow or widowhood – and offers ways of dealing with the situation.[39] Thus, in at least some cases, medicine lent recognition to nonmedical reasons for abstinence.

Aside from the specific situations just examined, however, there were few circumstances in which medical authors prescribed abstaining from intercourse. Warnings about the dangers of intercourse were not uncommon, but they were specific to a small number of cases and conditions. Continence, along with other elements of regime designed to avoid taxing the body, was prescribed in cases of general bodily weakness such as consumption,[40] and it was important to the treatments for particular sexual disorders.[41] One author recommended short periods of abstinence for phlegmatic couples as part of a treatment for sterility.[42] Many medical works include recipes for anaphrodisiacs – cucumbers, fish, and vinegar – but there are many more recipes for aphrodisiacs.[43]

Most medical warnings against intercourse fail to specify whether they apply to men, to women, or to both. In some cases the context suggests men only, and the general opinion that men use up natural heat in intercourse would support that interpretation. Even those authors who held that women as well as men produce seed and who drew upon Galenic sources tended to disregard the effects of coitus upon women. If coitus itself was not harmful to women in special conditions of weakness, its most serious result might be. *On the Diseases of Women* introduces a contraceptive with the observation that there are women for whom childbirth would be dangerous. Either because they have been injured in a previous birth or for other reasons, they would fear for their lives if pregnant. Abstinence is the obvious safeguard for these women, but, the author observes, they cannot all abstain.[44] We do not know if the impediment to abstinence was supposed to have resulted from women's inability to control their sexual appetites or from the impossibility of refusing their husbands (probably the latter).

The recipes for anaphrodisiacs in other texts likewise suggest that people (or perhaps men) need medical help in the pursuit of abstinence. One work is quite open about the problem and introduces remedies for those who are

39 [Ps.-]Trotula, *De passionibus mulierum*, Cambridge University Library, MS Dd.11.45, fol. 68v; British Library, MS Sloane 1124, fol. 172va. See also Cartelle, ed., *Liber minor de coitu*, pt. I, ch. 4, p. 64.

40 [*De coitu*], New York Academy of Medicine, MS "Collection of Surgical and Gynecological Texts," fol. 86vb.

41 Bernardus de Gordonio, *Lilium*, pt. VII, ch. ii, fol. 38ra.

42 *De impedimentis conceptionis* (Pagel, "Raymundus de Moleriis," p. 535).

43 Constantinus, *De coitu*, chs. 13–17, pp. 142–184. See also *Liber remediorum*, Munich, Bayerische Staatsbibliothek, MS CLM 77, fol. 16ra.

44 [Ps.-]Trotula, *De passionibus mulierum*, Cambridge University Library, MS Dd.11.45, fol. 63r.

not able to abstain or keep a vow.[45] The sympathetic helpfulness of these authors allows us to conclude, first (and not surprisingly), that abstinence was not easily achieved by ordinary people and, second, that medical works, in offering formulas for the suppression of sexual appetite, reflected the acceptance of a physical notion of sexual abstinence. As with virginity, so with abstinence and chastity more generally, the Augustinian view, increasingly invoked in late medieval theology, held that spiritual (not physical) state was paramount and that the essence of renouncing the world (including sex) was a spiritual act.[46] Making good behavior easy by providing medicines to minimize the tribulations was at least an evasion of the question of will. Indeed, it may even have presented an implicit challenge to that religious rationale for abstinence, since, like castration, it devalued the meaning of continence. Thus it illustrates the ambiguity and tenuousness of medicine's support for religiously motivated abstinence.

THE REINS ON RESTRAINT

There were, in fact, a significant number of forces undermining the value placed on virginity and on sexual abstinence more generally. The strongest objections came from medicine and natural philosophy, but there were also social and religious factors that limited the principles and practices of sexual continence. As the story of Christina of Markyate illustrates, the potential for conflict between the ascetic tendencies of the Christian religion and the social imperatives of the Christian laity was considerable. For that very reason, the incentives for accommodation were strong. Both the ideals of Christian community and the realities of interrelated lay and ecclesiastical elites favored the development of an integrated, if not entirely homogeneous, institution of marriage which would have a place for religious observances (including sexual abstinence) and a place for fulfilling social functions (including sexual and reproductive activity). The evolution of the concept of the marriage debt – the sexual obligation of husband and wife to each other – is an example of such accommodation, as is the bending of canon law to acknowledge the strength of lay opinion that a valid marriage must be sexually consummated.[47] The convergence of social practice and religious sensibility was a codification of social values, framed within the developing sacrament of marriage. If lust, lasciviousness, and overindulgence were particularly barred within marriage, so was continence, except in special cases by mutual agreement. Marriage was not the most exalted state,

45 Cartelle, ed., *Liber minor de coitu*, pt. I, ch. 4, p. 64.
46 Atkinson, " 'Precious Balsam,' " pp. 134–5.
47 Helmholz, *Marriage Litigation*, pp. 26–7, 32, 139–40. See also James A. Brundage, "The Treatment of Marriage in the *Questiones Londinenses* (MS Royal 9.E.VII)," *Manuscripta* 19 (1975): 86–97.

but it had developed into an *ordo*, a recognized status, and as such involved rights and responsibilities which helped define its function and place and which were incorporated into religious doctrine and canon law.

Within this coordination, however, tensions persisted. First, there are hints that some conflict was perceived between the observance of feast and fast days, on the one hand, and family life and the marriage debt, on the other. Second, although the doctrinal accommodation of the reproductive imperative found some support in the injunction to be fruitful and multiply, of the three "goods" of marriage – *fides* (mutual fidelity), *proles* (children), and *sacramentum* (the bond's indissolubility) – *proles* was not the most prominent in the late medieval ecclesiastical construct of marriage, and toward the end of the period didactic stories about happy and successful continent couples illustrated the view that it was not necessarily through reproduction that marriage provided a path to salvation.[48] Neither the injunction to be fruitful nor the concept of the marriage debt played an important role in sermons on marriage.[49] The ritual of marriage itself placed much more emphasis on such principles as consent and indissolubility than it did on progeny. Apart from fairly frequent references to the story of Sarah and the story of Tobias, and the prayer that the newlyweds live, grow old, and be multiplied in the love of God, there are strikingly few references to the marriage debt or to progeny in marriage rituals.[50] Even when the sexual dimension of marriage was at issue, especially in the blessing of the bed-chamber and bed, the rhetoric of the prayers and benedictions was aimed more at the promotion of marital chastity (fidelity, moderation, and pure intentions) than at the promotion of fecundity.[51] In some versions of the ritual, the word "seed" is even used metaphorically: "Bless these young people and sow the seeds of eternal life in their minds."[52] This echo of what must have been popular fertility practices is an indication that the incorporation of the sexual imperative within marriage into religious doctrine and canon law was in part an acquiescence to the needs and interests of the laity. The necessity to produce children and, in the case of families with substantial property, heirs was an essential aspect of the lay perspective on marriage,[53] but religious language muted the sexual and reproductive potency of

---

48 Leclercq, *Monks on Marriage*, pp. 43–8; Penny S. Gold, "The Marriage of Mary and Joseph in the Twelfth-Century Ideology of Marriage," in Vern L. Bullough and James A. Brundage, eds., *Sexual Practices and the Medieval Church* (Buffalo: Prometheus, 1982), pp. 102–17.

49 D'Avray and Tausche, "Medieval Marriage Sermons."

50 Jean-Baptiste Molin and Protais Mutembe, *Le rituel du mariage en France du Xᵉ au XVᵉ siècle*, Théologie historique 26 (Paris: Beauchesne, 1974). There is a prayer that cites God's intention to perpetuate the race through the institution of marriage and mentions the marriage debt (pp. 241 and 256).

51 Ibid., esp. ch. 12.

52 Ibid., p. 327: ". . . benedic adolescentes istos, et semina semen vite eterne in mentibus eorum. . . ."

53 Duby, *Medieval Marriage*, pp. 87–92.

the bed and the seed. In short, the Church acknowledged and lay society insisted that, in general, abstinence within marriage was problematic.

The social case against abstinence, weakly supported by the ecclesiastical recognition of the marriage debt, was strongly supported by philosophical and medical doctrine. Refraining from intercourse constituted a breach of the general principles of balance (which governed medieval concepts of what we would call physiology) and of moderation (which governed medieval concepts of the healthy regimen). The principle of moderation condemns not only overdoing but also underdoing and thus forms the basis for a medical disapprobation of sexual abstinence. Moderate amounts of sleep, waking, rest, exercise, food, drink, and sexual intercourse were necessary to sustain health.[54] In his treatise on intercourse, Constantine the African, the late eleventh-century medical writer and Benedictine monk, invoked the authority of Galen and Epicurus when he stated flatly that "no one who does not have intercourse will be healthy. Intercourse is truly useful and promotes health."[55] The endorsement of intercourse was not unqualified. Not only are men with specific disabilities enjoined from indulging, but – and here the theme of moderation is sounded – too much intercourse is harmful to anyone. Still, from the point of view of the matter at hand, the lesson is: there is indeed such a thing as too little sex.

An anonymous tract *On Intercourse* of the thirteenth century opens with a warning against immoderate venery.[56] But about halfway through the work the author changed course.[57] "There are those," he said, "who deny themselves this act and say it does nothing good for the body."[58] They are deceived.[59] If coitus were always harmful, it would not be part of nature.[60] On this point he invoked the authority of Hippocrates, Galen, and Nemesius, perhaps regarding the argument against abstinence that follows as more controversial and therefore more in need of the weight of authority than the argument against sexual excess. "We have seen some people who, for the love of chastity and the admiration of philosophy, did not wish to

---

54 This formulation of the categories of regimen was a commonplace from the Hippocratic period on. See, e.g., Constantinus, *De coitu*, ch. 8, p. 112; and [*De philosophia*], Munich, Bayerische Staatsbibliothek, MS CLM 8742, fol. 46.

55 Constantinus, *De coitu*, ch. 8, p. 112: ". . . nullus qui [non] coierit sanus erit – , veraciter utilis est coitus et proficiens ad salutem . . ." (my emendation).

56 Cartelle, ed., *Liber minor de coitu*, pt. I, ch. 1, p. 56.

57 [*De coitu*], New York Academy of Medicine, MS "Collection of Surgical and Gynecological Texts," fol. 87rb: "Nunc de eius edicatur utilitate." Cf. Cartelle, ed., *Liber minor de coitu*, pt. II, ch. 1, p. 78.

58 [*De coitu*], New York Academy of Medicine, MS "Collection of Surgical and Gynecological Texts," fol. 87rb: "Sunt qui eam operationem sibi denegant et nichil corpori prodesse affirmant." Cf. Cartelle, ed., *Liber minor de coitu*, pt. I, ch. 1, p. 78.

59 To the preceding quotation, Cambridge University, Gonville and Caius, MS 415, fol. 102r, adds ". . . quamvis eos esse mendaces sensus ipse comprobet." Cartelle, ed., *Liber minor de coitu*, pt. I, ch. 1, p. 78.

60 Ibid., pt. II, ch. 1, p. 80.

obey nature, and retained a lot of seed."[61] Dire consequences result from such restraint, ranging from headaches to weight loss to melancholia.

The physical mechanisms that cause these effects are bound up in the second, related principle upon which medical objections to abstinence were based: the concept of constitutional and temperamental balance. The retention of semen by men or women, like the retention of menses by women, creates an imbalance in the humors which carry out the operations of the body and govern its disposition. Those suffering from sciatica and arthritis are vulnerable to the ill effects of too much venery, as are men with fat, pale, humid bodies resembling women and phlegmatics.[62] They are already cold by nature and the loss of the heat inherent in the seed emitted during intercourse would only increase their coldness. But those with ample flesh and a hot, moist constitution will suffer if they avoid intercourse.[63] Unlike their phlegmatic neighbors, these people are not in danger of becoming too cold but would be harmed if they did not slough off some heat by emitting hot, moist seed. Although semen is a useful residue, a refined superfluity (unlike excrement), its accumulation could nevertheless unbalance the body and thus cause or exacerbate illness. And although people of different constitutions require different regimens, the release of seed by men and, according to many if not all medical writers, women serves a purgative function as part of a system of bodily intake and output. The specific problems associated with too much heat (from too little release of seed) and too little heat (from excessive release of seed) are less critical for women than for men, since their bodies in general and their seed in particular contain less heat, and since menstrual purgation draws off many superfluities. In other respects, however, women are quite susceptible to breaches of moderation and balance, and thus widows and nuns may "incur grave illness."[64]

Like overindulgence, abstinence is more harmful to some than to others. A thirteenth-century work counsels men with abundant *ventositas* (the windiness which causes erection) to avoid sexual abstinence, fasting, vigils, overwork, and beans.[65] Hildegard of Bingen, writing from a convent in the twelfth century, was of the opinion that sanguine men and dry women can abstain from sex without serious repercussions.[66] A person's sex is one of a number of factors that may influence the impact of continence. Hildegard believed that women, because they menstruate, are *healthier* than men in

61 [*De coitu*], New York Academy of Medicine, MS "Collection of Surgical and Gynecological Texts," fol. 87va: "Vidimus et nos aliquos qui castitatis amore et favore filosofie naturam noluerunt obsequi et copiam seminis detinuere." Cf. Cartelle, ed., *Liber minor de coitu*, pt. I, ch. 1, p. 78.

62 Cartelle, ed., *Liber minor de coitu*, pt. I, ch. 1, p. 56.

63 Ibid., p. 58; ch. 4, p. 68.

64 [Ps.-]Trotula, [*De passionibus mulierum*], British Library, MS Sloane 1124, fol. 172va: ". . . gravem incurrunt egritudinem."

65 *De impedimentis conceptionis* (Pagel, "Raymundus de Moleriis," p. 532).

66 Hildegard, *Causae et curae*, bk. II, pp. 72, 77.

some respects.[67] Female virgins are particularly susceptible to ill health,[68] and some held that abstinence is more unhealthy for women than for men. Hildegard held this to be so because men discharge more of their seed than women, perhaps a reference to nocturnal emissions and masturbation; Bernard of Gordon cited more generally women's constitution and way of life.[69] There is significant disagreement about which sex finds it more *difficult* to abstain, another question that extends beyond physiology to mores. Hildegard argued, for example, that women are more easily continent, both because their appetite is dissipated in the spaciousness of the womb and because they experience more shame and fear.[70] On the other hand, a commentary on the pseudo–Albertus Magnus *On the Secrets of Women* represents female desire as stronger and female morality as weaker.[71]

Most of the medical distinctions among groups of people as well as the general contraindication of abstinence were based on the principles of humoral balance and the assumption that release of seed maintains and restores balance. The remedies for the ill effects of abstinence suggested by medical authors confirm this understanding of the role of sexual activity in sustaining health: they are aimed either at restoring balance by the use of medicines and diets or, less frequently, at promoting the purgation of accumulated seed. For example, the "Trotula" treatise *On the Diseases of Woman* recommends that women whose circumstances or vows require continence treat the consequent pain and sickness by applying to the vulva a silk cloth soaked in a mixture of wine and herbs.[72] Some authors clearly expected that emissions of seed would occur naturally in the absence of sexual intercourse: men and women would experience nocturnal emissions.[73] Others prescribed masturbation. Galen and Avicenna had paved the way on this point by recommending masturbation for celibate men to avoid the detrimental effects of seed retention. For a widow or a virgin suffering from seed retention, they recommend that a midwife rub the genitals until seed is ejected.[74]

Insofar as they condemn virginity as essentially unhealthy, these medical

67 Ibid., pp. 99–100, 102.
68 *De impedimentis conceptionis* (Arlt, *Schule von Montpellier*, p. 23); [Excerpts from *Secreta secretorum*], British Library, MS Egerton 2852, fol. 112; some versions of "Trotula," e.g., Cambridge University Library, MS Dd.11.45, fol. 68v.
69 Hildegard, *Causae et curae*, bk. II, p. 77; Bernardus de Gordonio, *Lilium*, pt. VII, ch. i, fols. 87vb–88ra.
70 Hildegard, *Causae et curae*, bk. II, p. 76.
71 E.g., *De secretis mulierum*, Bibliothèque Nationale, MS lat. 7106, fol. 21r; *Propositiones de animalibus*, Cambridge University Library, MS Dd.3.16, fol. 75rb.
72 [Ps.-]Trotula, *De passionibus mulierum*, Cambridge University Library, MS Dd.11.45, fol. 68v.
73 Albertus Magnus, *De animalibus*, bk. X, tr. i, chs. 1 and 2. Cf. Aristotle, *Generation of Animals*, II, iv, 739a22–26.
74 On Galen, Avicenna, and some medieval Latin authors who agree, see Lemay, "William of Saliceto," pp. 177–8. See also the remedy for suffocation of the womb caused by retention of seed in *De impedimentis conceptionis* (Arlt, *Schule von Montpellier*, p. 23).

views present a limited challenge to family interests in guaranteeing marriage arrangements and legitimacy. More important, insofar as they oppose abstinence within marriage and provide nonreproductive solutions to health problems caused by abstaining from intercourse, they support the interests of secular society in the production of offspring within and only within marriage and perhaps also in attempts at family limitation. Medical opinion was slightly more problematic in relation to religious values. Although chastity was in some sense a virtue of moderation, the medical sense of moderation was offended by its more ascetic manifestations – virginity and continence.

The case of sexual abstinence shows medicine offering now support, now challenges (both in terms of rationale and in terms of practices), to the values of lay society and Christian institutions, themselves alternately harmonious and dissonant. Deriving from separate traditions and maintaining an independent existence, medicine was certainly not insulated from its context. Rather, medicine reflected a clear and sometimes uneasy awareness of its environment. Its position sometimes opposed the interests of religion and society, as with the disapprobation of a monk's continence or of a noble daughter's virginity, but its flexibility as manifested in the provision of remedies for the ill effects of abstention prevented the outbreak of open hostilities. There was no warfare between medicine and other values. Nor was there a cozy complicity. Although medicine might earnestly support the popular and scriptural condemnation of intercourse during pregnancy, its conclusions were sometimes more compatible than its reasoning, based often on physical rather than spiritual, individual rather than family, concerns. Indeed, the interactions are more complicated yet. When social and religious interests clashed, medicine might incline toward one or the other (usually the social), as in the prescription of nonreproductive sexual behaviors. And when there were tensions within the religious or the social domain, medicine might lend its voice to one position (preferring, for example, the fulfillment of the marriage debt to the observation of fast days) or to both (providing, for example, both the means to verify and the means to falsify a girl's virginity).

There is a consistency in the ways in which medical authors dealt with continence in men and women. Like sterility, sexual abstinence posed a set of concrete issues with which medical authors dealt frankly and directly in relation to both sexes. The result was a blurring of some of the distinctions between the sexes that tended to derive from and reinforce gender typology. Sexual release was necessary for both sexes; sexual abstinence was unhealthy for both. With respect to this symmetry, medical opinion was consonant with Christian doctrine, which in principle accorded similar value to the chastity of women and men, even though the medical and religious imperatives were in conflict – religion tending to promote and medicine tending to oppose strict sexual restraint as an ideal. In spite of the general principles establishing structural parallels between women and men, specific ecclesiastical and medical views converged with lay opinion, which placed significantly higher value upon female virginity, abstinence, chastity, and fidelity.

Each intellectual framework drew on its own circumstances, premises, and vocabulary. The Church was dealing not only with the legacy of Eve and Mary but also with emergent forms of feminine religious expression and with anxieties about them. Lay society entertained interests in orderly interactions within and among families, as well as in its more specific gender values. Medicine and, to a lesser extent, natural philosophy worked with distinctions of physiology and anatomy, as well as with the need to provide treatments and remedies for men and women with specific social and religious concerns. Medicine's contribution to the general problem of abstinence as it was formulated within these overlapping sectors of medieval culture, was ambiguous. Medical texts prescribed masturbation and herbal recipes to accommodate the promotion of abstinence but regularly recommended against the practice. More specifically, in connection with abstinence, medical opinion pointed up tensions and dangers associated with women's physiological, reproductive, and sexual natures. Support for abstinence came from the physical and moral dangers associated with menstruation and pregnancy. In that context, men's abstinence was not only a struggle for self-mastery but also a defense against a positive threat. Medical understanding also gave substance to that threat by suggesting its connection with women's sexual appetite, and thus in turn with the whole issue of sexual pleasure. As in the case of sexual pleasure, where physicians and canonists based their common condemnations of certain coital positions on incompatible assumptions, so in the case of sexual abstinence, agreement upon women's problematic and even dangerous sexual nature came from markedly different perspectives on the value of abstinence itself. Once again, where gender is concerned, neither complicity nor warfare characterizes the relationship between the outlook of learned physicians and natural philosophers and the values of other spheres of medieval culture. Sex difference as understood in terms of the natural characteristics of females and males did not inevitably entail a specific system of gender relations, but it did participate in the process by which a network of gender constructs was negotiated and sustained.

CONCLUSION

Latin medicine and natural philosophy manifested their flexibility and re-sourcefulness directly, when they dealt with specific problems like those posed by infertility or sexual abstinence, and indirectly, when they applied the language of sex difference to a broad array of subjects in a wide variety of contexts. They made use of the sorts of theories inherited from the ancients and taught in the universities – theories about coitus, sex determination, the purgation of superfluities, and the production of generative seed. They did not, however, adhere strictly to any one of these, much less to any system encompassing them all. This elusiveness or lack of dogmatism drew support from a number of sources and circumstances. First, their broad sense of basic sex distinctions, which went far beyond our notion of the biological to include disposition and mores, as well as the various extensions and applications of male–female terminology and thus of gender notions, made it difficult, if not impossible, for a single self-contained and consistent theory (or even set of theories) to suffice. Second, the concrete demands of specific problems of the sort encountered in the last two chapters encouraged eclectic or ad hoc approaches. Here medicine and natural philosophy were operating in territories also inhabited by social values and religious concerns, a situation that sometimes called for adjustment or negotiation. Third, the authors addressing these subjects were heirs to the diversity of traditions and genres which had accumulated from late antiquity on. Thus, they had a wealth of resources and methods upon which to draw. And finally, the theories themselves were not entirely settled. Scholastic philosophers and medical writers, for example, recognized that "female seed" could have any number of senses, which they discussed at length, but they did not come to any clear collective conclusion either about its meaning or about its role.

Some concepts of medicine and natural philosophy permeate most of the theories among which medieval authors could choose, but none was sufficiently strong to unify the field. In particular, heat was a component of a large number of explanations and prescriptions. It was one of the most fundamental factors in the distinction between females and males. It had a place in pharmacology, astrology, and ideas about the production of semen. It operated as a basis for the conceptualization of the masculine and the feminine both within and beyond reproduction – in the analysis of sexual appetites and in the explanation for different degrees of physical activity. But not all relevant dimensions of medicine and natural philosophy were regularly expressed in terms of the presence or lack of heat, even if some might be ultimately reducible to them. More important, to conclude that heat was the key to understanding sex difference and its gender implications would necessitate suppressing all the evidence rehearsed in this study of a multifaceted, multilayered, nonreductive way of working. Even in the rather abstract realms of natural philosophy and in the rationalistic and systematic environment of scholasticism, especially in the more practice-linked realms of medicine and in the complicated environment of social and religious forces, serious intellectuals could not have and did not practice their professions on the basis of a single principle, no matter how malleable and widely applicable it might be.

On the other hand, the description, explanation, and attribution of differences between the sexes was clearly not a free-for-all. Medicine and natural philosophy were not just offering up an undifferentiated and unstructured grab bag of miscellaneous components that other elements in the culture, say the Church or the aristocracy, could appropriate and use to enforce some gender agenda of their own. If nothing else, the fact that either medicine or natural philosophy sometimes differed from other perspectives is evidence that this was not the case. Their positions were guided by, but not reducible to, a cluster of principles which included not only the operations of heat but also the concepts of moderation and balance, with their attendant notion of purgation, and the sets of ideas associated with teleology and value hierarchies, such as the conviction that regular operations in nature are purposeful and good. Principles like these gave rise in turn to certain general ways of viewing sex difference, like the belief that sexual differentiation (in its reproductive and social manifestations) is a good thing, or the sense that women have less reproductive, physical, and intellectual strength and ability than men, and at the same time greater susceptibility to pleasure, disease, and reproductive failure than men.

Modern interests favor expressing such conclusions in terms of medieval views of women, but were women the issue to the authors whose works are represented here? Yes and no. Men were clearly central, primary, and standard. Two treatises entitled *On coitus*, for example, are almost entirely about men's anatomy, physiology, experiences, disorders, and regimens. In that respect, the woman is marginal, but she is certainly not invisible. Among the reasons for her marginality is her incompleteness, from which arises not only a social dependence on man but also a conceptual dependence on the masculine standard. This incompleteness also gives rise to specific female properties which *do* make her an issue, such as her sexual appetite when pregnant, her irascibility and unreliability, and her ability to prevent conception by jumping or dancing. Thus, the nature of woman was a serious preoccupation of medieval authors not so much in spite of as because of the reasons for her lack of importance.

The conceptual and social dependence of the female on the male and the woman on the man does not make medieval distinctions of sex and gender superficial; indeed, it *is* one of the important distinctions – one that medieval commentators called attention to in their readings of Genesis. In addition, the definition of the feminine in terms of the masculine was not all-encompassing. The womb is unique and the treatises on gynecology and obstetrics have a character of their own. The generative powers of the alchemical female and the physiognomic properties of the leopard belong to different systems of distinction. Furthermore, the efforts made by medieval authors both within and outside the disciplines of natural philosophy and medicine to explain and label things in the terms of a binary language confirm that the two sexes did mark a profound and significant division of the world. Lesbians and gays were accorded no existence, and homosexual behaviors were "masculine" or "feminine." A person with a mixture of traits was treated neither as an entity outside the duality nor as a synthesis in which the distinctness of the properties was submerged. On the contrary, such a person was explained in terms of the actions of two distinct forces (hot and cold or right and left) and labeled with combinations of two distinct sets of terms ("feminine male" or "virile woman"). The existence of hermaphrodites was both a logical consequence of the binary arrangement and a challenge to it, to which medieval authors' only partially satisfactory response was to lump them together with other problematic cases like bearded women, whose labels, if not lives, conformed to the two-sex division. Finally, the extension of the meanings of sex difference within creation but beyond the sphere of sexually reproducing animals, and even to the duality of the body and the soul, indicates how powerful those meanings were. The planets are masculine and feminine only partly because the gods whose names they bear are males and females (Saturn exerts a feminine influence). The terms and concepts are more than convenient analogies for the warm and cold powers of the heavenly bodies or the passive and active nature of a human being's body and soul. Their broad application suggests that the definitions and properties of female and male represented a principle which, at least partly, ordered the world.

WORKS CITED

MANUSCRIPTS

Authors and titles of works cited from manuscripts are listed as given in the manuscripts, usually according to the identification that appears most contemporaneous with the hand of the text. I have supplied additional identification in brackets, sometimes on the basis of collection catalogues or Thorndike and Kibre. In the case of several manuscripts, the material is miscellaneous and highly fragmented. Manuscripts marked "[Ph.]" were consulted in photoreproduction only.

Cambridge

Gonville and Caius College 415
 [Ps.-]C[onstantinus] A[fricanus], *De coitu*, fols. [100]r–[103]v.
Gonville and Caius College 593
 Bernardus de Gordonio, *De regimine vii etatum* [= *De regimine sanitatis* = *De conservatione vite humane*, bk. IV], fols. 30ra–56ra.
Trinity College O.2.5
 Secreta mulierum maior [= *De generatione humana*], fols. 75ra–85vb.
 Secreta mulierum minor, fols. 130va–132va.
Trinity College R.14.45
 [*Secreta mulierum minor*], fols. 24r–27r.
University Library Dd.3.16
 Propositiones de animalibus, fols. 73ra–76vb.
University Library Dd.11.45
 [Ps.-]Trotula, *De passionibus mulierum*, fols. 62v–80v.

Erfurt

Wissenschaftliche Bibliothek, Amplon. Q 299 (II) [Ph.: Columbia University Library, Lynn Thorndike Collection of Reproductions of MSS]
 [Johannes] Buridanus, *Questiones super* Secreta mulierum, fols. 167r–175v.

London

British Library, add. 37079
 [Petrus de Abano, *Physiognomia*], fols. 3r–81v.

British Library, Cotton. App. VI
  [astrology], fols. 8rb–20va.
British Library, Egerton 1984
  Thomas [Cantimpratensis?], *De partibus et membris corporis*, fols. 143r–144r.
British Library, Egerton 2852
  [gynecology], fols. 111r–114r.
British Library, Harley 5402
  Alkindrinus [nativities], fols. 1r–54v.
British Library, Sloane 282
  [medical questions], fols. 52v–53v.
British Library, Sloane 336
  Nicolaus Florentinus, *Capitulum de causa masculinitatis et femininitatis*, fols. 156r–
    159v.
British Library, Sloane 430
  [remedies], fols. 37v–60v.
British Library, Sloane 1124
  [Ps.-]Trotula, [*De passionibus mulierum*], fols. 172ra–178va.

Munich

Bayerische Staatsbibliothek, CLM 77
  Liber remediorum, fols. 1ra–17vb.
Bayerische Staatsbibliothek, CLM 444
  De ornatu mulierum, fols. 208rb–210rb.
Bayerische Staatsbibliothek, CLM 637
  Petrus de Padua [= de Abano], *Liber compilationis phisionomie.*
Bayerische Staatsbibliothek, CLM 3206
  [Thomas Cantimpratensis], *De proprietatibus et natura rerum*, fols. 1ra–145va.
Bayerische Staatsbibliothek, CLM 3875
  [Ps.-Albertus Magnus], *De secretis mulierum,* fols. 206va–215va.
Bayerische Staatsbibliothek, CLM 8742
  Johannes de Sancto Amando, *Concordantie artis medicine,* fols. 1r–42v.
  [philosophy, medicine], fols. 44r–49v.

New York

New York Academy of Medicine, "Collection of Surgical and Gynecological Texts"
  [*De coitu*], fols. 86vb–88rb.

Oxford

Bodleian Library, Ashmol. 399
  Physiognomia, fols. 1r–13r.
Bodleian Library, Ashmol. 1471
  [Ps.-]Galen, *Liber de xii portis*, fols. 68r–71v.
Bodleian Library, Bodley 484
  [Ps.-]Ysidorus, *De spermate*, fols. 45r–47r.

Bodleian Library, canon. misc. 350
  Guilhelmus de Mirica, *Physionomia*, fols. 1r–217v.
Bodleian Library, Digby 79
  [Trotula extracts, etc.], fols. 106r–119r.
Exeter College 35
  [Commentary on] *Versus Egidii*, fols. 52ra–85va.
  De ornatu mulierum, fols. 228vb–230ra.
New College 264
  Wilielmus de Wethelay, *De signis pronosticis sterilitatis*, fols. 253ra–264rb.

Paris

Bibliothèque Nationale, lat. 820
  [*Materia medica*], fol. 165ra.
Bibliothèque Nationale, lat. 6524
  Extractiones quedam de libris fratris Alberti Teutonici naturalibus.
Bibliothèque Nationale, lat. 6961
  Petrus Padubanensis [de Abano], *Conciliator discordiarum medicinalium*, fols. 1ra–269rb.
Bibliothèque Nationale, lat. 6964
  Thadeus [Florentinus], *Experimenta*, fols. 100ra–117ra.
Bibliothèque Nationale, lat. 7036
  [Constantinus Africanus, *De dietis universalibus*], fols. 1r–56v.
Bibliothèque Nationale, lat. 7066
  Jordanus de Turri, *De impregnatione mulieris*, fols. 6r–11r.
  De preparatione mulierum ad conceptum, fols. 11v–12v.
  Petrus de Nardillis, *De impregnatione mulieris*, fol. 13r–19v.
  De iuvantibus mulieres ad impregnandum, fol. 21r–v.
  Johannes Patavanus, *Regimen de conceptione*, fols. 24r–26v.
  Bernardus de Gordonio, *De sterilitate mulierum*, fols. 28r–32r.
Bibliothèque Nationale, lat. 7106
  De secretis mulierum, fols. 1r–62r.
Bibliothèque Nationale, lat. 7349
  [Ps.-]Albertus Magnus, *Anatomia*, fols. 16r–19v.
Bibliothèque Nationale, lat. 14809
  Philosophia sive De generatione humana, fols. 298v–312v.
Bibliothèque Nationale, lat. 16089
  Petrus de Padua [= de Abano], *Liber compilationis physionomie*, fols. 98ra–112vb.
  De ornatu mulierum, fols. 113ra–115rb.
Bibliothèque Nationale, lat. 16133
  Paulus, *De causa sterilitatis mulorum*, fols. 83ra–86rb.
Bibliothèque Nationale, lat. 16166
  Gerardus de Brolio, *Super librum* De animalibus, fols. 1ra–182vb.
Bibliothèque Nationale, lat. 16195
  [Ps.-]Th[omas], *De coitu*, fols. 23vb–25ra.
Bibliothèque Nationale, lat. nouv. acq. 693
  [*De generatione humana*], fols. 183r–184v.

Vienna

Nationalbibliothek, CVP 2532 [Ph.: Hill Monastic Manuscript Library 15,805]
  Experimenta, fols. 26r–55r.
  [medical formulary], fols. 67r–99v.
  Macer, *Experimenta*, fols. 106r–117r.

Zurich

Zentralbibliothek, Car. C. 172 [Ph.]
  [*De generatione humana*], fols. 3v–6v.

PRINTED WORKS

Because editions of texts in this field often contain significant critical and interpretive material, and monographs sometimes incorporate whole or partial editions of medieval texts, I have not divided the bibliography into separate lists of primary and secondary sources. Where one work contains sufficient material of both kinds to so warrant, I have given the full entry under the main author's name and included a cross-reference at the other author's name.

Medieval authors have been entered under their Latin names in order to keep works by the same author together. When their names appear in other forms on title pages or when they are commonly known by another name, I have provided cross-references. I have alphabetized medieval authors by first name, except as necessitated by established tradition, as with Geoffrey Chaucer, and have given cross-references where common usage might give rise to confusion, as with Johannes Buridanus.

Abelardus, Petrus, and Heloisa. *Lettres*. Edited by Victor Cousin; translated by Octave Gérard. 2d ed. Paris: Garnier Frères, 1875.
Adelardus. *Die Quaestiones Naturales des Adelardus von Bath*. Edited by Martin Müller. Beiträge zur Geschichte der Philosophie und Theologie des Mittelalters 31/2. Münster: Aschendorff, 1934.
Alan of Lille. *See* Alanus de Insulis; Häring, Nikolaus
Alanus de Insulis. *See* Häring, Nikolaus
Albertus Magnus. *De animalibus libri XXVI*. Edited by Hermann Stadler. Beiträge zur Geschichte der Philosophie des Mittelalters 15 and 16. Münster: Aschendorff, 1916 and 1920.
——— *Quaestiones super* De animalibus. Edited by Ephrem Filthaut. Vol. 12 of *Opera omnia*, edited by Bernhard Geyer. Münster: Aschendorff, 1955.
[Ps.-]Albertus Magnus. *De secretis mulierum item De virtutibus herbarum lapidum et animalium*. Amsterdam: Iodocus Ianstonius, 1643.
——— *Women's Secrets: A Translation of Pseudo-Albertus Magnus'* De secretis mulierum *with Commentaries*. Translated with introduction by Helen Rodnite Lemay. SUNY Series in Medieval Studies. Albany: State University of New York Press, 1992.
d'Alverny, Marie-Thérèse. "Comment les théologiens et les philosophes voient la femme," in [*La femme dans la civilisation des Xᵉ–XIIIᵉ siècles: Actes du colloque tenu á Poitiers les 23–25 septembre 1976*], *Cahiers de civilisation médiévale* 20 (1977): 105–29.

——— "Les traductions d'Avicenne (Moyen Age et Renaissance)." In *Avicenna nella storia della cultura medioevale: Relazioni e discussione (15 aprile 1955)*, pp. 71–87. Problemi attuali di scienzia e di cultura 40. Rome: Accademia Nazionale dei Lincei, 1957.

——— "Translations and Translators." In *Renaissance and Renewal in the Twelfth Century*, edited by Robert L. Benson and Giles Constable, pp. 421–62. Cambridge: Harvard University Press, 1982.

Andreas Capellanus. *De amore libri tres.* Edited by E. Trojel. Copenhagen: G. E. C. Gad, 1892. Reprint. Munich: Eidos, 1964.

Aquinas. *See* Thomas Aquinas.

Ariès, Philippe. *Centuries of Childhood: A Social History of Family Life.* Translated by Robert Baldick. New York: Random House, 1962.

Aristotle. *The Complete Works of Aristotle.* Edited by Jonathan Barnes. 2 vols. Rev. Oxford Translation, Bollingen Series 71/2. Princeton: Princeton University Press, 1984.

——— *Generation of Animals.* Edited and translated by A. L. Peck. Loeb Classical Library. Cambridge: Harvard University Press; London: William Heinemann, 1953.

——— *De generatione animalium translatio Guillelmi de Moerbeka.* Vol. XVII/2 of *Aristoteles Latinus.* Edited by H. J. Lulofs. Union académique internationale, Corpus philosophorum Medii Aevi. Bruges and Paris: Desclée de Brouwer, 1966.

——— *Historia animalium.* Edited and translated by A. L. Peck. 2 vols. Loeb Classical Library. Cambridge: Harvard University Press; London: William Heinemann, 1965.

——— *Aristotle's* De partibus animalium *I and* De generatione animalium *I with Passages from II.1–3.* Translated with commentary by David M. Balme. Clarendon Aristotle Series. Oxford: Clarendon Press, 1972.

——— *Parts of Animals.* Edited and translated by A. L. Peck. Loeb Classical Library. Cambridge: Harvard University Press; London: William Heinemann, 1937.

——— *The Physics.* Edited and translated by Philip H. Wicksteed and Francis M. Cornford. 2 vols. Loeb Classical Library. Cambridge: Harvard University Press; London: William Heinemann, 1957–60.

——— *On the Soul, Parva naturalia, On Breath,* edited and translated by W. S. Hett. Rev. ed. Cambridge: Harvard University Press; London: William Heinemann, 1957.

Arlt, Karl Eduard. *Neuer Beitrag zur Geschichte der medicinischen Schule von Montpellier.* Friedrich-Wilhelms-Universität. Berlin: Gustav Schade [Otto Francke], [1902].

Arnaldus de Villanova. *Aphorismi de gradibus.* Edited by Michael McVaugh. Vol. 3 of *Opera medica omnia.* Granada: Seminarium Historiae Medicinae Granatensis, 1975.

——— *De ornatu mulierum.* In *Opera omnia cum Nicolai Taurelli . . . annotationibus.* Basel: Conrad Waldkirch, 1585.

Atkinson, Clarissa W. " 'Precious Balsam in a Fragile Glass': The Ideology of Virginity in the Later Middle Ages." *Journal of Family History* 8 (1983): 131–43.

Augustine. *See* Aurelius Augustinus

Aurelius Augustinus. *De civitate dei.* 2 vols. Corpus Christianorum, Series Latina 47–8; Aurelii Augustini opera 14. Turnhout: Brepols, 1955.

Avicenna. *Liber canonis.* Venice: Pagininis, 1507. Reprint. Hildesheim: Georg Olms, 1964.

D'Avray, D. L., and M. Tausche. "Marriage Sermons in *ad status* Collections of the Central Middle Ages." *Archives d'histoire doctrinale et littéraire du Moyen Age* 47 (1980): 71–119.

Balme. *See also* Aristotle

Balme, David M. "Ανθρωπος ἄνθρωπον γεννᾷ: Human Is Generated by Human." In *The Human Embryo: Aristotle and the Arabic and European Traditions,* edited by G. R. Dunstan, pp. 20–31. Exeter: Exeter University Press, 1990.

Bartholomeus Anglicus. *De genuinis rerum coelestium, terrestrium inferarum* [sic] *proprietatibus libri XVIII.* Edited by Georgius Bartholdus Posanus. Frankfurt: Wolfgang Richter, 1601. Reprint. Frankfurt am Main: Minerva, 1964.

——— *De proprietatibus rerum.* [Translated by John of Trevisa]; revised with commentary by Stephen Batman. London: Thomas East, 1582.

Bazàn, B. C. "La *quaestio disputata.*" In *Les genres littéraires dans les sources théologiques et philosophiques médiévales: Définition, critique et exploitation: Actes du Colloque international de Louvain-la-Neuve, 25–27 mai 1981,* pp. 31–50. Publications de l'Institut d'etudes médiévales, 2d series. Textes, études, congrès 5. Louvain-la-Neuve: Institut d'études médiévales de l'Université Catholique de Louvain, 1982.

Bazàn, Bernardo C., John W. Wippel, Gérard Fransen, and Danielle Jacquart. *Les questions disputées et les questions quodlibétiques dans les facultés de théologie, de droit et de médecine.* Typologie des sources du Moyen Age occidental 44–5. Turnhout: Brepols, 1985.

Beccaria, Augusto. *I codici di medicina del periodo presalernitano (secoli IX, X e XI).* Storia e letteratura 53. Rome: Edizioni di Storia e Letteratura, 1956.

——— "Sulle trace di un antico canone latino di Ippocrate e di Galeno, I."; "II. Gli *Aforismi* di Ippocrate nella versione e nei commenti del primo medioevo"; "III. Quattro opere di Galeno nei commenti della scuola di Ravenna all'inizio del medioevo." *Italia medioevale e umanistica* 2 (1959): 1–56; 4 (1961): 1–75; 14 (1971): 1–23.

Benton, John F. "Trotula, Women's Problems, and the Professionalization of Medicine in the Middle Ages." *Bulletin of the History of Medicine* 59 (1985): 30–53.

Bernardus de Gordonio. *Practica dicta Lilium.* Venice: Bonetus Locatellus, 1498.

Bernardus Silvestris. *Cosmographia.* Edited with introduction by Peter Dronke. Textus minores in usum academicum 53. Leiden: E. J. Brill, 1978.

——— *The* Cosmographia *of Bernardus Silvestris.* Translated and introduced by Winthrop Wetherbee. New York: Columbia University Press, 1973.

Boswell, John. *Christianity, Social Tolerance, and Homosexuality: Gay People in Western Europe from the Beginning of the Christian Era to the Fourteenth Century.* Chicago: University of Chicago Press, 1980.

——— *The Kindness of Strangers: The Abandonment of Children in Western Europe from Late Antiquity to the Renaissance.* London: Allen Lane, Penguin Press, 1989 (c. 1988).

Bowersock, Glen W. *The Greek Sophists in the Roman Empire*. Oxford: Oxford University Press, 1969.

Boylan, Michael. "Galenic and Hippocratic Challenges to Aristotle's Conception Theory." *Journal of the History of Biology* 17 (1984): 83–112.

Brissaud, Y.-B. "L'infanticide à la fin du Moyen Age: Ses motivations psychologiques et sa répression." *Revue historique de droit français et étranger* 50 (1972): 229–56.

Brundage, James A. "Carnal Delight: Canonistic Theories of Sexuality." *Proceedings of the Fifth International Congress of Medieval Canon Law, Salamanca, 21–25 September 1976*. Vatican City: Biblioteca Apostolica Vaticana, 1980.

———— *Law, Sex, and Christian Society in Medieval Europe*. Chicago: University of Chicago Press, 1987.

———— "The Treatment of Marriage in the *Questiones Londinenses* (MS Royal 9.E.VII)." *Manuscripta* 19 (1975): 86–97.

Bugge, John. *Virginitas: An Essay in the History of a Medieval Ideal*. International Archives of the History of Ideas, ser. min., 17. The Hague: Martinus Nijhoff, 1975.

Bullough, Vern L. "Sex Education in Medieval Christianity." *Journal of Sex Research* 13 (1977): 185–96.

Bullough, Vern L., and Cameron Campbell. "Female Longevity and Diet in the Middle Ages." *Speculum* 55 (1980): 317–25.

Burguière, André. "De Malthus à Max Weber: Le mariage tardif et l'esprit d'entreprise." *Annales: Economies, sociétés, civilisations* 31 (1972): 1128–38.

Bynum, Caroline Walker. *Holy Feast and Holy Fast: The Religious Significance of Food to Medieval Women*. Berkeley and Los Angeles: University of California Press, 1987.

———— *Jesus as Mother: Studies in the Spirituality of the High Middle Ages*. Berkeley and Los Angeles: University of California Press, 1982.

Cadden, Joan. "*De elementis*: Earth, Water, Air and Fire in the 12th and 13th Centuries." Master's thesis, Columbia University, 1967.

———— "It Takes All Kinds: Sexuality and Gender Differences in Hildegard of Bingen's *Book of Compound Medicine*." *Traditio* 40 (1984): 149–74.

———— "A Matter of Life and Death: Water in the Natural Philosophy of Albertus Magnus." *History and Philosophy of the Life Sciences* 2 (1980): 241–52.

———— "The Medieval Philosophy and Biology of Growth: Albertus Magnus, Thomas Aquinas, Albert of Saxony and Marsilius of Inghen on Book I, Chapter v of Aristotle's *De generatione et corruptione*." Ph.D. diss., Indiana University, 1971.

———— "Medieval Scientific and Medical Views of Sexuality: Questions of Propriety." *Medievalia et Humanistica*, n.s., 14 (1986): 157–71.

———— "Wissenschaft, Sprache und Macht im Werk Hildegards von Bingen." *Feministische Studien* 9 (1991): 69–79.

Caelius Aurelianus. *Gynaecia: Fragments of a Latin Version of Soranus'* Gynaecia *from a Thirteenth-Century Manuscript*. Translated by Miriam F. Drabkin and Israel E. Drabkin. Supplements to the Bulletin of the History of Medicine 13. Baltimore: Johns Hopkins University Press, 1951.

Calcidius. *See* Plato

Carmody, Francis J., ed. "*Physiologus* latinus versio Y. *University of California Publications in Classical Philology* 12/7 (1941): 95–134.

Cartelle. *See also* Constantinus Africanus

Cartelle, Enrique Montero, ed. *Liber minor de coitu: Tratado menor de andrología anonimo salernitano.* Lingüística y filología 2. Valladolid: Universidad de Valladolid, 1987.

Celsus. *De medicina.* Edited and translated by W. G. Spencer. 3 vols. Loeb Classical Library. Cambridge: Harvard University Press; London: William Heinemann, 1935–8.

Chaucer, Geoffrey. *The Complete Works.* Edited by Walter W. Skeat. 6 vols. Oxford: Clarendon Press, 1894.

Cohen, Jeremy. *The Friars and the Jews: The Evolution of Medieval Anti-Judaism.* Ithaca: Cornell University Press, 1982.

———— "Scholarship and Intolerance in the Medieval Academy: The Study and Evaluation of Judaism in Medieval Christendom." *American Historical Review* 91 (1986): 592–613.

Coleman, Emily. "L'infanticide dans le Haut Moyen Age." *Annales: Economies, sociétés, civilisations* 29 (1974): 315–35.

Coloman, Viola. "Manières personnelles et impersonnelles d'aborder un problème: Saint Augustin et le XIIᵉ siècle. Contribution à l'histoire de la *quaestio.*" In *Les genres littéraires dans les sources théologiques et philosophiques médiévales: Définition, critique et exploitation: Actes du Colloque international de Louvain-la-Neuve, 25–27 mai 1981*, pp. 11–30. Publications de l'Institut d'études médiévales, 2d series. Textes, études, congrès 5. Louvain-la-Neuve: Institut d'études médiévales de l'Université catholique de Louvain, 1982.

Constantinus Africanus. *See also* Delany, Paul; Green, Monica H.

Constantinus Africanus. *De humana natura vel De membris principalibus corporis humani.* In Albucasis, *Methodus menendi . . .* , pp. 313–21. Basel: Henricus Petrus, 1541.

———— *Liber de coitu: El tratado de andrología de Constantino el Africano.* Edited and translated by Enrique Montero Cartelle. Monografias de la Universidad de Santiago de Compostela 77. Santiago de Compostela: Universidad de Santiago, 1983.

———— *Pantegni.* In Isaac [Israeli], *Opera omnia*, 2d foliation. Fols. 1ra–144ra. Lyon: Andreas Turinus, 1515.

———— *Viaticum.* In Isaac [Israeli], *Opera omnia*, 2d foliation. Fols. 144rb–171vb. Lyon: Andreas Turinus, 1515.

Coopland, G. W. *Nicole Oresme and the Astrologers: A Study of His* Le livre des divinacions. Liverpool: University of Liverpool Press, 1952.

Corner, G. W. *Anatomical Texts of the Earlier Middle Ages: A Study in the Transmission of Culture.* Carnegie Institute of Washington, Publication 364. Washington: National Publishing, 1927.

Cornford. *See* Plato

Coudert, Allison. *Alchemy: The Philosopher's Stone.* Boulder, Colo.: Shambahala, 1980.

Crompton, Louis. "The Myth of Lesbian Impunity: Capital Laws from 1270–1791." *Journal of Homosexuality* 6 (1980/81): 11–25.

Dales. *See* Marius

Dante Alighieri. *The Divine Comedy*. Edited and translated with commentary by Charles S. Singleton. 6 vols. Bollingen Series 80. Princeton: Princeton University Press, 1970–5.

—— *The Divine Comedy of Dante Alighieri the Florentine*. Translated with commentary by Dorothy Sayers. 3 vols. Harmondsworth: Penguin, 1949.

Daston, Lorraine, and Katharine Park. "Hermaphrodites in Renaissance France." *Critical Matrix* 1/5 (1985).

Davis, Natalie Zemon. "Women on Top." In *Society and Culture in Early Modern France: Eight Essays*, pp. 124–51. Stanford: Stanford University Press, 1975.

Delany, Paul. "Constantinus Africanus' *De coitu*: A Translation." *Chaucer Review* 4 (1969): 55–65.

Delorme, Ferdinand Marie. "Quodlibets et questions disputées de Raymond de Rigaut, maître franciscain de Paris, d'après le Ms. 96 de la Bibl. Comm. de Todi." In *Aus der Geisteswelt des Mittelalters: Studien und Texte Martin Grabmann . . . gewidmet*, edited by Albert Lang, Joseph Lechner, and Michael Schmaus. 2 vols. Beiträge zur Geschichte der Philosophie und Theologie des Mittelalters, suppl. 3, vol. 2, pp. 826–41. Münster: Aschendorff, 1935.

Demaitre, Luke. *Doctor Bernard de Gordon: Professor and Practitioner*. Toronto: Pontifical Institute of Mediaeval Studies, 1980.

—— "The Idea of Childhood and Child Care in Medical Writings of the Middle Ages." *Journal of Psychohistory* 4 (1977): 461–90.

Demaitre, Luke, and Anthony A. Travill. "Human Embryology and Development in the Works of Albertus Magnus." In *Albertus Magnus and the Sciences: Commemorative Essays, 1980*, edited by James A. Weisheipl, pp. 405–40. Studies and Texts 49. Toronto: Pontifical Institute of Mediaeval Studies, 1980.

Depauw, J. "Amour illégitime et société à Nantes au XVIIIᵉ siècle." *Annales: Economies, sociétés, civilisations* 31 (1972): 1155–82.

Diels, Hermann. *Die Handschriften der antiker Arzte*. 2 pts. Philosophische und historische Abhandlungen. Berlin: Akademie der Wissenschaften, 1905–6.

Diepgen, Paul. *Frau und Frauheilkunde in der Kultur des Mittelalters*. Stuttgart: Georg Thieme, 1963.

—— "Studien zu Arnald von Villanova: Zweite Folge." *Archiv für Geschichte der Medizin* 6 (1913): 380–91.

Dino del Garbo. *See* Dinus de Florentia

Dinus de Florentia. *Expositio supra capitulo* De generatione embrionis *cum questionibus eiusdem* and *Recollectiones super libro Hypocratis* De natura fetus. In *De generatione embrionis*, compiled Bassanius Politus. Venice: Bonetus Locatellus, 1502.

Doane, Winifred W., and Barbara K. Abbott. *Pocketbook Profiles: (Sexism Satirized:) Quotes from the Biological Literature*. N.p.: Society for Developmental Biology, 1976.

Dronke, Peter. "Problemata Hildegardiana." *Mittellateinisches Jahrbuch* 16 (1981): 97–131.

—— *Women Writers of the Middle Ages: A Critical Study of Texts from Perpetua (†203) to Marguerite Porete (†1310)*. Cambridge: Cambridge University Press, 1984.

Duby, Georges. *L'économie rurale et la vie des campagnes dans l'occident médiéval (France,*

Angleterre, Empire, IXe–XVe siècles): Essai de synthèse et perspectives de recherches. 2 vols. Collections historiques. Paris: Aubier, Editions Montaigne, 1962.

——— *Medieval Marriage: Two Models from the Twelfth Century.* Translated by Elborg Forster. Baltimore and London: Johns Hopkins University Press, 1978.

Duhem, Pierre. *Le système du monde.* 10 vols. Paris: Librairie Scientifique A. Hermann, 1913–59.

Durling, Richard J. "Corrigenda and Addenda to Diels' Galenica, I: Codices Vaticani." *Traditio* 23 (1967): 463–76.

Egert, Ferdinand Paul. *Gynäkologische Fragmente aus dem frühen Mittelalter nach einer Petersburger Handschrift aus dem VIII.–IX. Jahrhundert.* Abhandlungen zur Geschichte der Medizin und der Naturwissenschaften 11. Berlin: Emil Ebering, 1936. Reprint. Nedeln, Liechtenstein: Kraus, 1977.

Erikson, Carolly. *The Medieval Vision: Essays in History and Perception.* New York: Oxford University Press, 1976.

Ferckel, Christoph. *Die Gynäkologie des Thomas von Brabant: Ein Beitrag zur Kenntnis der mittelalterlichen Gynäkologie und ihrer Quellen: Ausgewählte Kapitel aus Buch I* [De anatomia corporis humani] *De naturis rerum beendet um 1240.* Alte Meister der Medizin und Naturkunde 5. Munich: C. Kuhn, 1912.

——— "Zur Gynäkologie und Generationslehre im *Fasciculus medicinae* des Johannes de Ketham." *Archiv für Geschichte der Medizin* 6 (1913): 205–22.

——— "Die *Secreta mulierum* und ihr Verfasser." *Sudhoffs Archiv für Geschichte der Medizin und der Naturwissenschaften* 38 (1954): 267–74.

Fisher, John Douglas Close. *Christian Initiation: Baptism in the Medieval West, a Study in the Disintegration of the Primitive Rite of Initiation.* London: S. P. C. K., 1965.

Flandrin, Jean-Louis. "Contraception, mariage et relations amoureuses dans l'occident chrétien." *Annales: Economies, sociétés, civilisations* 24 (1969): 1370–90.

——— *Families in Former Times: Kinship, Household and Sexuality.* Translated by Richard Southern. Cambridge: Cambridge University Press, 1976.

——— "Mariage tardif et vie sexuelle: Discussions et hypothèses de recherche." *Annales: Economies, sociétés, civilisations* 27 (1972): 1351–78.

——— "Sex in Married Life in the Early Middle Ages: The Church's Teaching and Behavioural Reality." In *Western Sexuality: Practice and Precept in Past and Present Times,* edited by Philippe Ariès and André Béjin; translated by Anthony Forster, pp. 114–29. Oxford: Basil Blackwell, 1985.

——— *Un temps pour embrasser: Aux origines de la morale sexuelle occidentale (VIe–IXe siècle).* L'univers historique. Paris: Editions du Seuil, 1983.

Foerster, Richard, ed. *Scriptores physiognomonici Graeci et Latini.* 2 vols. Bibliotheca scriptorum Graecorum et Romanorum Teubneriana. Leipzig: B. G. Teubner, 1893.

——— ed. *De translatione Latina* Physiognomicorum *quae ferentur Aristotelis.* Kiel: Libraria Academica, 1884.

Foucault, Michel. *The Use of Pleasure.* Translated by Robert Hurley. Vol. 2 of *The History of Sexuality.* New York: Random House, 1985.

von Franz, Marie-Louise, ed. and comm. *Aurora consurgens: A Document Attributed to Thomas Aquinas on the Problem of Opposites in Alchemy.* Translated by R. F. C. Hull and A. S. B. Glover. Bollingen Series 77. New York: Random House, Pantheon Books, 1966.

French, Roger K. "*De juvamentis membrorum* and the Reception of Galenic Physiological Anatomy." *Isis* 70 (1979): 96–109.

du Fresne du Cange, Charles. *Glossarium mediae et infimae Latinitatis.* Suppl. D. P. Carpenter and G. A. L. Henschel; new ed. Léopold Favre. Niort and London: L. Favre and David Nutt, 1882–7.

Galen. *Opera omnia.* Edited by Carl Gottlob Kühn. 20 vols. in 22. Leipzig: C. Cnobloch, 1821–33. Reprint. Hildesheim: Georg Olms, 1964–5.

——— "On the Anatomy of the Uterus." Translated by Charles Mayo Goss. *Anatomical Record* 144 (1962): 77–83.

——— *On the Natural Faculties.* Edited and translated by Arthur John Brock. Loeb Classical Library. Cambridge: Harvard Univerity Press; London: William Heinemann, 1916.

——— *On the Usefulness of the Parts of the Body.* Translated with an introduction by Margaret Tallmadge May. 2 vols. Cornell Publications on the History of Science. Ithaca: Cornell University Press, 1968.

García-Ballester, Luis, Michael R. McVaugh, and Agustín Rubio-Vela. *Medical Licensing and Learning in Fourteenth-Century Valencia.* Transactions of the American Philosophical Society 79/6. Philadelphia: American Philosophical Society, 1989.

Gerlach, Wolfgang. "Das Problem des 'Weiblichen Samens' in der antiken und mittelalterlichen Medizin." *Sudhoffs Archiv für Geschichte der Medizin und der Naturwissenschaften* 30 (1938): 177–93.

Gerson, Johannes. *De pollutione.* Cologne: Ludwig von Renchen, n.d.

Gilbertus Anglicus. *Compendium medicine.* Lyon: Jacobus Saccon, 1510.

Gillispie, Charles Coulston, ed. *The Dictionary of Scientific Biography.* 16 vols. New York: Charles Scribner for The American Council of Learned Societies, 1970–80.

Glorieux, Palémon. *La littérature quodlibétique de 1260–1320.* 2 vols. Bibliothèque thomiste 5 and 21, Section historique 18. Le Saulchoir, Kain: Revue des Sciences Philosophiques et Théologiques, 1925. Paris: Librairie Philosophique J. Vrin, 1935.

Gold, Penny S. "The Marriage of Mary and Joseph in the Twelfth-Century Ideology of Marriage." In *Sexual Practices and the Medieval Church*, edited by Vern L. Bullough and James A. Brundage, pp. 102–17. Buffalo: Prometheus, 1982.

Green, Monica H. "Constantinus Africanus and the Conflict between Religion and Science." In *The Human Embryo: Aristotle and the Arabic and European Traditions*, edited by G. R. Dunstan, pp. 47–69. Exeter: University of Exeter Press, 1990.

——— "Female Sexuality in the Medieval West." *Trends in History* 4 (1990): 127–58.

——— "The *De genecia* Attributed to Constantine the African." *Speculum* 62 (1987): 299–323.

——— "The Transmission of Ancient Theories of Female Physiology and Disease through the Early Middle Ages." Ph.D. diss., Princeton University, 1985.

——— "Women's Medical Practice and Health Care in Medieval Europe." *Signs* 14 (1989): 434–73.

Guilelmus de Conchis. *Dialogus de substantiis physicis ante annos ducentos confectus à Vuilhelmo Aneponymo philosopho . . .* [= *Dragmaticon*]. Edited by Guilielmus Gratarolus. Strasburg: Iosias Rihelius, 1567. Reprint. Frankfurt-am-Main: Minerva, 1967.

——— *Glosae super Platonem*. Edited by Edouard Jeauneau. Textes philosophiques du Moyen Age 13. Paris: Librairie Philosophique J. Vrin, 1965.

——— *Philosophia*. Edited and translated (into German) by Gregor Maurach with Heidemarie Telle. Pretoria: University of South Africa, 1980.

Guillaume de Conches. *See* Guilelmus de Conchis

Guillaume de Lorris, and Jean de Meun. *Le roman de la rose*. Edited by Ernest Langlois. Société des anciens textes français. 5 vols. Paris: Firmin-Didot, 1914.

Hanson, Anne, trans. "Hippocrates: *Diseases of Women, I.*" *Signs* 1 (1975): 567–84.

Häring, Nikolaus M., ed. "Alan of Lille, *De planctu naturae*." *Studi medievali*, 3d ser., 19 (1978): 797–879.

Harvey, William. *Anatomical Exercises on the Generation of Animals*. In *Works*, translated by Robert Willis. London: Sydenham Society, 1847.

Haskins, Charles Homer. *Studies in the History of Mediaeval Science*. 2d ed. Cambridge: Harvard University Press, 1927. Reprint. New York: Frederick Ungar, 1960.

Heer, Friedrich. *The Medieval World: Europe, 1100–1350*. Translated by Janet Sondheimer. Cleveland: World, 1962.

Helmholz, R. H. *Marriage Litigation in Medieval England*. Cambridge Studies in English Legal History. London: Cambridge University Press, 1974.

Heloise. *See* Abelardus, Petrus, and Heloisa

Henkel, Nikolaus. *Studien zum* Physiologus *im Mittelalter*. Hermaea: Germanistische Forschungen, n.s., 38. Tübingen: Max Niemayer, 1976.

Herlihy, David. "The Generation in Medieval History." *Viator* 5 (1974): 333–64.

——— "Life Expectancies for Women in Medieval Society." In *The Role of Women in the Middle Ages: Papers of the Sixth Annual Conference of the Center for Medieval and Renaissance Studies, State University of New York at Binghamton, 6–7 May 1972*, edited by Rosemarie Thee Morewedge, pp. 1–22. Albany: State University of New York Press, 1976.

——— "The Making of the Medieval Family: Symmetry, Structure, and Sentiment." *Journal of Family History* 3 (1983): 116–30.

Hewson, M. Anthony. *Giles of Rome and the Medieval Theory of Conception: A Study of the* De formatione corporis humani in utero. University of London Historical Studies 38. London: Athelone Press, University of London, 1975.

Hildegard. *See also* Schipperges, Heinrich

Hildegard [of Bingen]. *Causae et curae* [= *Liber compositae medicinae*]. Edited by Paul Kaiser. Bibliotheca scriptorum Graecorum et Romanorum Teubneriana. Leipzig: B. G. Teubner, 1903.

——— *Liber divinorum operum simplicis hominis* [= *De operatione dei*]. Edited by Joannes Dominicus Mansi. In *Opera omnia*, edited by Friedrich Anton de Reuss, cols. 739–1038. *Patrologia Latina* 197 (1853).

——— *Liber simplicis medicinae* [= *Physica*]. Edited by C. Daremberg. In *Opera omnia*, edited by Friedrich Anton Reuss, cols. 1117–1353. *Patrologia Latina* 197 (1853).

——— *Scivias*. Edited by Adelgundis Führkötter with Angela Carlevaris. 2 vols. Corpus Christianorum, Continuatio mediaevalis, 43–43A. Turnhout: Brepols, 1978.

Hippocrates. *See also* Hanson, Anne; Lonie, Iain M.

Hippocrates. *De la génération, De la nature de l'enfant, Des maladies IV, Du foetus de huit mois*. Edited and translated by Robert Joly. Vol. 11 of *Oeuvres*. Collection des Universités de France. Paris: Société d'Edition "Les Belles Lettres," 1970.

――― *Hippocrates on Intercourse and Pregnancy: An English Translation of* On Semen *and* On the Development of the Child. Translated by Tage U. H. Ellinger. New York: Henry Schuman, 1952.

――― *Les oeuvres complètes d'Hippocrate*. Edited by Emile Littré. 10 vols. Paris: J. B. Baillière, 1839–61.

――― *Du régime*. Edited and translated by Robert Joly. Vol. 6/2 of *Oeuvres*. Collection des Universités de France. Paris: Société d'Edition "Les Belles Lettres," 1972.

――― *Works*. Edited and translated by W. H. S. Jones, E. T. Witherington, and Paul Potter. 6 vols. Loeb Classical Library. Cambridge: Harvard University Press; London: William Heinemann, 1923–88.

Holmyard, E. John. *Alchemy*. Harmondsworth: Penguin, 1957.

Horowitz, Maryanne Cline. "Aristotle and Women." *Journal of the History of Biology* 9 (1976): 183–213.

Husband, Timothy. *The Wild Man: Medieval Myth and Symbolism*. With Gloria Gilmore-House. New York: Metropolitan Museum of Art, 1980.

Isidore of Seville. *See* Isidorus Hispalensis

Isidorus Hispalensis. *Etymologiarum sive originum libri XX*. Edited by W. M. Lindsay. 2 vols. Scriptorum classicorum bibliotheca Oxoniensis. Oxford: Oxford University Press, 1911.

Jacobus Forliviensis. *Expositio supra capitulum* De generatione embrionis *cum questionibus eiusdem*. In *De generatione embrionis*, compiled by Bassanius Politus, fols. 2ra–17va. Venice: Bonetus Locatellus, 1502.

Jacquart, Danielle. *Le milieu médical en France du XIIᵉ au XVᵉ siècle: En annexe 2ᵉ supplément au* Dictionaire d'Ernest Wickersheimer. Centre de recherches d'histoire et de philologie de la IVᵉ section de l'Ecole pratique des hautes études V, Hautes études médiévales et modernes 46. Geneva: Droz, 1981.

――― "La question disputée dans les facultés de médecine." In *Les questions disputées et les questions quodlibétiques dans les facultés de théologie, de droit et de médecine*, by Bernardo C. Bazàn, John W. Wippel, Gérard Fransen, and Danielle Jacquart, pp. 281–315. Typologie des sources du Moyen Age occidental, 44–5. Turnhout: Brepols, 1985.

――― "La réception du *Canon* d'Avicenne: Comparaison entre Montpellier et Paris aux XIIIᵉ et XIVᵉ siècles." In *Histoire de l'école médicale de Montpellier*, vol. 2 of *Actes du 110ᵉ* Congrès national des sociétés savantes, Montpellier, 1985: Section d'histoire des sciences et des techniques, pp. 69–77. Paris: Ministère de l'Education Nationale, Comité des Travaux Historiques et Scientifiques, 1985.

Jacquart, Danielle, and Claude Thomasset. "Albert le Grand et les problèmes de la sexualité." *History and Philosophy of the Life Sciences* 3 (1981): 73–93.

――― "L'amour 'héroïque' à travers le traité d'Arnaud de Villeneuve." In *La folie et le corps*, edited by Jean Céard, pp. 143–58. Paris: Presses de l'Ecole Normale Supérieur, 1985.

――― *Sexuality and Medicine in the Middle Ages*. Translated by Matthew Adamson. Princeton: Princeton University Press, 1988.

James of Forlì. *See* Jacobus Forliviensis

Johannes Anglicus. *Rosa Anglica practica medicine*. Venice: Bonetus Locatellus, 1516.

Johannes de Sancto Amando. *Die* Concordanciae *des Johannes de Sancto Amando nach einer Berliner und zwei Erfurter Handschriften . . . herausgegeben*. Edited by Julius Leopold Pagel. Berlin: Georg Reimer, 1894.

John of Gaddesden. *See* Johannes Anglicus

John of Saint Amand. *See* Johannes de Sancto Amando

Johnson, Michael. "Science and Discipline: The Ethos of Sex Education in a Fourteenth-Century Classroom." In *Homo Carnalis: The Carnal Aspect of Medieval Human Life*, edited by Helen Rodnite Lemay, pp. 157–72. Center for Medieval and Early Renaissance Studies, Acta, 14, for 1987. Binghamton, N.Y.: State University of New York, 1990.

Kibre, Pearl. *Hippocrates Latinus: Repertorium of Hippocratic Writings in the Latin Middle Ages*. Rev. ed. New York: Fordham University Press, 1985.

——— "Hippocratic Writings in the Middle Ages." *Bulletin of the History of Medicine* 18 (1945): 371–412.

Klibansky, Raymond. *The Continuity of the Platonic Tradition during the Middle Ages: Outlines of a Corpus Platonicum Medii Aevi*. London: Warburg Institute, 1939.

Klibansky, Raymond, Erwin Panofsky, and Fritz Saxl. *Saturn and Melancholy: Studies in the History of Natural Philosophy and Art*. London: Thomas Nelson and Sons, 1964.

Kristeller, Paul Oskar. "Bartholomaeus, Musandinus and Maurus of Salerno and Other Early Commentators of the *Articella* with a Tentative List of Texts and Manuscripts." *Italia medioevale e umanistica* 19 (1976): 57–87.

——— "Bartolomeo, Musandino, Mauro di Salerno e altri antichi commentatori dell' *Articella*, con un elenco di testi e di manoscritti." In *Studi sulla Scuola medica salernitana*, pp. 95–151. Naples: Instituto Italiano per gli Studi Filosofici, 1986.

——— "Beitrag der Schule von Salerno zur Entwicklung der scholastischen Wissenschaft im 12. Jahrhundert: Kurze Mitteilung über handschriftliche Funde." In *Artes liberales von antiken Bildung zur Wissenschaft des Mittelalters*, edited by Josef Koch, pp. 84–90. Studien und Texte zur Geistesgeschichte des Mittelalters 5. Leiden: E. J. Brill, 1959.

——— "The School of Salerno: Its Development and Its Contribution to the History of Learning." *Bulletin of the History of Medicine* 17 (1945): 138–94. Reprinted in his *Studies in Renaissance Thought and Letters*, vol. 1, pp. 495–551. Storia e letteratura 54. Rome: Edizioni di Storia e Letteratura, 1956.

——— *La Scuola Medica di Salerno secondo ricerche e scoperte recenti*. Quaderni del Centro studi e documentazione della Scuola Medica Salernitana 5. Salerno: Centro studi e documentazione della Scuola Medica Salernitana, 1980.

Kudlein, Fridolf. "The Seven Cells of the Uterus: The Doctrine and Its Roots." *Bulletin of the History of Medicine* 49 (1965): 415–23.

Kurdziałek, Marian. "Anatomische und embryologische Aeusserungen Davids von Dinant." *Sudhoffs Archiv für Geschichte der Medizin und der Naturwissenschaften* 45 (1961): 1–22.

Kusche, Brigitte. "Zur *Secreta mulierum* – Forschung." *Janus* 62 (1975): 102–23.

Lachs, Johann. *Die Gynaekologie des Galen: Eine geschichtlich-gynaekologische Studie*. Abhandlungen zur Geschichte der Medicin 4. Wrocław: J. U. Kerns, 1903.

Lacombe, Georges, Aleksander Birkenmajer, and Lorenzo Minio-Paluello. *Aristoteles Latinus: Codices.* 3 vols. Vol. 1, rev. ed. Union académique internationale, Corpus philosophorum Medii Aevi. Bruges and Paris: Desclée de Brouwer, 1957. Vol. 2. Cambridge: Academia, 1955. [Vol. 3], *Supplementa altera.* Bruges and Paris: Desclée de Brouwer, 1961.

Laqueur, Thomas. *Making Sex: Body and Gender from the Greeks to Freud.* Cambridge: Harvard University Press, 1990.

Lawn, Brian, ed. *The Prose Salernitan Questions Edited from a Bodleian Manuscript (Auct. F.3.10).* Auctores Britannici Medii Aevi 5. London: British Academy at Oxford University Press, 1979.

Lawn, Brian. *I Quesiti Salernitani: Introduzione alla storia della letteratura problematica medica e scientifica nel Medio Evo e nel Rinascimento.* Translated by Alessandro Spagnuolo. [Salerno]: Di Mauro, 1969.

———— *The Salernitan Questions: An Introduction to the History of Medieval and Renaissance Problem Literature.* Oxford: Clarendon Press, 1963.

Le Roy Ladurie, Emmanuel. *Montaillou: The Promised Land of Error.* Translated by Barbara Bray. New York: Random House, 1978.

Leclercq, Jean. *Monks on Marriage: A Twelfth-Century View.* New York: Seabury Press, 1982.

Leff, Gordon. *Paris and Oxford Universities in the Thirteenth and Fourteenth Centuries: An Institutional and Intellectual History.* New York: John Wiley and Sons, 1968. Reprint. Huntington, N.Y.: Robert E. Krieger, 1975.

Lemay. *See also* [Ps.-]Albertus Magnus

Lemay, Helen Rodnite. "William of Saliceto on Human Sexuality." *Viator* 12 (1981): 165–81.

Levy, Jean-Philippe. "Officialité de Paris et les questions familiales à la fin du XIVe siècle." In *Etudes d'histoire du droit canonique dediées à Gabriel Le Bras*, vol. 2, pp. 1265–94. Ouvrage publié avec le concours du Centre national de la recherche scientifique. Paris: Sirey, 1965.

Liebeschütz, Hans. *Das allegorische Weltbild der heiligen Hildegard von Bingen.* Studien der Bibliothek Warburg 16. Leipzig and Berlin: B. G. Teubner, 1930.

Lindberg, David C., ed. *Science in the Middle Ages.* Chicago History of Science and Medicine. Chicago: University of Chicago Press, 1978.

Lohr, Charles H. "Medieval Latin Aristotle Commentaries." *Traditio* 23 (1967): 313–413; 24 (1968): 149–245; 26 (1970): 135–216; 27 (1971): 251–351; 28 (1972): 281–396; 29 (1973): 91–197; 30 (1974): 119–44.

Lonie, Iain M. *The Hippocratic Treatises* On Generation, On the Nature of the Child, Diseases IV: *A Commentary.* Ars medica: Texte und Untersuchungen zur Quellenkunde der alten Medizin 2. Abteilung, Griechisch-lateinische Medizin 7. Berlin: Walter de Gruyter, 1981.

Lulofs. *See* Aristotle

McKee, Lauris. "Sex Differential in Survivorship and the Customary Treatment of Infants and Children." *Medical Anthropology* 8 (1984): 91–108.

McLaughlin, Eleanor Commo. "Equality of Souls, Inequality of Sexes: Women in Medieval Theology." In *Religion and Sexism: Images of Women in the Jewish and Christian Traditions*, edited by Rosemary Radford Reuther, pp. 213–66. New York: Simon and Schuster, 1974.

McLaughlin, Mary Martin. "Survivors and Surrogates: Children and Parents from the Ninth to the Thirteenth Centuries." In *The History of Childhood*, edited by Lloyd deMause, pp. 101–81. New York: Psychohistory Press, 1974.

Mclean, Ian. *The Renaissance Notion of Woman: A Study in the Fortunes of Scholasticism and Medical Science in European Intellectual Life*. Cambridge Monographs on the History of Medicine. Cambridge: Cambridge University Press, 1980.

McVaugh. *See also* Arnaldus de Villanova

McVaugh, Michael. Review of *Giles of Rome and the Medieval Theory of Conception*, by M. Anthony Hewson. *Speculum* 52 (1977): 987–89.

Makowsky, Elizabeth M. "The Conjugal Debt and Medieval Canon Law." *Journal of Medieval History* 3 (1977): 99–114.

Marius. *Marius on the Elements*. Edited and translated by Richard C. Dales. Publications of the Center for Medieval and Renaissance Studies, UCLA, 10. Berkeley and Los Angeles: University of California Press, 1976.

Meier, Ludger. "Les disputes quodlibétiques en dehors des universités." *Revue d'histoire ecclesiastique* 53 (1958): 401–42.

Michaelis Scotus. *De secretis naturae*. In *Alberti Magni De secretis mulierum. Item De virtutibus herbarum, lapidum et animalium. De mirabilibus mundi. Michaelis Scoti Libellus de secretis naturae*. Amsterdam: I. Ianssonius, 1643.

Mitterer, Albert. "*Mas occasionatus* oder zwei Methoden der Thomasdeutung." *Zeitschrift für katholische Theologie* 72 (1950): 80–103.

Molin, Jean-Baptiste, and Protais Mutembe. *Le rituel du mariage en France du Xe au XVe siècle*. Théologie historique 26. Paris: Beauchesne, 1974.

Money, John W. "Sex Hormones and Other Variables in Human Eroticism." In *Sex and Internal Secretions*, edited by William C. Young. vol. 2, pp. 1383–400. 3d ed. Baltimore: Williams and Wilkins, 1961.

Moore, R. I. *The Formation of a Persecuting Society: Power and Deviance in Western Europe, 950–1250*. Oxford: B. Blackwell, 1987.

Murdoch, John Emory. *Album of Science: Antiquity and the Middle Ages*. Albums of Science. New York: Charles Scribner's Sons, 1984.

—— "From Social into Intellectual Factors: An Aspect of the Unitary Character of Late Medieval Learning." In *The Cultural Context of Medieval Learning: Proceedings of the First International Colloquium on Philosophy, Science and Theology in the Middle Ages – September, 1973*, edited by John Emory Murdoch and Edith Dudley Sylla, pp. 271–339. Synthèse Library 76; Boston Studies in the Philosophy of Science 26. Dordrecht and Boston: D. Reidel, 1975.

Murray, Alexander. "Religion among the Poor in Thirteenth-Century France: The Testimony of Humbert de Romans." *Traditio* 30 (1974): 285–324.

Muscio. *Sorani Gynaeciorum vetus translatio latina*. Edited by Valentine Rose. Leipzig: B. G. Teubner, 1882.

Needham, Joseph. *A History of Embryology*. 2d ed., rev. with Arthur Hughes. History, Philosophy and Sociology of Science. Cambridge: Cambridge University Press, 1959. Reprint. New York: Arno, 1975.

Nemesius Emesenus. *De natura hominis: Traduction de Burgundio de Pise*. Edited by G. Verbeke and J. R. Moncho. Corpus Latinum commentariorum in Aristotelem Graecorum, suppl. 1. Leiden: E. J. Brill, 1975.

Niebyl, Peter H. "Old Age, Fever, and the Lamp Metaphor." *Journal of the History of Medicine* 26 (1971): 351–68.

Noonan, John T., Jr., *Contraception: A History of Its Treatment by the Catholic Theologians and Canonists.* Cambridge: Harvard University Press, Belnap Press, 1965.

Oresme. *See* Coopland, G. W.

Otis, Leah L. *Prostitution in Medieval Society: The History of an Urban Institution in Languedoc.* Women in Western Culture and Society. Chicago: University of Chicago Press, 1985.

Pack, Roger A., ed. "Auctoris incerti *De physiognomonia libellus.*" *Archives d'histoire doctrinale et littéraire du Moyen Age* 41 (1974): 113–38.

Pagel, Julius. "Raymundus de Molieriis und seine Schrift *De impedimentis conceptionis.*" *Janus* 8 (1903): 530–37.

Paniagua, Juan A. *El Maestro Arnau de Vilanova médico.* Cuadernos valencianos de la historia de la medicina y de la ciencia, ser. A, 8. Valencia: Catedra e Instituto de Historia de la Medicina, 1969.

Paris, Gaston, ed. *La vie de saint Alexis: Poème du XIe siècle.* Les classiques français du Moyen Age. Paris: Librairie Ancienne Honoré Champion, 1911.

Payer, Pierre J. *Sex and the Penitentials: The Development of a Sexual Code, 550–1150.* Toronto: University of Toronto Press, 1984.

Pelzer, Auguste. "Un traducteur inconnu: Pierre Gallego, franciscain et premier évêque de Carthagène (1250–1267)." In *Per la storia della teologia e della filosofia,* pp. 407–56. Vol. 1 of *Miscellanea Francesco Ehrle: Scritti di storia e paleografia.* Studi e testi 37. Rome: Biblioteca Apostolica Vaticana, 1924.

Peter of Abano. *See* Petrus de Abano Pativinus

Peter the Venerable. *See* Petrus Venerabilis

Petrus de Abano Pativinus. *Conciliator differentiarum philosophorum et precipue medicorum.* Venice: Gabriele de Tarvisio for Thomas Tarvisio, 1476.

——— *Expositio* Problematum *Aristotelis.* Edited by Stephanus Illarius. Mantua: Paulus Johannis de Puzpach, 1475.

Petrus Gallegus. *See* Pelzer, Auguste

Petrus Venerabilis. *The Letters of Peter the Venerable.* Edited by Giles Constable. 2 vols. Harvard Historical Studies 78. Cambridge: Harvard University Press, 1967.

Physiologus. *See* Carmody, Francis J.; White, T. H.

Plato. *Le banquet* [*Symposium*]. Edited and translated by Léon Robin. Vol. 4, pt. 2 of *Oeuvres complètes.* Collection des Universités de France, Association Guillaume Budé. Paris: Société d'Edition "Les Belles Lettres," 1962.

——— *Plato's Cosmology: The* Timaeus *of Plato.* Translated with commentary by Francis MacDonald Cornford. London: Routledge and Kegan Paul, 1937.

——— *Timée, Critias.* Edited and translated by Albert Rivaud. Vol. 10 of *Oeuvres complètes.* Collection des Universités de France, Association Guillaume Budé. Paris: Société d'Edition "Les Belles Lettres," 1963.

——— Timaeus *a Calcidio translatus commentarioque instructus.* Vol. 4 of *Plato Latinus.* Edited by J. H. Waszink. Rev. ed. Corpus Platonicum Medii Aevi. London: Warburg Institute; Leiden: E. J. Brill, 1975.

Plinius Caecilius Secundus, C. *Epistolarum libri decem.* Edited by R. A. B. Mynors.

Scriptorum classicorum bibliotheca Oxoniensis. Oxford: Oxford University Press, 1963.

——— *Natural History.* Edited and translated by H. Rackham, W. H. S. Jones, and D. E. Eicholz. 10 vols. Loeb Classical Library. Cambridge: Harvard University Press; London: William Heinemann, 1938–62.

Pliny. *See* Plinius Caecilius Secundus, C.

Preus, Anthony. "Galen's Criticism of Aristotle's Conception Theory." *Journal of the History of Biology* 10 (1977): 65–85.

Priscianus, Theodorus. *Euporiston libri III cum Physicorum fragmento et additamentis pseudo-Theodoreis.* Edited by Valentin Rose. Bibliotheca scriptorum Graecorum et Latinorum Teubneriana. Leipzig: B. G. Teubner, 1894.

Rashdall, Hastings. *The Universities of Europe in the Middle Ages.* New ed. by F. M. Powicke and A. B. Emden. 3 vols. Oxford: Clarendon Press, 1936.

Reisert, Robert. *Der siebenkammerige Uterus: Studien zur mittelalterlichen Wirkungsgeschichte und Entfaltung eines embryologischen Gebärmuttermodells.* Würzburger medizinhistorische Forschungen 39. Pattensen: Horst Wellm, 1986.

Riddle, John M. "Oral Contraceptives and Early-Term Abortifacients during Classical Antiquity and the Middle Ages." *Past and Present* 132 (1991): 3–32.

Riquet, Michel. "Christianity and Population." In *Popular Attitudes toward Birth Control in Pre-industrial France and England,* edited by Orest Ranum and Patricia Ranum, pp. 21–44. New York: Harper and Row, 1972.

Robbins, Frank. *The Hexaemeral Literature: A Study of the Greek and Latin Commentaries on Genesis.* Chicago: University of Chicago Press, 1912.

Rossiaud, Jacques. "Prostitution, jeunesse et société dans les villes du Sud-Est au XVᵉ siècle." *Annales: Economies, sociétés, civilisations* 31 (1976): 289–325.

Saffron, Morris Harold, ed. and trans. *Maurus of Salerno: Twelfth-Century "Optimus Physicus" with His Commentary on the Prognostics of Hippocrates.* Transactions of the American Philosophical Society, n.s., 62/1. Philadelphia: American Philosophical Society, 1972.

Salisbury, Joyce E. "The Latin Doctors of the Church on Sexuality." Paper presented at The Annual Meeting of the American Historical Association, December 1985.

——— *Medieval Sexuality: A Research Guide.* Garland Medieval Bibliographies 5; Garland Reference Library of Social Science 565. New York: Garland, 1990.

Sayers. *See* Dante Alighieri

Schipperges, Heinrich. *Die Assimilation der arabischen Medizin durch das lateinische Mittelalter.* Sudhoffs Archiv für Geschichte der Medizin und der Naturwissenschaften 48, suppl. 3. Wiesbaden: F. Steiner, 1964.

Schipperges, Heinrich, trans. and intro. *Hildegard von Bingen, Heilkunde: Das Buch von dem Grund und Wesen und der Heilung der Krankheiten.* Salzburg: Otto Müller, 1957.

Schleissner, Margaret Rose. "Pseudo–Albertus Magnus: *Secreta mulierum cum commento,* Deutsch: Critical Text and Commentary." Ph.D. diss., Princeton University, 1987.

Scholz, Bernhard W. "Hildegard von Bingen on the Nature of Women." *American Benedictine Review* 31 (1980): 361–83.

Sears, Elizabeth. *The Ages of Man: Medieval Interpretations of the Life Cycle.* Princeton: Princeton University Press, 1986.

Shahar, Shulamith. *The Fourth Estate: A History of Women in the Middle Ages.* Translated by Chaya Galai. London: Methuen, 1983.

Shatzmiller, Joseph. *Médicine et justice en Provence: Documents de Manosque, 1262–1348.* Aix-en-Provence: Publications de l'Université de Provence, 1989.

Shaw, James R. "Scientific Empiricism in the Middle Ages: Albertus Magnus on Sexual Anatomy." *Clio Medica* 10 (1975): 53–64.

Sigerist, Henry E. "Early Mediaeval Medical Texts in the Manuscripts of Vendôme." *Bulletin of the History of Medicine* 14 (1943): 68–113.

Singer, Charles. "The Scientific Views and Visions of Saint Hildegard." In *Studies in the History and Method of Science,* vol. 1, pp. 1–55. 2d ed. London: William Dawson, 1955.

Siraisi, Nancy G. *Arts and Sciences of Padua: The Studium of Padua before 1350.* Studies and Texts 25. Toronto: Pontifical Institute of Mediaeval Studies, 1973.

———— *Avicenna in Renaissance Italy: The Canon and Medical Teaching in Italian Universities after 1500.* Princeton: Princeton University Press, 1987.

———— "The *Expositio* Problematum *Aristotelis* of Peter of Abano." *Isis* 61 (1970): 321–339.

———— "The Medical Learning of Albertus Magnus." In *Albertus Magnus and the Sciences: Commemorative Essays, 1980,* edited by James A. Weisheipl, pp. 379–404. Studies and Texts 49. Toronto: Pontifical Institute of Mediaeval Studies, 1980.

———— *Taddeo Alderotti and His Pupils: Two Generations of Italian Medical Learning.* Princeton: Princeton University Press, 1981.

Smith, Daniel Scott. "Family Limitation, Sexual Control, and Domestic Feminism in Victorian America." In *Clio's Consciousness Raised: New Perspectives on the History of Women,* edited by Mary S. Hartman and Lois Banner. Harper Colophon Books. New York: Harper and Row, 1974.

Soranus. *Gynaeciorum libri iv, De signis fracturarum, De fasciis, Vita Hippocratis secundum Soranum.* Edited by Johannes Ilberg. Corpus medicorum Graecorum 4. Leipzig and Berlin: B. G. Teubner, 1927.

———— *Soranus' Gynecology.* Translated by Owsei Temkin with Nicholson J. Eastman, Ludwig Edelstein, and Alan F. Guttmacher. Publications of the Institute of the History of Medicine, Johns Hopkins University, 2d ser., Texts and Documents 3. Baltimore: Johns Hopkins University Press, 1956.

———— *See also* Caelius Aurelianus; Muscio

Stahl, William Harris. *Roman Science: Origins, Development, and Influence to the Later Middle Ages.* Madison: University of Wisconsin Press, 1962.

Steinschneider, Moritz. *Die europäischen Uebersetzungen aus dem arabischen bis Mitte des 17. Jahrhunderts.* Sitzungsberichten der Kaiserlichen Akademie der Wissenschaften, philosophisch-historische Klasse 149 (1904) and 151 (1905). Vienna: Kaiserliche Akademie der Wissenschaften, 1905–6. Reprint. Graz: Akademische Druck- und Verlagsanstalt, 1956.

Steneck, Nicholas H. *Science and Creation in the Middle Ages: Henry of Langenstein (d. 1397) on Genesis.* Notre Dame and London: University of Notre Dame Press, 1976.

Stock, Brian. *Myth and Science in the Twelfth Century: A Study of Bernard Silvester.* Princeton, N.J.: Princeton University Press, 1972.

Stuard, Susan Mosher, ed. *Women in Medieval Society.* [Philadelphia]: University of Pennsylvania Press, 1976.

Sudhoff, Karl. "Drei noch unveröffentlichte Kindslagenserien des Soranos-Muscio aus Oxford und London." *Archiv für Geschichte der Medizin* 4 (1911): 109–28.

——— "Salerno, eine mittelalterliche Heil- und Lehrstelle am Tyrrhenischen Meere." *Archiv für Geschichte der Medizin* 21 (1929): 43–62.

Sylla, Edith. "Medieval Quantifications of Qualities: The 'Merton School.' " *Archive for History of the Exact Sciences* 8 (1971): 9–39.

Taddeo Alderotti. *See* Thaddeus Florentinus

Talbot, Charles, ed. and trans. *The Life of Christina of Markyate, a Twelfth Century Recluse.* Oxford: Clarendon Press, 1959.

——— "Medical Education in the Middle Ages." In *The History of Medical Education: An International Symposium Held February 5–9, 1968,* edited by C. D. O'Malley, pp. 73–87. U.C.L.A. Forum in Medical Sciences 12. Berkeley and Los Angeles: University of California Press, 1970.

Taube, Eduard, ed. *Aristoteles de arte physiognomonica ad Alexandrum scriptor.* Programm königlichen katholischen Gymnasiums zu Gleiwitz. Gleiwitz: Gustav Neumann, 1866.

Tavone Passalacqua, Vera, trans. and comm. *Microtegni seu De spermate.* Rome: Instituto di Storia della Medizina dell'Università di Roma, 1959.

Temkin, Owsei. *Galenism: Rise and Decline of a Medical Philosophy.* Cornell Publications in the History of Medicine. Ithaca: Cornell University Press, 1973.

Thaddeus Florentinus. *In* Isagogas *Joannitianas expositio.* In *Expositiones in arduum* Aphorismorum *Ipocratis, in divinum* Prognosticorum *Ipocratis librum, in preclarum* Regiminis acutorum *Ipocratis opus, in subtilissime Joannitii* Isagogarum *libellum.* Edited by Joannis Baptista Nicollinus. Venice: Luca Antonius, 1527.

Thomas Aquinas. *Summa theologiae.* Rev. ed. 5 vols. Bibliotheca de auctores cristianos, seccion 2, Teología y canones 77, 80, 81, 83, 87. Madrid: La Editorial Catolica, 1955–58.

Thomas Cantimpratensis. *See also* Ferckel, Christoph

Thomas Cantimpratensis. *Liber de natura rerum.* Pt. I. *Texte.* Edited by H. Boese. Berlin and New York: Walter de Gruyter, 1973.

Thomasen, Anne-Liese. "*Historia animalium* contra *Gynaecia* in der Literatur des Mittelalters." *Clio Medica* 15 (1980): 5–23.

Thorndike, Lynn. "Buridan's Questions on the Physiognomy Ascribed to Aristotle." *Speculum* 18 (1943): 99–103.

——— "Further Consideration of the *Experimenta, Speculum astronomiae* and *De secretis mulierum* ascribed to Albertus Magnus." *Speculum* 30 (1955): 413–43.

——— *A History of Magic and Experimental Science.* 8 vols. New York: Macmillan and Columbia University Press, 1923–58.

——— "Translations of Works of Galen from the Greek by Niccolô da Reggio (c. 1308–1345)." *Byzantina Metabyzantina* 1 (1946): 213–35.

Thorndike, Lynn, and Pearl Kibre. *A Catalogue of Incipits of Mediaeval Scientific Writings in Latin.* Rev. ed. Mediaeval Academy of America 29. Cambridge: Mediaeval Academy of America, 1963.

Thrupp, Sylvia L. *The Merchant Class of Medieval London (1300–1500)*. Chicago: University of Chicago Press, 1948.

Trexler, R. "Foundlings of Florence." *History of Childhood Quarterly* 1 (1973): 259–75.

Vindicianus Afrus. *Gynaecia*. In Theodorus Priscianus, *Euporiston libri III cum Physicorum fragmento et additamentis pseudo-Theodoreis*, edited by Valentin Rose, pp. 428–62. Bibliotheca scriptorum Graecorum et Latinorum Teubneriana. Leipzig: B. G. Teubner, 1894.

Vorwahl, H. "Die Sexualität im Hoch-Mittelalter." *Janus* 37 (1933): 293–99.

Wack, Mary Frances. "The *Liber de heroes morbo* of Johannes Afflacius and Its Implications for Medieval Love Conventions." *Speculum* 62 (1987): 324–44.

——— *Lovesickness in the Middle Ages: The* Viaticum *and Its Commentaries*. Middle Ages Series. Philadelphia: University of Pennsylvania Press, 1990.

Walum, Laurel Richardson. *The Dynamics of Sex and Gender: A Sociological Perspective*. Chicago: Rand McNally College Publishing, 1977.

Wetherbee. *See* Bernardus Silvestris

White, T. H. *The Book of Beasts, Being a Translation from a Latin Bestiary of the Twelfth Century*. New York: G. Putnam's Sons, 1954.

Wickersheimer, Ernest. *Commentaires de la faculté de médecine de l'université de Paris (1395–1516)*. Collection de documents inédits sur l'histoire de France. Paris: Imprimerie Nationale, 1915.

——— *Dictionaire biographique des médecins en France au Moyen Age*. 2 vols. Paris: Droz, 1936.

——— "Henri de Saxe et le *De secretis mulierum*." In *3ᵉ Congrès de l'histoire de l'art de Guérir, Londres, 17–22 juillet, 1922*, pp. 253–8. Antwerp, 1923.

William of Conches. *See* Guilelmus de Conchis

Wippel, J. F. "The Quodlibetal Question as a Distinctive Literary Genre." In *Les genres littéraires dans les sources théologiques et philosophiques médiévales: Définition, critique et exploitation: Actes du Colloque international de Louvain-la-Neuve 25–27 mai 1981*, pp. 67–84. Publications de l'Institut d'études médiévales, 2d series. Textes, études, congrès 5. Louvain-la-Neuve: Institut d'études médiévales de l'Université Catholique de Louvain, 1982.

Wolfson, Harry Austryn. *Studies in the History of Philosophy and Religion*. Edited by Isadore Twersky and George H. Williams. 2 vols. Cambridge: Harvard University Press, 1973.

Wood, Charles T. "The Doctors' Dilemma: Sin, Salvation, and the Menstrual Cycle in Medieval Thought." *Speculum* 56 (1981): 710–27.

Ziolkowski, Jan. *Alan of Lille's Grammar of Sex: The Meaning of Grammar to a Twelfth-Century Intellectual*. Speculum Anniversary Monographs 10. Cambridge, Mass.: Medieval Academy of America, 1985.

INDEX

The names of medieval authors and works are entered here as they appear in the text, that is, usually in their English form. I have alphabetized medieval authors by first name, except as necessitated by established tradition, as with Geoffrey Chaucer.

Where medieval language is at least sometimes inclusive, I have subsumed specific terms under general. Thus "seed, females' " includes references to women's seed. Where the medieval material, taking the male and heterosexual cases to be standard, identifies "special" cases, this is indicated by the presence of separate subheadings (or occasionally headings), as in "desire, sexual, homosexual." Where medieval usage is exclusive, the headings reflect this, as in "intercourse, heterosexual."

A page number followed by an "f" indicates that the reference is to to a figure.

Cambridge History of Medicine